www.harcourt-interna[tional.com]

Bringing you products from all Harcou[rt]
companies including Baillière Tindall, C[hurchill Livingstone,]
Mosby and W.B. Saunders

University

- ▶ **Browse** for latest information on new books, journals and electronic products

- ▶ **Search** for information on over 20 000 published titles with full product information including tables of contents and sample chapters

- ▶ **Keep up to date** with our extensive publishing programme in your field by registering with **eAlert** or requesting postal updates

- ▶ **Secure online ordering** with prompt delivery, as well as full contact details to order by phone, fax or post

- ▶ **News** of special features and promotions

If you are based in the following countries, please visit the country-specific site to receive full details of product availability and local ordering information

USA: www.harcourthealth.com

Canada: www.harcourtcanada.com

Australia: www.harcourt.com.au

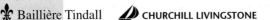 Baillière Tindall    CHURCHILL LIVINGSTONE   Mosby   W.B. SAUNDERS

Human Movement

For Churchill Livingstone:

Editorial Director, Health Professions: Mary Law
Project Manager: Gail Murray
Project Development Manager: Dinah Thom
Designer: George Ajayi

Human Movement

An Introductory Text

Edited by

Marion Trew BA MSc DipTP MCSP
Head of the School of Health Professions, University of Brighton, Eastbourne, UK

Tony Everett BA MEd DipTP MCSP
Senior Lecturer and Course Leader, Department of Physiotherapy Education, School of Healthcare Studies, University of Wales College of Medicine, Cardiff, UK

FOURTH EDITION

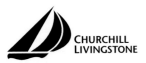
CHURCHILL
LIVINGSTONE

EDINBURGH LONDON NEW YORK PHILADELPHIA ST LOUIS SYDNEY TORONTO 2001

CHURCHILL LIVINGSTONE
An imprint of Harcourt Publishers Limited

First edition 1981
Second edition 1987
Third edition 1997
Fourth edition 2001

ISBN 0 443 07068 7

British Library Cataloguing in Publication Data
A catalogue record for this book is available from the British Library

Library of Congress Cataloging in Publication Data
A catalog record for this book is available from the Library of Congress

Note
Medical knowledge is constantly changing. As new information
becomes available, changes in treatment, procedures, equipment and
the use of drugs become necessary. The editors, contributors and the
publishers have taken care to ensure that the information given in this
text is accurate and up to date. However, readers are strongly advised
to confirm that the information, especially with regard to drug usage,
complies with the latest legislation and standards of practice.

The
publisher's
policy is to use
**paper manufactured
from sustainable forests**

Printed in China

Contents

Contributors vii

Preface ix

1 **Introduction** 1
Tony Everett, Marion Trew

2 **Musculoskeletal basis for movement** 7
Di J. Newham, Anne-Marie Ainscough-Potts

3 **Biomechanics of human movement** 37
Robert W. M. van Deursen, Tony Everett

4 **The neural control of human movement** 69
J. Lesley Crow, Bernhard Haas

5 **Joint mobility** 85
Tony Everett

6 **Strength, power and endurance** 105
Di J. Newham

7 **Motor learning** 129
Nicola Phillips

8 **Measuring and evaluating human movement** 143
Marion Trew, Tony Everett

9 **Scales of measurement** 161
Susan Corr

10 **Function of the lower limb** 173
Marion Trew

11 **Function of the upper limb** 193
Allen Hinde

12 **Function of the spine** 203
Ann Moore, Nicola J. Petty

13 **Posture and balance** 225
Tracey Howe, Jacqueline Ann Oldham

14 **Tension and relaxation** 241
Marion Trew

15 **Human movement through the life span** 253
Marion Trew

Index 269

Contributors

Anne-Marie Ainscough-Potts MSc MCSP DipHE
Lecturer, Physiotherapy Division, Guy's, King's
and St Thomas' School of Biomedical Sciences,
King's College London, London, UK

Susan Corr MPhil DipMedEd DipCOT SROT
Reader, Division of Occupational Therapy,
Centre for Healthcare Education, University
College Northampton, Northampton, UK

J. Lesley Crow MSc GradDipPhys MCSP CertEd(FE/HE)
DipTP
Former Senior Lecturer, School of Physiotherapy,
University of Brighton, Eastbourne, UK;
Research Physiotherapist, Department of
Physiotherapy, University Hospital
Rotterdam/Dijkzigt, Rotterdam, Netherlands

Robert W. M. van Deursen MSc PhD MCSP
Lecturer/Research Co-ordinator, Director of the
Research Centre for Clinical Kinaesiology,
Department of Physiotherapy Education, School
of Healthcare Studies, University of Wales
College of Medicine, Cardiff, UK

Tony Everett BA MEd DipTP MCSP
Senior Lecturer and Course Leader,
Department of Physiotherapy Education,
School of Healthcare Studies, University of
Wales College of Medicine, Cardiff, UK

Bernhard Haas BA(Hons) MSc MCSP
Senior Lecturer in Physiotherapy, School of
Health Professions, University of Brighton,
Eastbourne, UK

Allen Hinde BA MA MCSP DipTP SRP CertEd MISM
Former Senior Lecturer and MSc Health Studies
Programme Leader, University College
Northampton, Northampton, UK

Tracey Howe MSc PhD CertEd MCSP
Research Associate, School of Nursing Studies,
University of Manchester, Manchester, UK

Ann Moore PhD GradDipPhys FCSP CertEd MMACP
Director, Clinical Research Centre, School of
Health Professions, University of Brighton,
Eastbourne, UK

Di J. Newham MPhil PhD MCSP SRP
Head of Physiotherapy Division, Guy's, King's
and St Thomas' School of Biomedical Sciences,
King's College London, London, UK

Jacqueline Ann Oldham BSc(Hons) PhD RGN
Reader, School of Nursing Studies, University of
Manchester, Manchester, UK

Nicola J. Petty MSc GradDipManipTh MCSP MMPA
MMACP
Senior Lecturer, School of Health Professions,
University of Brighton, Eastbourne, UK

Nicola Phillips MSc MCSP SRP
Lecturer, Department of Physiotherapy
Education, School of Healthcare Studies,
University of Wales College of Medicine,
Cardiff, UK

Marion Trew BA MSc DipTP MCSP
Head of the School of Health Professions,
University of Brighton, Eastbourne, UK

Preface

The fourth edition of *Human Movement* continues the process of providing referenced, evidence-based material for those studying human movement for therapeutic and other disciplines. The material in this book forms the anatomical, physiological and biomechanical basis for the understanding of human movement in everyday contexts.

Many of the chapters in the fourth edition have undergone changes in their content and presentation, and most have been updated in their referencing. The order of presentation of the chapters has been changed to reflect a more logical sequence. The basic concepts and different approaches are covered in the earlier chapters and their application to regions of the body is covered in the later chapters.

'Biomechanics of human movement' still retains the basic physical principles but has been extended to enable the reader to use these principles in calculating the forces and moments generated and experienced by the body during movement.

'Motor learning' has been completely rewritten to reflect a more concrete application, with many examples from the sporting field used to illustrate the basic principles.

The new chapter in this edition, 'Scales of measurement', introduces the reader to the assessment of the functional implications of movement, particularly when there has been a pathological overlay.

The presentation and format of this edition have, in the main, been retained unaltered from the previous edition to give the reader an easy-to-read, comprehensive introduction to the study of human movement. The activities throughout the text, together with the objectives in each chapter, should provide a means by which understanding is tested.

Although some of the principles described in this book form the basis of many therapeutic techniques, any student whose profession involves the study of human movement should find this text of use.

Marion Trew
Tony Everett

Eastbourne and Cardiff 2001

CHAPTER CONTENTS

The study of human movement 1
Self-awareness and observational skills 4
Knowledge of human movement through direct
experience 4

**Understanding human movement and its clinical
application 5**

Using this book 5

1

Introduction

T. Everett   M. Trew

OBJECTIVES

**When you have completed this chapter you
should be:**

1. **Enthusiastic about the study of human
   movement**

2. **Aware of the range of factors that
   influence the initiation, production and
   control of human movement**

3. **Conscious of the difficulties of
   simultaneously considering all aspects of
   human movement, yet at the same time
   aware of the need to maintain a holistic
   approach**

4. **Beginning to develop awareness of your
   own body at rest and when moving**

5. **Starting to develop the skills of
   observation of human movement.**

THE STUDY OF HUMAN MOVEMENT

The study of human movement is fascinating for
two main reasons. Firstly, because it is about our-
selves and how we are able to go about our everyday lives performing a vast range of functional
activities, sporting activities and other pastimes. It
is natural to have a curiosity about oneself and the
study of human movement inevitably leads to a
sense of amazement at the wide variety of intricate tasks that we are able to perform with ease,
and often without thought. The second fascination
lies in the complexity of human movement and
the challenges that arise out of this. There are still

1

a surprising number of gaps in our knowledge not only about the fine details of how movement is initiated and controlled but even in the apparently simple areas of exactly what happens when we perform basic everyday tasks. Whilst there have been a substantial number of scientific studies of walking and running, there are only a few research papers on other major lower limb functions and very few detailed studies of the everyday activities we perform with our upper limbs.

Observation of human movement reveals a complex and seemingly infinite variety of positional changes which involve or are controlled by a wide range of internal and external factors. To begin to understand how the systems of the body interact to produce finely controlled and purposeful movement it is essential that some order is introduced into the study. It is necessary to know how human movement is initiated, performed and controlled and such knowledge forms the basis of those professions working in this area.

Human movement can be viewed from a number of different standpoints (see Fig. 1.1):

● Anatomical: describing the structure of the body, the relationship between the various parts

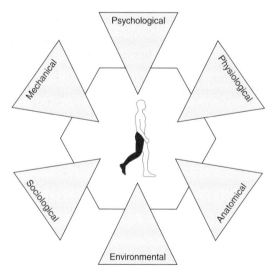

Figure 1.1 There are a number of ways in which the study of human movement can be approached; each approach is valid in its own right but, on its own, limited. For a holistic understanding of how the human body moves and why the component parts work as they do, a multidimensional approach has to be taken.

and the body's potential for movement. Incorrect alignment or disruption of anatomical structures will clearly affect movement.

● Physiological: concerned with the way in which the systems of the human body function and the initiation and control of movement. In many cases incorrect functioning or failure of integration between systems will lead to movement abnormalities.

● Mechanical: involving the force, time and distance relationships in movement.

● Psychological: examining the sensations, perceptions and motivations that stimulate movement and the neurological and chemical/hormonal mechanisms which control them.

● Sociological: considering the meanings given to various movements in different human settings and the influence of social settings on the movements produced.

● Environmental: considering the influence of the environment on the way in which movement occurs.

The following chapters expand the anatomical, physiological and mechanical basis of human movement. This does not lessen the importance of the other approaches and readers should familiarise themselves with this information which can be obtained from other well recognised sources.

By studying the musculoskeletal basis of movement it is possible to have an anatomical framework on which movement can be referenced and described in an unambiguous manner. An intact musculoskeletal system is essential for correct movement to take place. Joints need to possess sufficient freedom of movement to perform the required activities and to be able to move in a smooth and unrestricted manner. Muscles provide the means of achieving this movement and they must possess the necessary strength, power and endurance to carry out this function. They must also be controlled in an extremely delicate and sensitive way and the efficient functioning and correct integration of the central and peripheral nervous system is essential.

Whilst some movements arise out of a conscious decision and require active thought processes, most have been previously learned and are automatic. The neural processes that store, adapt and use these learned movements are complex and demonstrate well the interdependence of all the systems of the body in the production of movement.

Movement does not take place in isolation from the external environment. There is a complex interaction of forces acting on the body including the constant force of gravity and the changing frictional forces. The force of gravity may have the effect of initiating or producing actual movements but it is always a force which the body has to counter to achieve and maintain an upright position. Friction, on the other hand, changes as the body comes into contact with a variety of surfaces, thus causing different reactions of the body's internal environment in response to these changing conditions.

Forces from many other sources such as wind, water, animate and inanimate objects all have their effect on the way movement is carried out. It is important that the physical laws of the external environment are understood so that the prediction of, and compensation for, these forces can be implemented by the controlling systems.

It is obvious that each of these aspects is interrelated and that between them they give a framework and a direction for the study of movement. However, any attempt to consider all possible factors simultaneously would result in a very lengthy and complex process and this inevitably means that research into movement rarely encompasses more than one or two aspects. In this book the initial chapters examine some of the different theoretical backgrounds to the description of human movement and in the later chapters there is a more holistic evaluation of some common everyday activities and consideration of how movement can be affected by factors such as ageing or stress. There are also two chapters addressing the measurement of human movement, emphasising the difficulties which arise from attempting to measure and evaluate complex, multidimensional activities. One chapter focuses on the collection of the objective physical markers of human movement whilst the other looks at the use of measurement scales to study the impact of movement on everyday life.

It is essential for the reader to remember that, in the practical or clinical situation, most approaches to considering human movement will look at only one or two of the many aspects. This is obviously a limited approach and may give a false or distorted picture of the individual's ability. Sadly, it is not possible to achieve the ideal situation and take simultaneous measurements of all components of a complex functional activity, but providing there is an awareness of the limitations of the way in which human movement is measured and assessed, the right conclusions about how an individual's performance may be corrected or improved may still be reached.

Case Study 1.1

A premier division soccer team were undergoing a series of tests of 'fitness' which, it was hoped, would provide information which could be used to build an improved training programme. These tests included anthropometric measurements, tests for elasticity of soft tissue, muscle length and the strength and endurance capacity of their lower limb muscles. Towards the end of the day one of the players, Mr F, was having the peak torque ratio of his knee and hip flexors and extensors tested on the isokinetic dynamometer.

When the results for the team were analysed, it was found that the torque generated by the non-dominant limb was always greater or equal to that of the dominant limb, except in the case of Mr F, where his dominant limb appeared to have generated substantially more torque than expected. There was concern that either there had been an error in the data collection procedure or that Mr F had an injury to his non-dominant limb which he had not mentioned to the laboratory staff and which was being reflected in abnormally low torque levels. It was decided to call him back in for review.

On reattendance, discussion with Mr F revealed that he had begun to lose interest in the testing procedures by the end of the day when his isokinetic test was scheduled. He speculated that he had not been putting as much effort as he might into the test until, just as the peak torque in his dominant limb was being measured, his team manager and coach walked into the laboratory. He clearly remembered trying to impress them with his keenness and fitness by working as hard as he could and as a consequence had distorted the data.

In this case the laboratory staff were looking for physiological or mechanical reasons why the data for Mr F should be aberrant. In the end, the reason was psychological.

Self-awareness and observational skills

Case study 1 was used to illustrate how movement and performance can be affected by a number of factors, which may not always be those that are most obvious. Another interesting fact that became apparent during the testing procedures undertaken on these professional soccer players was that their balance and spatial awareness was surprisingly poor. This information came to light inadvertently during a plyometric testing procedure, when the players found the test hard to complete and lost their balance repeatedly. Despite the fact that their profession required a high level of physical ability, none of the players had a good level of awareness of the way in which their body moved and they all found it difficult to work out how to modify their approach to the plyometric test in order to remain in balance. This lack of consciousness of movement is common in the general population, with most people never considering how they are able to undertake everyday tasks until they lose that ability.

Take yourself: do you know exactly what movements occurred in the joints of your upper limb as you picked up this book and opened it? Were you even aware of the process or did it happen automatically? All people, during their waking hours, are constantly moving and yet they rarely stop to analyse these movements and have no idea how complicated most of them are.

In the later chapters of this book, common activities such as walking or getting out of a chair will be considered and their complexity will become apparent. However, most people are oblivious to the way in which they perform tasks, and many daily activities occur at a subconscious, reflex level. This frees the brain to undertake other tasks at the same time, for example it becomes possible for a musician to play a guitar, sing and move about the stage simultaneously.

If a detailed analysis of everyday activities is carried out, it is clear that there are patterns of joint movement and muscle action which are common to several activities. For example, going up stairs uses the same basic pattern of movement as standing up from a chair or walking up a slope. Swinging the upper limbs in walking is similar to taking food to the mouth, though the range of movement is different. The brain works in terms of patterns of movement rather than movement of individual joints and contractions of individual muscles. It is probably because of this that tasks performed frequently become reflex. As long as the ability to perform tasks automatically exists, most familiar movements can be undertaken in a smooth and efficient manner. When this ability is lost, perhaps through injury or disease, movement becomes noticeably slower and less coordinated.

Anyone whose work involves the moving human body needs to become aware of the way normal movement occurs and which patterns of movement are frequently used. Once an understanding and awareness of normal movement is acquired, it becomes possible to recognise deviations from normal and to plan rehabilitation or training programmes with precision.

Knowledge of human movement through direct experience

Few people consciously explore their full potential for movement, but students of human movement must become very aware of themselves and the way they move before they can consider others. It is as important to be aware of movement and to 'feel' or consciously experience joints moving and muscles contracting as it is to observe others.

In addition to developing self-awareness it is also essential to learn observational skills, as these are the mainstay of clinical practice. Every opportunity should be taken to observe the movements of other people. Look at the different ways they walk or stand and try to identify exactly what makes one person move differently to another. Be precise in this, observing not only which joint moves, but by how much or how fast. As you develop the skills of observation you should try to compare groups of people.

Task 1.1

You need to develop personal self-awareness and the skills of observation if you are to have a full understanding of normal movement. This can be done in a number of ways, all of which require you to put in some effort.

1. Try to become aware of all parts of your body. For example, think about the position of your shoulder girdle: is it elevated or depressed? Be aware of your vertebral column: are the various components flexed, extended or laterally flexed? Constantly re-evaluate how your body is aligned and notice how your body changes the alignment of its parts for different activities. Become aware of the differing ranges of joint movement that can occur between individuals; compare yourself with others to see if your joints are more or less mobile. Notice what it feels like when you reach the limit of a movement. Is it the same feeling for all joints?
2. Think about what your body feels like when it moves in contrast to when it is still. If some movements cause discomfort, ask yourself why and try to work out exactly which structures are involved. Is it because you have moved too near to the limit of your normal range of movement or because you are working a muscle particularly hard?
3. Notice the difference in feeling when a muscle is contracted or relaxed by making a very tight fist and holding it tight for 30 seconds. Then relax and notice the changing sensations as relaxation occurs: is the process of relaxation instantaneous?
4. Try to become aware of the way in which your body weight is distributed during activities which require balance ability. Is your weight equally distributed between both feet, or is it more on one foot than the other? Consider whether your weight is distributed across the whole foot evenly or if there is more taken through the ball of the foot than the heel. What advantages come from different alignments of body weight across one or both feet?

Task 1.2

Do elderly people move differently from the young, or women from men? If you think the answer is yes, then you should try to identify the differences.

UNDERSTANDING HUMAN MOVEMENT AND ITS CLINICAL APPLICATION

To develop the skills of human movement analysis it is first important to become more self-aware and this, combined with a knowledge of relevant research, will lead gradually to a firsthand understanding of many of the factors of 'normal' movement. This needs to be combined with the ability to observe, in a structured and purposeful manner, the way other people perform everyday activities. In the professional setting it is possible to use the senses of hearing, sight and touch to collect information about individuals and their problems. The skills of interviewing, listening with understanding, looking and seeing, palpating and testing, all contribute towards a pool of knowledge and modern measurement techniques will enable some quantifiable data to be collected.

When working with patients, it is necessary to identify the skills they require to perform activities of daily living and to analyse the way in which they actually try to undertake these activities. With this knowledge it becomes possible to consider how certain tasks might be made more efficient or how a person with a disability might be helped towards greater independence. Specific problems can be identified, goals set and a realistic programme designed. Finally, the patient's progress will need to be regularly evaluated and goals altered when necessary. By systematically approaching each individual's movement problems in this way, clinical judgement can be developed and clinical practice becomes more effective.

USING THIS BOOK

Use the early chapters, in conjunction with other specialised textbooks, to gain a grounding in the theories underpinning how human movement is planned, initiated and controlled. This basic knowledge is essential to an understanding of what is happening when movement occurs and why it happens. Use the later chapters as introductions to the way in which various parts of the body contribute to functional movement and as an introduction to how complex movements are analysed. These chapters will also consider some of the common factors that lead to deviations from normal movement patterns.

Throughout the book there are case studies which form the link between theory and actuality, illustrating why the acquisition of knowledge and understanding will lead to better results. If you are already working with patients or clients, then you should try to see how the content of the chapters relates to your experience.

In all the chapters there are tasks which are designed to encourage thought or help you develop skills. If you are to benefit from the learning process you should undertake each task, attempting to fulfil all its requirements. Some of the tasks are short, but a number will develop into skills which you will use for the rest of your working life. Most of these tasks are easy and do not require answers to be provided within the book; if you are unsure of any of the answers then reread the relevant parts of the chapter, discuss the problem with your colleagues and talk to more experienced staff.

When you use this book you must be aware that it is a basic text designed as an introduction to the study of human movement. It is not a definitive repository of all knowledge in the subject area but should help in the understanding of more advanced research. If you are to be excellent in your work then you must constantly strive to further your knowledge through reading and enquiry. This should not be a burdensome task because human movement is a fascinating subject, intriguing in its complexity and of direct interest to every one of us.

CHAPTER CONTENTS

Introduction   7

Muscles   7
Skeletal muscle structure   8

Muscle contraction   11
Factors affecting force generation   11
Types of muscle contraction   13
Velocity of contraction   14
Power   16
Frequency of stimulation   16

The motor unit   17
Gradation of muscle force   17

Fibre types   18

Gross muscle structure   19
Determinants of force   19
Determinants of velocity   20
Muscle length, strength and power   21
Muscle attachments   21

Roles of muscles   21

Range of movement   22
Active and passive insufficiency   22

Human movement   23
Forces and stresses   24
The hip joint   24
The knee joint   26
The ankle joint   28
The foot   29
The vertebral column   29
The shoulder complex   31
The elbow joint   33
Wrist and hand   33

Conclusion   34

2

Musculoskeletal basis for movement

D. J. Newham
A.-M. Ainscough-Potts

OBJECTIVES

At the end of this chapter you should be able to:

1. **Describe the structure and function of muscle**

2. **Discuss the physiological processes for the different types of contraction**

3. **Discuss the different types of muscle activity**

4. **Explain the role of the muscle in different activities.**

INTRODUCTION

In order to be able to analyse movement it is essential to have a good understanding of muscle function, anatomy and biomechanics. This chapter does not attempt to reproduce the basic textbook material in these areas. Its aim is to bring together the components of knowledge necessary for movement analysis and help the reader integrate them.

The first section describes skeletal muscle structure and function. The second section incorporates this knowledge into the consideration and analysis of human movement.

MUSCLES

There are three major types of muscle: skeletal (striated), cardiac and smooth muscle. The latter is found in the walls of blood vessels and gut.

Skeletal muscle is that which enables the maintenance of posture and movement and will be considered in this section. It is under both voluntary and reflex control.

Skeletal muscle structure

An understanding of how skeletal muscle works requires knowledge of its structure from the level of gross anatomy to molecular organisation. There is a hierarchical structure seen in Table 2.1 and illustrated in Figure 2.1. Muscle structure and function are discussed in more detail in specialised works (e.g. Jones & Round 1990, Lieber 1992).

Skeletal muscle is composed of contractile and non-contractile components. The contractile components are the actin and myosin filaments that are responsible for the generation of active force (tension).

The non-contractile components are elastic structures such as tendons, connective tissue sheaths and structural proteins which contribute to the development of passive tension.

Muscle fibres

These long, multinucleated muscle cells may extend over the whole length of the muscle or may be much shorter, depending on the arrangement of fibres within the muscle. A network of capillaries, many of which will be closed at rest, surrounds them. During activity the capillaries become patent and muscle blood flow can be greatly increased.

The muscle cells contain many mitochondria that are responsible for aerobic metabolism. Their presence allows the muscle to function continuously in the presence of oxygen and their number varies with fibre type and also endurance train-

Table 2.1 The hierarchy of muscle organisation

Whole muscle	Bundles of fascicles	Surrounded by connective tissue sheath (epimysium)
Muscle fascicles	Groups of muscle fibres	Surrounded by connective tissue sheath (perimysium)
Muscle fibres	Bundles of myofibrils (about 2000) arranged in parallel	Surrounded by connective tissue sheath (sarcolemma) 10–100 μm diameter, multinucleated
Myofibrils	String of sarcomeres arranged in series	Surrounded by sarcoplasmic reticulum and T tubules about 1 μm diameter
Sarcomeres	Functional unit of muscle contraction	Composed of myofilaments and structural, non-contractile proteins
Myofilaments	Actin (thin) and myosin (thick) filaments	

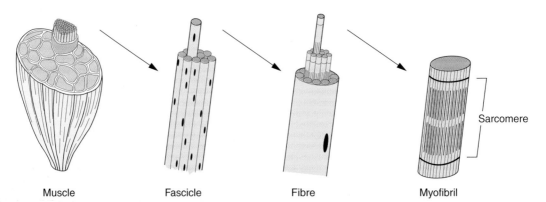

| Muscle | Fascicle | Fibre | Myofibril |

Sarcomere

Figure 2.1 Representation of the relationship between muscle, muscle fibres and myofibrils. The striations in the myofibrils are the result of the arrangement of the actin and myosin filaments. Each myofibril consists of adjacent sarcomeres connected to each other in series. These run the length of the fibre.

ing. The cells also contain glycogen and lipid droplets.

Myofibrils

A membranous network called the sarcoplasmic reticulum (SR) surrounds each myofibril. The interior of the SR is quite separate from the contents of the fibre and contains the calcium that is necessary for the interaction of actin and myosin and the generation of force. The signal for calcium release from the SR is the arrival of the action potential from the nerve via the neuromuscular junction. This travels over the surface of the fibres and is transmitted into the interior by a series of invaginations in the surface membrane called the T (tubular) system. The SR is in close proximity with the T tubules and ensures an effective calcium release, as shown in Figure 2.2. Once the action potential has passed,

calcium is pumped back into the SR and the muscle relaxes.

The sarcomere

These are the structural units for muscle, which repeat along the length of each fibril. They are bound at each end by a Z line that connects adjacent sarcomeres as shown in Figure 2.3. The actin (thin) myofilaments are a structural part of the Z line and the myosin (thick filaments) interdigitate with the actin filaments, but are not connected directly to the Z line. The alignment of the actin and myosin filaments give the striations to skeletal muscle.

However, the myosin filaments do not lie free in the sarcomere. They, and the architecture of the entire sarcomere, are maintained by a number of structural proteins. They include some for which the purpose is unclear while

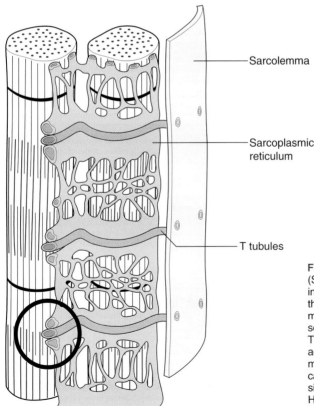

Sarcolemma

Sarcoplasmic reticulum

T tubules

Figure 2.2 The relationship between sarcoplasmic reticulum (SR), T tubules and muscle fibres. The T tubules are invaginations of the sarcolemma and allow transmission of the action potential into the interior of the fibre. The membranous bags forming the SR are wrapped around sections of each myofibril and have a T tubule on either side. They contain calcium that is released on the arrival of an action potential, and cause the interaction between actin and myosin that results in force generation. The area circled is called a triad and is a T tubule with a portion of SR on either side. (Reproduced with permission from 'Skeletal Muscle in Health and Disease' by D A Jones and J M Round, 1990, Manchester University Press, Manchester, UK.)

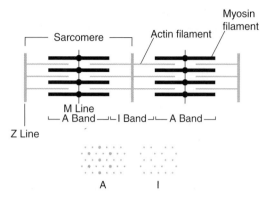

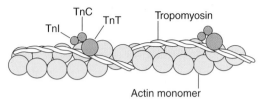

Figure 2.4 A section of an actin filament. The double strands of actin monomers form a groove into which the regulatory protein tropomyosin fits. The protein troponin is made of three subunits and is located at intervals along the tropomyosin. Tropomyosin blocks the binding sites for myosin until caused to move by the binding of calcium to troponin C. Troponin T binds troponin to tropomyosin and troponin I inhibits tropomyosin when there is no calcium release. (Reproduced with permission from 'Skeletal Muscle in Health and Disease' by D A Jones and J M Round, 1990, Manchester University Press, Manchester, UK.)

Figure 2.3 Two adjacent sarcomeres. This pattern is repeated along the length of the fibre. The actin (thin) and myosin (thick) filaments are arranged precisely and give the striations to skeletal muscle. The A band contains both types of filament, while the I band contains only actin filaments. Cross sections through the A and I bands are shown below.

others have an identified role. An example of the latter is dystrophin which is absent or reduced in muscular dystrophy.

The *actin filament* is a globular protein that appears as double helical strands with tropomyosin and three troponin (Tn) subunits TnC, TnT and TnI (Fig. 2.4). The regulatory protein tropomyosin blocks the myosin binding sites until it is caused to move and uncover them, when calcium binds to TnC. TnT binds troponin

and tropomyosin and TnI inhibits tropomyosin in the absence of calcium.

Myosin filaments are two identical chains arranged in an antiparallel fashion. The globular head of the S1 fragment is attached to the S2 fragment. This is a flexible neck region that connects with the long tail of the molecule. The S1 fragment forms the cross bridge with the actin filament and causes force generation. Individual myosin molecules pack together to form the thick filament with the heads projecting out around the filament which has a central area free of cross bridges. This is shown in Figure 2.5.

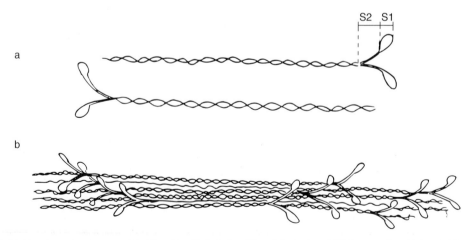

Figure 2.5 (a) Myosin molecules consist of two identical chains. The globular head (SI fragment), which combines with actin, and the extensible neck region (S2 fragment) are connected to a long tail or backbone. (b) The molecules are packed together to form the thick filaments. They are rotated so that the heads are arranged around the filament.

MUSCLE CONTRACTION

Figure 2.6 is a diagrammatic representation of a muscle contraction. When a muscle contracts, the filaments themselves do not change length. However, the sarcomeres, and therefore fibres, may change length because of changes in the amount of overlap between actin and myosin filaments (Huxley & Simmons 1971). The myosin head attaches to a binding site on the actin fila-

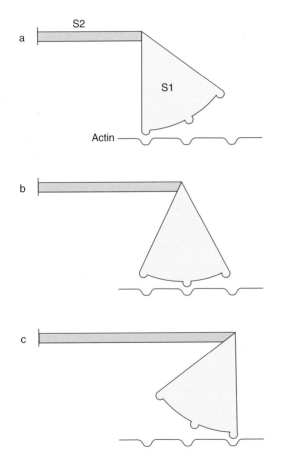

Figure 2.6 During muscle contraction the cross bridge or S1 fragment of the myosin molecule attaches to a binding site on the actin filament (a). During an isometric contraction the myosin head rotates (b and c) and pulls the actin filament (to the left), but the relative position of the actin and myosin filaments remains constant and the S2 portion of the myosin molecule is stretched and force is generated. If the muscle shortens during contraction, phases a, b and c occur as above. Then the actin filament is pulled towards the myosin molecule and the stretch on the S2 fragment decreases.

ment and rotates, thus pulling the actin filament toward the centre of the sarcomere and exerting a passive extension force on the S2 fragment. The myosin heads are released and attempt to attach to another binding site and the cross bridge cycle continues as long as the muscle is activated and the energy requirements are met.

Factors affecting force generation

Studies on isolated muscle preparations have shown that the force that can be generated by a fully activated muscle fibre, or even a single sarcomere, is affected by a number of factors. These are intrinsic properties of skeletal muscle and also apply to intact human muscles.

Length

There are two components which affect the force that is generated at different muscle lengths. These components are active and passive tension.

Active tension is the force generated by the cross bridges and is illustrated in Figure 2.7. The muscle has been moved through the full range and stimulated electrically at numerous different lengths while tension is measured as each length remains constant. It can be seen that there is an optimum length for force generation. Force declines when the muscle is activated at either longer or shorter lengths (Gordon et al 1966) and at the extremes of length no force is generated.

The explanation for this lies in the amount of overlap between the actin and myosin filaments and underlies the sliding filament theory of contraction (Huxley & Simmons 1971). At optimal length there is sufficient overlap for numerous cross bridges to form and the length of the sarcomere does not impair force generation. At lengths shorter than optimal, the actin filaments from the two ends of the sarcomere come closer together and progressively interfere with force generation. At lengths longer than optimal, the amount of overlap between actin and myosin filaments decreases, reducing the number of cross bridges that can be formed. Muscles in intact animals and humans do not reach the extremes

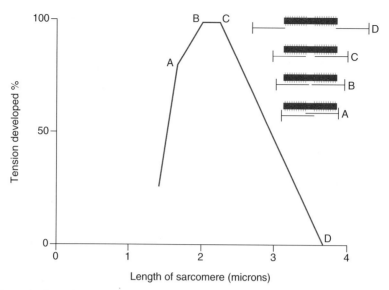

Figure 2.7 The length tension for a single sarcomere, measured during a series of isometric contractions at different sarcomere lengths. On the ascending limb, force increases with length. At sarcomere lengths shorter than 2 μm (B), the thin filaments begin to overlap and at still shorter lengths (A) they come into contact with the Z lines. These factors both reduce the force that can be generated. On the descending limb (C–D), force declines as length is increased. As length increases the amount of overlap between thick and thin filaments decreases and so fewer connections can be made between them. The optimal conditions for force generation occur on the plateau (B–C). (After Gordon et al 1966, reproduced with permission.)

of length shown in Figure 2.7 because of anatomical constraints. However, a number of intact human muscles demonstrate a length:tension relationship which clearly shows an optimal length and decreasing force as length changes in either direction. Other muscles show flatter curves and this is probably due to biomechanical changes and also orientation of fibres within the muscle (described later).

Some muscles in the intact human body develop maximal active tension at approximately the midpoint of joint range, but relatively few muscles have been studied systematically in this respect.

Passive tension is developed during stretch of even a resting muscle. The origin of passive tension lies in the connective tissue that is both in series and parallel with the myofilaments. The tendons and structural proteins, particularly titin, form the series elastic component, while the surrounding connective tissue represents the parallel component.

Total tension can be calculated when active and passive tensions are both measured, as illustrated

in Figure 2.8. This initially reduces the effects of active tension lost on the ascending limb of the length:tension relationship. However, further increases in length cause a rapid increase in total tension and can be sufficient to cause muscle rupture.

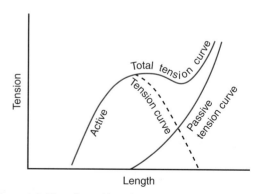

Figure 2.8 The effect of length on total tension. The active length tension relationship of a single sarcomere is shown here and in Figure 2.7. In intact preparations the non-contractile components start to exert passive tension, at approximately mid-length, which increases with length.

Task 2.1

Why and how does muscle length affect the active tension that can be generated?

Is the effect of length the same for active and passive tension?

In the living body most muscles which cross a single joint cannot be stretched to the point where passive tension contributes significantly to total tension. However, muscles acting over more than one joint may be stretched sufficiently for passive tension to limit joint range.

It is important to remember that the length:tension relationship describes the effect of length on isometric (static) tension. In order to describe movement it is necessary to understand the effect on force of contraction type and also velocity.

Types of muscle contraction

The sliding filament theory of muscle contraction dictates that an active muscle will attempt to shorten. Whether or not length changes occur depends on the external resistance offered. It is important to realise that the term 'contraction' is used to describe an active muscle and relays no information about whether or not it changes length during activity:

- An *isometric* (static) contraction occurs when there is no external movement, because the internal tension generated by the muscle is equal to the external force.
- When there is movement a *dynamic* contraction takes place and the muscle may become longer or shorter.

- A muscle will shorten and perform a *concentric* contraction if the force generated is greater than the external force.
- An *eccentric* contraction occurs when a muscle generates a lower force than the external load and is lengthened by it.

The characteristics of isometric, concentric and eccentric contractions and the forces generated by each type of activity are very different, as shown in Table 2.2 (Jones & Round 1990, Lieber 1992).

Isometric contractions occur when there is no movement and thus the muscle does no external work. The maximal force that can be generated and the energy cost required for a given amount of force are intermediate between concentric and eccentric contractions.

Although the muscle does not change length in gross terms, there is some internal shortening as the sarcomeres shorten slightly due to filaments sliding past each other. In the intact body, the elastic tendons are slightly stretched.

Concentric contractions occur when the muscle shortens, movement occurs and external work is done. A muscle contracting concentrically will always generate less force than when contracting isometrically. The actin binding sites are moving past the myosin cross bridges and it takes a certain amount of time for cross bridges to attach to, and detach from, the actin binding sites. Therefore, the number of attached cross bridges, and thus the force generated, is less than during an isometric contraction. This rapid cycling of cross bridges has a high energy cost and, therefore, the highest oxygen demand and heat production occurs during concentric contractions.

Eccentric contractions occur when an external resistance lengthens active muscle. Work is done on the muscle, rather than by it, and so negative

Table 2.2 The characteristics of the three types of muscle contraction. The determining factor for movement is whether the internal force generated by a muscle is the same, lower or higher than the external forces

Type of contraction	Function	External force (relative to internal)	External work by muscle	Force generated	Energy cost (O_2 demand)
Concentric	Acceleration	Less	Positive	Lowest	Highest
Isometric (static)	Fixation	Same	None	Intermediate	Intermediate
Eccentric	Deceleration	Greater	Negative	Highest	Lowest

work is said to be done. During an eccentric contraction a muscle generates a force higher than it is capable of under isometric or concentric conditions. This is thought to be partly because the tension generated by cross bridge formation is increased by the additional component of elastic force caused by the stretch of the neck of the myosin molecule (S2 fragment). The cross bridges remain attached to the actin binding site unless ripped away by the stretching force.

Curiously, in view of their high force generation, eccentric contractions are performed at a very low energy cost. This is thought to be because the myosin head is mechanically pulled from the binding site, rather than requiring ATP as in other types of contraction, and when the myosin head is pulled away from the actin filament, it is in the correct position for subsequent reattachment to another binding site and does not require energy to move into the attachment position.

The high force generation and low energy cost of eccentric exercise is still not fully understood. The performance of unaccustomed, high force eccentric activity will cause muscle fatigue, pain and damage in excess of that caused by isometric or concentric contractions and this is thought to be due to mechanical damage (Clarkson & Newham 1995).

Functional examples

The rather complicated concept of the different types of muscle contraction can be illustrated by considering the right quadriceps muscle. If a person stands on his right leg, his quadriceps will be working isometrically to prevent the knee flexing. If he stands from sitting, the muscle will work concentrically to straighten the knee. If he sits down in a controlled manner then the muscle will be working eccentrically as it controls movement velocity by opposing the force of gravity.

Thus, isometric contractions are generally used for fixation, concentric ones for acceleration and eccentric for deceleration.

Isokinetic/isotonic contractions

Muscle contractions may also be isotonic or isokinetic in nature. An *isotonic* contraction is one in which the force remains constant throughout. An *isokinetic* contraction is dynamic and is performed at a constant velocity throughout. These are considered in more detail in Chapter 6.

Functional activity

It is relatively unusual for a muscle to perform only one type of contraction in any particular activity. Most activities involve a mixture of varying proportions of the different types and all have important functional roles. An eccentric contraction often precedes a concentric one and it is thought that this utilises the energy stored during eccentric activity and increases mechanical efficiency (Komi 1986). A common example of this 'stretch–shortening' cycle is in the calf muscles where the active muscles are stretched prior to shortening during the push off phase of walking, running and jumping, as illustrated in Figure 2.9.

Velocity of contraction

The amount of tension that a fully activated muscle can generate also varies with the velocity of contraction. If an active muscle is either allowed to shorten, or is stretched, at a range of different velocities and the force generated is measured at each velocity, then the force:velocity relationship can be determined (Fig. 2.10). This also shows the effect of contraction type on force as discussed above.

It can clearly be seen that, while eccentric force remains above and concentric force below isometric (zero velocity) force, velocity has a marked and different effect on the two types of dynamic contraction. Concentric force decreases with velocity while eccentric force increases.

Concentric contractions

The higher the velocity of shortening, the shorter is the time available for the myosin cross bridges to attach to the actin binding sites moving past them. The proportion of cross bridges that manage to attach to the actin filament in the region in which the cross bridges can exert a useful force decreases as velocity increases. Therefore, the number of

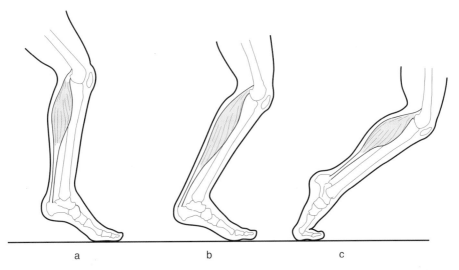

Figure 2.9 The stretch–shortening cycle of the calf muscles during walking, jumping and running. Just before contact the muscles are activated (a) in order to resist the forces of impact during which they are stretched and perform an eccentric contraction (b). This is immediately followed by a shortening (concentric) contraction during push off (c).

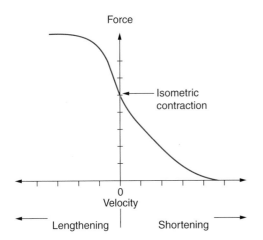

Figure 2.10 The force:velocity relationship of a maximally activated muscle. Concentric force is always greater than isometric and decreases as velocity increases. Eccentric force is always greater than isometric, it initially increases with velocity, then remains relatively constant.

attached cross bridges, and the force they can exert, decreases with velocity.

Maximal velocity of shortening (V_{max})

Eventually a velocity is reached at which no force can be sustained; this is the maximal velocity of shortening (V_{max}). The V_{max} differs between individuals and also in different muscles in the same person or animal. It is largely determined genetically by the fibre types within muscle and is little affected by physical training (Jones & Round 1990).

Eccentric contractions

In contrast, eccentric force increases with velocity and plateaus at about 1.8 times the isometric force. As the velocity of stretch increases, the extensible S2 portions of the cross bridges produce more passive, elastic force. The plateau of the eccentric force:velocity relationship suggests that skeletal muscles are relatively resistant to stretch and this is useful in many normal movement patterns.

Functional implications

Activities of daily life frequently demonstrate the practical consequences of the effects of velocity on force generation. The heavier a weight is, the slower we are able to move or lift it using concentric contractions. However, eccentric contractions such as those involved in lowering heavy weights,

---

Task 2.2

Why are different forces generated by a fully activated muscle depending on whether it stays the same length (isometric) gets shorter (concentric) or longer (eccentric)?

Is the effect of velocity similar for concentric and eccentric force?

---

whether an inanimate object or the weight of the body, become faster with heavier weights.

Power

In many activities the functional requirement is for power, i.e. the rate of doing work, rather than force. Power is the product of force and velocity, therefore during isometric contractions (zero velocity), and at maximal velocity (zero force) dynamic contractions, the power output is zero. Figure 2.11 shows the power output at different velocities of concentric contraction.

Maximal power output usually occurs at about two-thirds of the maximal velocity.

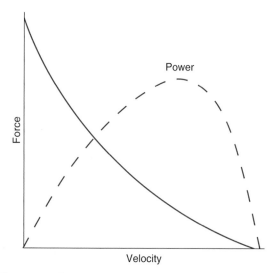

Figure 2.11 The power output at different velocities of concentric contraction. This is derived from the force:velocity relationship (solid line) as shown in Figure 2.10.

Frequency of stimulation

When a muscle fibre is stimulated at an intensity above the threshold for motor activation it will generate force. The force generated is strongly influenced by the frequency of stimulation. A single impulse will result in a mechanical response called a twitch. If stimulation frequency is increased, the force initially increases and then remains relatively constant despite substantial increases in force, as shown in Figure 2.12.

As the stimulation frequency initially increases, two observations can be made. The first is that the contraction becomes smoother because the muscle has less time to relax between consecutive stimuli. The second observation is that the force increases with stimulation frequency because the next impulse arrives before the muscle has completely relaxed and the impulse is superimposed on the remaining tension. This is known as the summation of force. When stimulated at a sufficiently high frequency (termed the *fusion frequency*), the muscle will produce a smooth, tetanic force in which there is no relaxation between individual stimuli. The frequency at which this occurs depends on the fibre type and is discussed later in this chapter. An increase in stimulation frequency above the fusion frequency does not increase the force of contraction.

Functional implications

Recordings from muscles during voluntary contractions have shown that the physiological

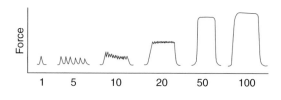

Stimulation frequency (Hz)

Figure 2.12 The relationship between force and the frequency of external electrical stimulation. Note that increased frequency initially increases force and reduces oscillations. However, increasing the frequency above that which produces a fused tetanic contraction does not increase force.

firing rates are usually at a frequency lower than the fusion frequency found when muscles are stimulated electrically (Binder-Macleod 1992). However, we can easily make a smooth voluntary contraction using stimulation frequencies that would show marked oscillation using external electrical stimulation. This is because during external stimulation the active fibres are being stimulated synchronously, but in voluntary activity they are all firing asynchronously, smoothing out force oscillations.

THE MOTOR UNIT

Each individual muscle fibre generates a force so small as to be impractical for even the most delicate movements. Therefore, the system is designed such that a group of muscle fibres share common innervation from a single alpha motor neurone (gamma motor neurones innervate the intrafusal fibres within the muscle spindle). This functional grouping is called a motor unit and is composed of the cell body of the alpha motor neurone (the anterior horn cell in the spinal cord), the motor neurone itself and the muscle fibres innervated by it. Figure 2.13 illustrates the motor unit. If a motor neurone fires, all the muscles in that unit will contract at the same time, producing a synchronised

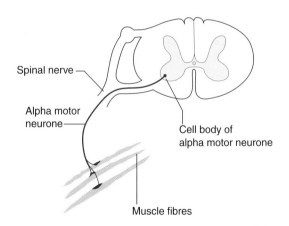

Figure 2.13 A single motor unit is composed of the motor neurone and the muscle fibres which it innervates. The cell body of the motor neurone is in the anterior horn cell in the spinal cord and its axon is one of the motor nerves in a mixed peripheral nerve.

electrical discharge (action potential) which can be measured by electromyography and also the generation of force. The size of both action potential and force are proportional to the number of muscle fibres within the motor unit. There is a range of motor unit size within a single muscle and also between muscles. Muscles requiring the precise regulation of small forces, such as the small hand muscles, have smaller motor units that may contain only 10 fibres. Large postural muscles, such as the quadriceps, have much larger motor units that may have several thousand fibres.

The fibres belonging to an individual motor unit are scattered throughout a muscle, thus adjacent fibres are unlikely to belong to the same motor unit. All the fibres within a single unit are the same fibre type.

Gradation of muscle force

It is clear that both voluntary and reflex muscle force can be precisely controlled. There are two ways in which force can be varied, motor unit recruitment and rate coding. Both have been shown to be used in voluntary contractions of human muscle, but it is unclear to what extent they are employed. It is possible that large postural muscles, which do not require fine control of force, predominantly use motor unit recruitment. Those needing fine control, such as the hand muscles, may rely more on rate coding.

Motor unit recruitment

Activating more motor units will increase the force generated and this is termed motor unit recruitment. The smaller motor units have the most excitable motor neurones and therefore are recruited first. As more force is required, the larger, and progressively less excitable, motor neurones are recruited in an orderly fashion. This has become known as the size principle (Hennemann et al 1974).

Rate coding

The force of active motor units can also be varied by the frequency of stimulation of the motor

> **Task 2.3**
>
> What is a motor unit? What is their role in the generation of different levels of force?

neurone and by utilising the force:frequency characteristics. Recordings from single motor units have shown that the firing rate varies considerably even within a constant low force contraction. Initially, a short burst of firing may be used to generate relatively high forces by the motor unit, but this rapidly decreases to maintain force.

FIBRE TYPES

The observation that some muscles are dark and others light, as in the leg and breast muscle of a chicken, is an indication that not all muscle fibres are the same. It was thought previously that discrete fibre types existed, but it seems that there is a spectrum of fibre types. Considerable variations in histochemistry, contractile properties and the type of metabolic fuel used have been identified. This is shown in Table 2.3. The colour differences exist because of the different levels of myoglobin which is red. It can be seen from Table 2.3 that Type I fibres are specialised to use oxidative metabolism and are resistant to fatigue. They contain a lot of myoglobin and are relatively slow to contract and relax. They are recruited early in low force muscle activity due to their small axon size and therefore fatigue resistance is an important feature. The number of

muscle fibres in slow motor units is small and so motor unit recruitment can result in fine gradations of force. They rely on oxidative (aerobic) metabolism and are developed so that the delivery and utilisation of oxygen is maximised.

Type II fibres are subdivided into Types IIa, b and c. The Type IIb fibres contrast sharply to Type I fibres in almost all respects. They are fast to contract and relax and rely on anaerobic metabolism and intramuscular stores of fuel. Due to the large axon diameter they are recruited only during high force contractions and fatigue rapidly. This is illustrated in Figure 2.14. The

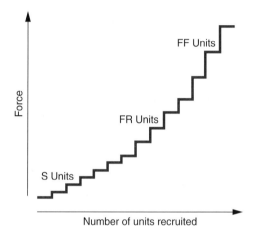

Figure 2.14 The regulation of force by recruitment of motor units. At low forces only the small, slow (S) units are recruited. As force increases, the larger, fatigue-resistant (FR) and then the largest fast, fatigable (FF) units are recruited. The S units have relatively few muscle fibres and the FF units have the most. Therefore the increment in force as a new unit is recruited also varies.

Table 2.3 Examples of differences between fibre types. Note that different terminology exists for types of muscle fibre and motor unit

Property	Type I	Type IIa	Type IIb
Muscle fibre type	Slow oxidative (SO)	Fast oxidative glycolytic (FOG)	Fast glycolytic (FG)
Motor unit type	Slow (S)	Fast fatigue resistant (FR)	Fast fatigable (FF)
Motor unit size	Small	Medium	Large
Twitch tension	Low	Moderate	High
Mechanical speed	Slow	Fast	Fast
Fatigability	Low	Low	High
Mitochondrial enzyme activity	High	Medium	Low
Glycogenolytic enzyme activity	Low	Medium	High
Myoglobin content	High	Medium	Low
Capillary density	High	Medium	Low

motor units contain relatively large numbers of fibres and so recruitment of additional units causes relatively large force increases.

Type IIa fibres and their motor units are intermediate between Types I and IIb and span a broad range of the characteristics of both. The subgroup IIc is found mainly in regenerating fibres and in the embryo.

Functional aspects

During a low force contraction only the Type I fibres are recruited. Therefore, they are used mainly for normal activity which does not require maximal or high force contractions. They are well suited to this role by their fatigue resistance. As the force of contraction increases, the Type IIa and then IIb fibres are progressively recruited and during maximal contractions all the motor units are active. However, maximal force rapidly declines due to the high rate of fatigue in the fast fibres.

Fibre type is largely determined genetically and is governed by the activity in the motor neurone. Training with voluntary activity may shift the characteristics of motor units and their muscle fibres, but does not actually transform motor units and muscle fibres into different types.

GROSS MUSCLE STRUCTURE

Within a single muscle, groups of fibres are organised into fascicles. Figure 2.15 shows that the arrangement of the fascicles varies considerably in different muscles and this has an impact on muscle function. Muscles arranged with the fibres in parallel with the line of pull (strap and also fusiform structure to a large extent) usually have a tendon at each end that inserts into bone. In these muscles the fibre length is long and similar to the muscle length. In muscles with a pennate structure, the fibres are inserted into a longitudinal tendon and lie at an angle to the line of pull of the muscle. In this case the muscle fibres are much shorter than the whole muscle and also shorter than the fibres in a strap or fusiform alignment.

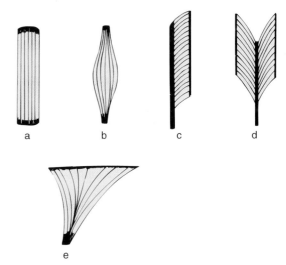

Figure 2.15 Some of the common arrangements of muscles. Strap (a) and fusiform (b) muscles have a tendon at either end and relatively long muscle fibres which run between the tendons. The muscle fibres are arranged in parallel, or are very similar to, the angle of pull of the tendon. Unipennate (c) and bipennate (d) muscles have a central tendon into which short muscle fibres are inserted. The fibre direction is different to the angle of pull of the tendon. Triangular muscles (e) display mixed characteristics.

Effect of fibre alignment on muscle performance

An important concept is that we basically require muscles for two purposes: one is to produce power and cause movement, the other is to generate relatively static force for the maintenance of posture. Therefore, force and power are the key requirements and power is the product of force and velocity. It can be seen that force is necessary for all muscle activity, but power, and thus velocity, are essential for rapid movement. Parallel fibres are usually seen in muscles which are fast acting, such as sartorius, whereas pennate arrangements are seen more in muscles required for strength, such as gluteus maximus.

Determinants of force

The force a muscle can generate in any given situation is proportional to its cross-sectional area, i.e. the number of sarcomeres in parallel.

Along the length of a fibre the tension generated by adjacent sarcomeres is equal and opposite at the central Z line and therefore they cancel each other. The only forces transmitted through the muscle attachments are those generated by the sarcomeres at either end of the muscle. Therefore, force is independent of fibre length (Fig. 2.16).

Muscles that are mainly required for static activity tend to have a large cross-sectional area. A pennate structure has the advantage that more fibres can be packed into the same cross-sectional area (compare Fig. 2.15a and c). The disadvantage is that the force transmitted to the tendon is the cosine of the angle between the angle of pull of the tendon and the fibres and therefore some of the generated force is lost.

Muscle cross-sectional area can be increased by strength training (see Ch. 6) and this increases force generation. However, in pennate muscles with a large angle between the line of pull and fibre alignment, an increased cross-sectional area may result in an increased angle of pennation and therefore a relatively small increase in force.

Determinants of velocity

The maximal velocity at which a muscle can contract is determined by its length, i.e. the number of sarcomeres arranged in series, and is independent of the cross-sectional area. At the start of muscle activity all the sarcomeres begin to contract at about the same time and velocity. If a

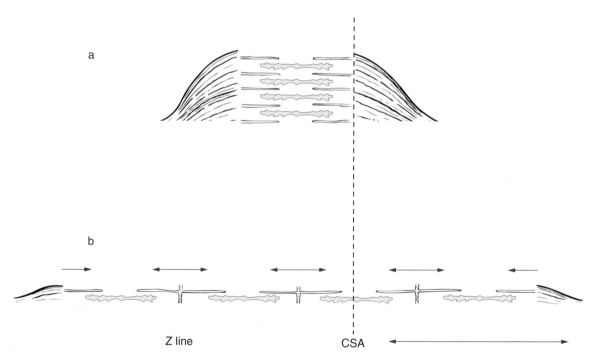

Figure 2.16 Illustration of four sarcomeres arranged in parallel (a) and in series (b). When they are arranged in series, the forces from adjacent sarcomeres at each Z line are equal and opposite. Therefore the only force transmitted by the muscle is that from the outside half of the two sarcomeres at the end of the fibre. The same force is generated by each fibre, irrespective of its length. With a parallel arrangement the force of each sarcomere is transmitted to the tendon. Therefore the same four sarcomeres will generate four times as much force as when they are arranged in series. Note that the cross-sectional area (CSA) is proportional to the force that is produced.

muscle contained only one sarcomere which shortened by 1 mm in 0.1 seconds (s), the shortening velocity would be 10 mm/s. If the muscle contained 100 sarcomeres in series, each would shorten at the same time and velocity, so the total velocity of shortening of the whole muscle would be 1 mm/s.

The maximal velocity of shortening of a single cross bridge and sarcomere is governed by the fibre type and activity of the enzyme myosin ATPase and appears to be relatively unaffected by training.

Muscle length, strength and power

We have already seen that strength is proportional to the cross-sectional area and velocity to length of a muscle. Therefore a short, fat muscle will generate more force and have a lower velocity of shortening than a long, thin one. However, as power is the product of force (cross-sectional area) and velocity (length), it is proportional to volume.

Muscle attachments

Most muscles are connected at each end to at least two bones through a tendinous attachment. One of the bones remains relatively steady and anchors one end of the muscle. Therefore, the force of the contracting muscle moves the bony lever attached to the other end of the muscle.

The traditional anatomical description of muscle attachments is for the more proximal one to be called the *origin* and the distal one the *insertion*. The proximal attachment is usually the more stationary, but there are instances where this is not the case. To avoid confusion in movement analysis, the attachments are often referred to as either *fixed* or *moving*.

ROLES OF MUSCLES

An individual muscle rarely works alone. Usually several different muscles are active simultaneously in even the simplest movement. The forces generated by the active muscles may vary considerably throughout a movement. Each muscle can fulfil several roles in different movements or patterns of movement. These roles are discussed below.

- The *prime mover* or *agonist* is the muscle that plays the major role in initiating, carrying out and maintaining a particular movement. An example is the biceps brachii during elbow flexion.
- *Assistant movers* are those muscles which perform a movement similar to the prime mover, but which play a less significant role in a particular movement. This is the role played by the brachialis in elbow flexion.
- *Stabilisers* or *fixators* are muscles that contract to control the position of a bone so that it may act as a steady base from which the agonist can act. They thus provide a fixed attachment for another muscle. During elbow flexion the shoulder girdle muscles act as fixators to control the position of the arm.
- A *synergist* is a muscle that acts simultaneously with one or more muscles to produce a movement that neither could produce alone. All muscles in the team are called synergists. There are two types of synergists, true and helping.
  — *True synergists* act, for example, when using the long finger flexors as agonists to grip an object in the hand. The unwanted action of these muscles in flexing the wrist needs to be controlled or opposed. This is done by the simultaneous contraction of the wrist extensors acting as true synergists.
  — *Helping synergists* act simultaneously. Flexor carpi radialis and extensor carpi radialis longus are usually antagonistic to each other in producing wrist flexion and extension, respectively. However, they can act simultaneously as helping synergists to produce radial deviation at the wrist.
- *Antagonists* are muscles that act in a direction that is opposite to the agonist. They are often inhibited by a reflex mechanism originating from the agonist and known as reciprocal inhibition. However, during reciprocal and rapid movements they are often activated at the end of joint range and perform an eccentric contraction to

decelerate the movement. This aids movement control and can offer protection against musculo-skeletal damage. During elbow flexion the triceps are antagonists and may be either relaxed or active.

RANGE OF MOVEMENT

During a dynamic contraction muscles move through a range of movement. This is called full range when the muscles move throughout the full anatomical position from the shortest to longest possible length. The extremes of both short and long length in an intact body are much less than those that would be possible if the muscle were freed from its bony attachments. This is because of the limitations imposed by the anatomical arrangement of joints and soft tissue such as joint capsules and ligaments.

Movement through the range will be from long to short length for the agonist during a concentric contraction. Conversely, during an eccentric contraction the agonist will move from short to long length.

The full range of muscle excursion can be subdivided, as shown diagrammatically in Figure 2.17. In *the outer range* the muscle length moves between its longest length and the mid-point of the range. The *inner range* is between the shortest length and the midpoint of range. In the *middle range* the muscle changes its length from the middle positions of the inner and outer ranges.

It is important not to confuse this terminology with that of the range of joint motion since muscle and joint range may not be the same, particularly in muscles acting over more than one joint.

Active and passive insufficiency

Muscles which cross only one joint are usually capable of shortening and lengthening suffi-ciently to allow full range of anatomical move-ment, but this is not necessarily the case for muscles crossing one or more joints. Multiple joint muscles causing simultaneous movement at all the joints crossed may reach a length at which they can no longer generate a useful active tension. At this point the muscle is said to be actively insufficient. This occurs when the ham-strings are used to simultaneously flex the knee whilst extending the hip.

If a multiple joint muscle is unable to stretch across the joints enough to allow their full anatomical range, they are said to be passively insufficient. An example of this is when the length

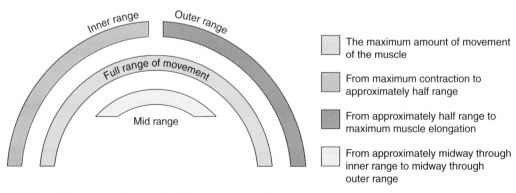

Figure 2.17 A muscle can move through its full range or parts of it.

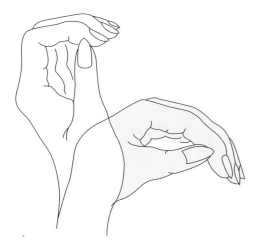

Figure 2.18 The tenodesis action of the long finger flexors causes finger flexion to increase as the wrist is extended.

of the hamstrings prevents touching the toes or floor with extended knees, as they are stretched over both hip and knee (Gowitzke & Milner 1980, Lehmkuhl & Smith 1983). Increasing the passive tension in a multiple joint muscle may cause joint movement called tenodesis. This occurs when moving from flexion to extension of the wrist when the fingers are relaxed. The fingers automatically extend during wrist flexion and flex during wrist extension as shown in Figure 2.18.

HUMAN MOVEMENT

The reader should have some knowledge of human anatomy as found in numerous basic textbooks. Further information on movement analysis and biomechanics can be found in Kapandji (1978), Basmajian & Deluca (1979), Broer & Zernicke (1979) and Palastanga et al (1990). In this section the movements possible at each body segment, and how they are brought about, are considered in biomechanical terms. The body is a series of long and short bones connected at junctions or joints. For movement to occur, the junctions must allow for free movement in the directions that their design allows. The internal forces generated by muscle contraction or by external forces such as gravity and manual or mechanical forces produce movement. It occurs at joints and is contained by ligaments.

In order to understand the way in which the body moves it is necessary to understand how it is constructed and formally described (Fig. 2.19).

The skeleton is designed to absorb and attenuate stress and comprises the long bones of the limbs and short bones of the vertebral column. The hand and foot have short irregular bones proximally and long bones distally. The scapula and pelvis are irregular flat bones. The purpose

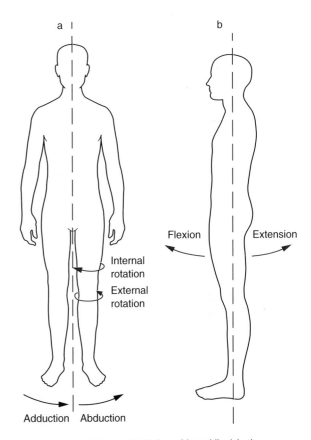

Figure 2.19 (a) The sagittal plane (dotted line) is the midline of the body and divides it into right and left halves. Abduction and adduction are movements away from and towards the sagittal plane respectively. Rotation may be toward (internal rotation) or away from (external rotation) this plane. (b) The frontal plane (dotted line) divides the body into front and back halves. Flexion is a movement about this plane in which the angle between two adjacent surfaces decreases as the joint is bent. Extension is the opposite movement and causes the angle to increase (except in the thumb where these movements occur in a frontal plane). The arrows show the direction of movement for the hip joint. They are not the same for all joints and, for example, are reversed for the knee.

of these bones is to provide shape to the body, to provide attachments for muscles, ligaments and joint capsules and also to dissipate stress generated by movement.

Another function of bone is to protect delicate structures. The skull and vertebral canal protect the brain and spinal cord respectively, the rib cage protects the heart and lungs.

Muscles provide movement at joints and are anchored to bone via connective tissue. In most cases there is one (often proximal) aponeurotic attachment to bone which leaves a roughened surface, and a tendinous (often distal) attachment to bone which is invariably onto a raised tubercule or a depression. Rounded tendons leave a smooth surface.

Forces and stresses

Each time we take a step and the heel strikes the floor, the shock wave that occurs has to be transmitted through the body. Therefore, at heel strike the heel pad initially attenuates some of the shock wave along with the bony joint surfaces and cartilage. The presence of some knee flexion also helps to attenuate it (Payne 1998).

Stress forces travel in straight lines. Every time they meet an interface some are absorbed and others are reflected. Those absorbed will be transmitted to the soft tissues outside the bone. As the tibia is not straight, the stress force will meet at least one interface before arriving at the knee and therefore lose some of its strength. This continues through the body segments so that only a relatively small stress force remains to cause a jarring at the junction of the skull and the vertebral column. All long bones are slightly curved and this enhances the dissipation of stress within the body (Leveau & Bernhardt 1984).

Movement occurs in the limbs at synovial joints. The joint surfaces are lined with hyaline cartilage, and a strong fibrous capsule lined with a synovial membrane that produces synovial fluid surrounds the joint. The combination of fluid and the shiny cartilaginous surfaces produces an almost friction-free environment that enables the muscles to direct their energies to moving the body levers, rather than to over-

coming friction. However, when the joint surfaces become worn with age or disease this is no longer the case. Patients with arthritis find it much more difficult and tiring to move; one of the reasons is the friction that they have to overcome when moving an affected joint.

All synovial joints have only one position where the surfaces fit precisely together and there is maximal contact between the opposing surfaces (MacConaill & Basmajian 1977). This is called the close packed position and it permits no movement. When not in this position, the joint is said to be in the loose packed position and movements of spin, roll and glide may occur. Each joint has a least packed position in which the capsule is at its most lax. Joints tend to assume this position when there is inflammation in order to accommodate the increased volume of synovial fluid.

Through stresses and strains imposed on the bony skeleton by muscle contraction and impact forces, the final adult skeleton shapes are formed and maintained; in later life these same forces may lead to degeneration (see Ch. 5 on stiffness, p. 97). During everyday activity the spinal, hip and shoulder joints are moved in their mid-ranges, the elbow and knee move through a wider range just avoiding the extremes, whereas the wrist and ankles are moved about their mid-ranges. The long bones of the limbs allow the body to make use of momentum for everyday activities, which is a labour saving device for the muscles.

The hip joint

The hip is a ball and socket joint with the rounded head of the femur fitting into the deep socket of the acetabulum on the pelvis.

Movements

The anatomical movements that can occur at this joint are flexion, extension, abduction, adduction, external (lateral) rotation and internal (medial) rotation. When these are combined a circular arc of movement, known as circumduction, occurs. These movements are performed by large muscle groups that work in a coordinated way to produce the anatomical movements. They are large and strong because (for much of the time) they have to counter the effects of gravity (Fig. 2.19).

Functional anatomy

In order to flex the hip when standing, the flexor muscles have to counter the effects of gravity acting on the lower limb. The centre of gravity of a straight lower limb is approximately halfway along its length, i.e. at the knee joint.

With the hip acting as a fulcrum, the force that the body needs to overcome is the product of the lower limb weight and the perpendicular distance between the muscle attachment and the fulcrum centre (Fig. 2.20). The forces exerted are referred to as *turning moments*. Consider the performance of the same limb action as above when lying supine (straight leg raise).

In the first example the perpendicular distance is very close to the centre of the fulcrum (hip joint) so little effort is required to initiate hip flexion. In the second example the perpendicular distance has greatly increased so the forces required to initiate hip flexion are much greater.

During a straight leg raise, the lumbar spine tends to develop a lordosis due to the vertebral attachments of the hip flexors. This action should be countered by the strong deep stabilising back muscles, such as transversus abdominis, or can be prevented if the contralateral knee is flexed and the foot rested on the supporting surface, allowing the muscles to work at a more effective length.

Patients with weak hip flexors may have a well-preserved gait on level ground as they can use momentum to aid forward propulsion. However, climbing up stairs may present a problem due to the increased anti-gravity forces required as the lever arm moves further from the fulcrum. The abductors and adductors are most commonly used to stabilise the pelvis, an action that requires considerable strength. A part or all of the body weight is transmitted through each hip, depending on whether one or two limbs are being used for weight bearing. This is shown in Figure 2.21.

The main role of the hip extensors is to propel the body upwards against gravity as when walking upstairs. The hip flexors raise the leg so

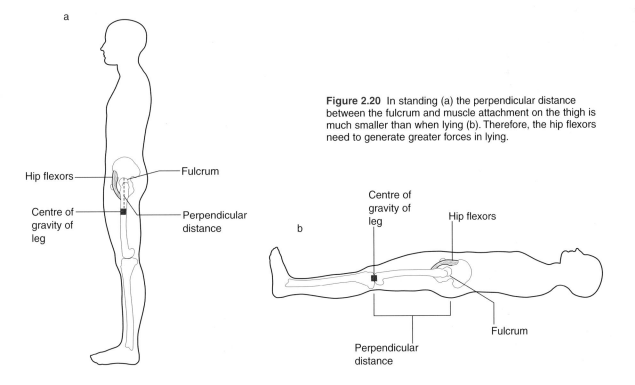

Figure 2.20 In standing (a) the perpendicular distance between the fulcrum and muscle attachment on the thigh is much smaller than when lying (b). Therefore, the hip flexors need to generate greater forces in lying.

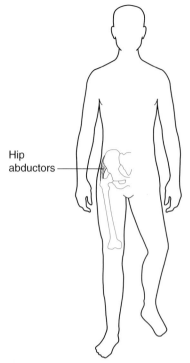

Figure 2.21 The pelvis is stabilised during single leg weight bearing by the action of the hip abductors. When standing on the right leg, the pelvis tends to drop on the left. This is prevented by an isometric contraction of the hip flexors on the right.

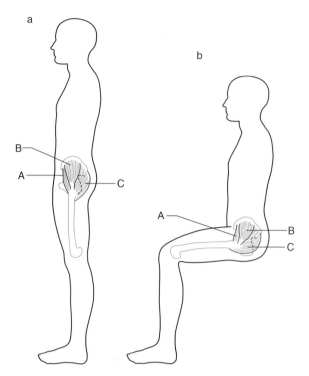

Figure 2.22 The glutei are fan shaped and their action depends on the relative position of the hip and thigh due to the angle of pull. (a) In standing gluteus minimus (A) causes medial rotation, gluteus medius (B) causes abduction and the horizontal fibres of gluteus maximus (C) produce lateral rotation of the femur. (b) In sitting the angle of pull is different and gluteus medius (B) produces medial rotation.

that the foot can be placed and then the hip extensors raise the body over the foot. In this situation both muscle groups are working concentrically and need to be strong.

The muscles around the hip are shaped like a fan. Depending on the position of the hip in relation to the torso, different muscles are mechanically better suited to produce rotation; the abductors and gluteus maximus produce a great deal of rotation (Fig. 2.22).

Task 2.5

Consider the differences between the activity of the agonists during hip abduction when (a) standing on one leg and (b) side lying.

What are the actions of the hip extensors during ascending and descending a flight of stairs?

The knee joint

In sharp contrast to the hip, the knee joint is inherently unstable due to the nature of its bony construction. Two fibrocartilaginous menisci greatly aid stability between the rounded femoral condyles, which sit on an almost flat tibia. Much of the stability of the knee comes from the ligaments. The back of the patella articulates with the femur and is covered in hyaline cartilage. This allows it to move freely over the femur during movements at the knee. The anterior capsule is attached to the sides of the patella.

Movements

The main movements that occur at the knee are extension and flexion. As flexion increases it is possible to gain rotation. The amount of rotation possible slowly increases as the knee flexes, reaches a peak at 90° and thereafter declines.

While the hamstring muscles produce flexion and the quadriceps produce extension of the knee, many of the daily knee movements are caused by the quadriceps. They do this by working concentrically to produce extension and then eccentrically to control flexion speed which is usually caused by gravity.

Functional anatomy

The presence of the patella improves the mechanical advantage of the quadriceps by increasing the distance from the patella tendon to the centre of axis of the knee joint.

In daily life the quadriceps muscles nearly always work in their inner to mid-range. During climbing the foot is placed on the step and the quadriceps work in order to propel the body upwards onto an upright knee (Fig. 2.23).

The hamstring muscles often work in conjunction with the quadriceps. The hamstrings flex the knee but extend the hip. When the quadriceps

work to extend the knee, the hamstrings may be working simultaneously to bring about hip extension. The hamstring tension aids knee stability by helping to prevent the tibial shift that would otherwise stress the cruciate ligaments. The opposing forces of the two muscle groups at the knee allow the rolling action of the femoral condyles on the flat tibial condyles and so through co-contraction there is improved stability. This muscular stability is important to those with permanent damage or loss of knee ligaments, particularly the cruciates.

The medial and lateral hamstrings produce medial and lateral rotation of the knee, respectively. This action of the hamstrings, and their ability to rotate the knee, is particularly important as the knee is frequently used in a semi-flexed position, which permits rotation. Rotation cannot occur when the knee is extended or locked. If we step forward onto a flexed left leg and turn to the left, the foot and tibia are fixed and the lateral hamstrings cause lateral rotation.

Often a twist or a turn at the knee occurs very rapidly. If not controlled, the sudden forced rotation can injure menisci or ligaments.

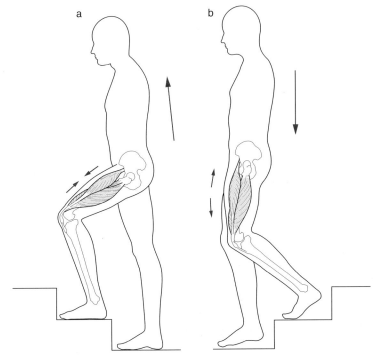

Figure 2.23 The quadriceps are important for activities such as ascending and descending stairs, but their action is different in the two situations. When going up stairs (a) they work concentrically to extend the knee of the leading leg. They work eccentrically when going down stairs (b) as they control the knee of the trailing leg. Without this eccentric contraction, the body weight would cause the knee to flex in an uncontrolled manner.

The popliteus muscle plays a part in knee rotation. The tension it generates in a fully extended knee allows the medial femoral condyles to slide against the tibia. This moves the knee out of the locked position and allows flexion to occur.

Functionally, the knee is very rarely held in the fully extended, locked or close packed position, where no movement can occur and there is maximum congruence between the bony surfaces. To achieve this position, rotation occurs in the final few degrees of extension by the action of the horizontal fibres of vastus medialis.

During weight bearing the lateral condyles of the tibia and femur reach full congruence with the lateral meniscus a few degrees before the medial edge. The action of vastus medialis oblique pulls the patella medially and allows the medial femoral condyle to slide posterolaterally on the medial tibial condyle, bringing the medial structures into total congruence. The popliteus muscle reverses this action.

Weakness in the action of vastus medialis in particular gives rise to what is termed quadriceps lag. In this situation the passive range of movement at the knee joint is full, but the patient cannot achieve the last few degrees of extension actively. When the knee is locked in full extension, the bony congruence prevents the soft tissues being stressed and, therefore, clinical knee examinations are usually carried out in slight flexion.

The ankle joint

The ankle joint is the articulation of the lower end of the tibia and fibula with the superior surface of the talus. The tibia, the more medial of the two bones, is wider across the talus, the fibula being simply a strut on the lateral side. The two bones are strongly held together at the lower tibiofibular joint.

The capsule has two ligament components to reinforce it. On the medial side it has a very strong ligament, triangular in shape, and on the lateral aspect a weaker ligament, originating from the fibula, consisting of three bands.

Immediately distal to the talus is the calcaneus and the articulation of these two bones, the subtalar joint. It is inappropriate to consider the ankle without this joint, which is strongly reinforced by a capsule and an interosseous ligament, which permit very little movement.

Movements

At the ankle joint there is active dorsiflexion, plantar flexion and some inversion and eversion when the foot is plantar flexed. At the subtalar joint, very slight inversion and eversion are regarded as accessory, rather than active, movements. It is important that this tolerance to movement exists to allow for the dissipation of stress and also for accommodation in the fore foot during weight bearing. An excess of movement at this joint would lead to an unstable platform for the ankle joint.

The muscles that operate the ankle joint are in four groups. The dorsiflexors, or anterior tibial muscles, cause pure dorsiflexion only when acting simultaneously. Acting separately the tibialis anterior has a secondary action of foot inversion. The two lateral peronei are primarily evertors of the foot while dorsiflexion and plantar flexion are assisted by peroneus brevis and longus respectively. The posterior deep flexors primarily assist plantar flexion. Tibialis anterior and posterior assist each other to produce inversion. The power of the plantar flexion comes from the gastrocnemius and soleus muscles, whereas flexion of the fore foot on the hind foot is from the deep flexors.

Functional anatomy

Most daily activity requires that our bodies are propelled forwards. The plantar flexors work strongly, and often simultaneously, as an anti-gravitational force. The gastrocnemius and soleus muscles, therefore, work powerfully together concentrically to produce plantar flexion at the ankle joint. Gastrocnemius is used more when power and speed are required in activities such as running, jumping or climbing stairs. During the push off phase in walking and running these two muscles can be seen to work strongly. Gentle walking may use only the soleus muscle, but as speed and power requirements increase, the gastrocnemius becomes more active. In dorsiflexion, achieved by the combined action of the anterior tibial muscles, power is usually less important than in the calf muscles. Frequently the foot is simultaneously dorsiflexed and inverted, as when clearing the foot off the ground during walking. Tibialis anterior plays a very important role in achieving this activity. Reduced strength and power from these muscles causes a drop foot. Often these muscles work eccentrically to control plantar flexion against gravity.

In routine activity the foot rarely operates in full dorsiflexion, the close pack position. Therefore, there is some surface incongruity at the ankle joint, the muscles acting like guy ropes around a ship's mast to create stability. Each muscle has its counterpart, e.g. tibialis anterior and posterior. This enables the fast stabilising reactions required on uneven ground when the foot is pronated and there is a lack of joint congruence.

The reaction speed of the peronei is thought to be important in preventing lateral ankle sprains. Following a ligament sprain at the ankle, the muscular response time is decreased (Lentell et al 1990). For this reason, balance and proprioception should be assessed during rehabilitation.

The foot

Strong ligaments and capsules hold the tarsal and metatarsal bones together. Numerous synovial junctions exist between the various bones.

Movements

Between each junction some movement occurs. It is normally thought of as an accessory movement where one bone can move against its neighbour, rather than an active, volitional movement.

Functional anatomy

These subtle movements are essential to allow the foot to mould and operate effectively on uneven ground.

Task 2.6

Compare the actions of moving from sitting to standing and walking. Consider the range of movement of the lower limb joints and which muscles produce both movement and stability.

The vertebral column

The adult lumbar and cervical spine are characterised by a lordosis, which is due to a slight wedge shape in both vertebral bodies and intravertebral discs.

The vertebral column is designed to accept the vertical stresses and strains of everyday life and also to protect the very delicate spinal cord and neural structures that run down its centre. Strands of bone fibres run across the width of the vertebral body and give strength and enhance the ability to resist compressive forces. The ability to dissipate stress is important in preventing the skull from jarring down onto the top of the neck. The vertical stresses are passed posteriorly throughout the lamina to the pedicles and finally to the spinous processes and into the soft tissues. The pedicles, acting almost vertically compared with the horizontal lamina, comprise hard cortical bone around a hollow centre. The design of the pedicles allows for stresses and strains to be transmitted along their edges and, therefore, distortion may occur without causing fractures (Bogduck & Twomey 1991). The discs are equally designed to accept stresses and allow distortion to accommodate for movement of the column.

Strong ligaments run between the bones throughout the entire length of the vertical column. The ligamentum flavum is particularly important as it contains a high number of elastic fibres that are never fully relaxed. In natural standing the ligament exerts a vertical compressive force at each level.

The major muscles producing extension of the vertical column are the posterior erector spinae muscles. These vary enormously in length and are arranged in layers. The muscles on the anterior abdominal wall, collectively known as the abdominals, produce spinal flexion.

Movement

Movement is dependent on the shape of the interlocking facets of the synovial joints of the articulating vertebral pillar, which occur at every level. In the lumbar spine these joints allow the movements of flexion, extension and lateral flexion and little or no rotation occurs. The thoracic region is much more rigid, particularly the upper thoracic cage which protects the heart and the lungs. The movement that does occur is mostly that of rotation. In the neck, with the exceptions of C1 and C2, the articulating pillar allows for flexion, extension, rotation and lateral flexion. The movement between C1 and C2 is mostly rotation, while movement between the skull and C1 is mostly flexion and extension as in nodding.

Functional anatomy

Once again gravity is important in this area. The muscles, which produce or control the movement, depend on the starting position. If a person standing upright bends forward at a rate slower than that dictated by gravity, the erector spinae work eccentrically to control the movement and prevent the torso from falling forward. When returning to the upright position, the same muscles act concentrically as extensors.

However, when moving from supine lying to sitting, the abdominals, particularly rectus abdominis, work concentrically to bring the thoracic cage closer to the pelvis and cause spinal flexion against gravity. When returning to supine lying, these muscles work eccentrically to control the movement against gravity.

The internal and external oblique muscles work to produce trunk rotation. Transversus abdominis controls and restrains the abdominal contents. It has been found that when the arm moves transversus abdominis activates, even before the muscles at the shoulder, so acting to stabilise the spinal joints (Hodges & Richardson 1996). The diaphragm, which is under semiautomatic control, separates the thoracic and abdominal cavities. As it contracts and relaxes, it alters the pressures within the thoracic and abdominal cages. When contracting, it descends towards the abdomen, increasing the size of the thoracic cage and allowing the lungs to expand, so increasing the intake of air. When relaxing, the muscle rises in the thorax, forcing air out of the lungs. This accounts for the majority of the work of breathing at rest. The rib cage moves in conjunction with the movement of the diaphragm.

Question 2.1

Consider the actions of quiet breathing and coughing. Which muscles are more involved in coughing than in natural breathing, and why do you think that this occurs?

In coughing, an increase in expulsion of the thoracic content is required. Therefore, the abdominal pressure is maximised by the simultaneous activity of the diaphragm, abdominal and pelvic muscles.

The weak link in the lumbar spine appears to be the fibrocartilaginous disc. In midlife the nucleus dries, the annulus becomes fairly brittle and is subjected to greater stresses thus becoming prone to microfractures (Bogduck & Twomey 1991). Studies of the stresses likely to cause damage in the lumbar spine indicate that disc pressure is greatest during sitting and flexion, least during lying and intermediate during standing and walking (Nachemson & Morris 1964).

Many activities require movement of the hands towards the floor, thus increasing the lever, or moment arm, across the lower back. The weight of the torso, acting approximately halfway along its length, increases its perpendicular distance from the fulcrum at L5 and also increases the pressure in the lumbar spine. Therefore, during lifting or hip flexion with extended knees, the pressure on the lumbar spine is high. If a load is added at the hands, the perpendicular distance from the centre of gravity of the torso to the fulcrum increases.

Keeping the moment arm as short as possible, i.e. keeping the hands close to the trunk, helps to decrease the affective stresses in the lumbar spine. Studies using electromyography and biomechanical modelling techniques using the pressure data of Nachemson & Morris (1964) have led to the recommendation of crouch lifting to reach the floor and lift objects. This literature is well reviewed by Basmajian & Deluca (1979), Singleton (1986) and Chaffin & Anderson (1990). In practice, however, the recommended posture is often impractical and creates an increased leverage over the knee joint, which can make the lifting of certain shaped objects difficult. It is often suggested that increasing the power and strength of the muscles surrounding the abdominal cavity will assist and protect the lumbar spine. By increasing the pressure and strength of these muscles, it should be possible to increase the pressure exerted on the abdominal cavity. Since the pressure on contained fluids increases in all directions, this would assist in decompression of the loaded lumbar spine and decrease the stresses upon it. However, it is generally recommended that the muscle strengthening exercises should not involve spinal movement. Static muscle contractions help increase strength without distorting the disc.

Question 2.2

Imagine lying flat on the floor with the knees bent and feet resting on the floor. Gently tuck in the chin and raise the shoulders only off the floor. Hold this position and then return slowly to the start position. Which muscles are contracting and how are they working?

Rectus abdominis works concentrically when raising the shoulders, isometrically to hold them and eccentrically when returning to the start position.

Question 2.3

Consider the same starting position, lying flat on the floor with the knees bent, but this time take your right arm over to your left knee. Which muscles are working and how?

The right external oblique and left internal oblique work concentrically when rising and eccentrically when returning to the start position.

The shoulder complex

The upper limb comprises a collection of complex joints, which are often thought to start with the glenohumeral joint. However, the sternoclavicular and acromioclavicular joints need to be considered along with the shoulder.

Movements

The clavicle is able to elevate, depress and rotate. The greatest movement is elevation and depres-sion at the distal (acromioclavicular) end. At the medial (sternal) end, small gliding movements occur against the sternum. If the sternal end depresses, the acromial end will elevate. The clavicle is also capable of protraction and retraction; if the sternal end protracts the acromial end will retract and vice versa. The scapula, strongly associated with the clavicle, is also capable of elevation and depression, protraction, retraction and rotation and the scapula mimics any movement that occurs at the acromial end of the clavicle.

Movements of the scapula and clavicle are closely associated with those of the glenohumeral joint. The glenohumeral joint has a strong fibrous capsule that is loose inferiorly so this joint is fundamentally designed to supply mobility, rather than stability, to the upper limb. The joint is capable of the same six anatomical movements available at the hip. Circumduction allows for a huge excursion and combination of movements.

In conjunction with movement of the elbow and hand, the glenohumeral joint, along with scapula and clavicular movements, enables the hand to be placed practically anywhere on the body.

It is mostly the muscles attached to the scapula that perform movements of the scapula and clavicle. The rhomboids retract and serratus anterior protracts the scapula. The large, triangular trapezius operates the scapula by working in several ways. If it acts as a single unit, the scapula retracts. If the upper fibres alone contract, the scapula will rise at the acromial end and external rotation occurs. If the lower fibres act independently, the reverse happens, the scapula is depressed at the acromial end and the inferior angle is internally rotated. The middle fibres acting alone cause retraction. Levator scapula assists the upper fibres of trapezius in scapula elevation and the fibres of latissimus dorsi assist the lower fibres of trapezius in scapula depression.

There are two types of muscle that control movement of the glenohumeral joint. Small muscles travelling from the scapula to the humerus control the position of the head of the humerus in the glenoid cavity. There are also large and powerful muscles which run from the torso to the humerus.

Functional anatomy

The small muscles are known collectively as the rotator cuff and consist of supraspinatus, infraspinatus, subscapularis, teres major and minor and are assisted by the long heads of triceps and biceps. Their role is vital in controlling and stabilising the head of the humerus.

The alignment of supraspinatus enables it to initiate abduction, while infraspinatus is at a good angle for initiating lateral rotation and assisting adduction. It is also able to assist in depressing the head of the humerus within the glenoid during abduction. Subscapularis is at the correct angle for medial humeral rotation and assisting infraspinatus in controlling the descent of the humeral head during movement and keeping it in contact with the glenoid cavity. These actions are reinforced by teres major and minor, along with the long heads of biceps and triceps. In stabilisation of the shoulder joint, the long heads of biceps and triceps assist them. These muscles also initiate flexion and extension respectively, and help to keep the humeral head in contact with the glenoid cavity. Together they are vital in maintaining stability of the humeral head and provide a fixed point of attachment for the prime movers.

The head of the humerus glides down within the glenoid cavity during arm abduction, backwards during flexion and forwards during extension. The rotator cuff muscles are responsible for this fine control. They act in a coordinated way like guy ropes to control the humeral head, and alter its position in relation to the glenoid to keep maximum congruity. They can be seen in many instances almost as elastic ligaments because of their subtle control, which provides stability for the anatomically unstable joint. As the tendons of supraspinatus, infraspinatus and teres minor travel underneath the acromion, they are protected by one of the largest fluid bursa in the body. This bursa prevents the tendons becoming trapped as the humeral head rises in abduction.

The main power muscle across the glenohumeral joint is the deltoid, which forms the shape of the shoulder and causes abduction, flexion and extension. This muscle can act in unison as an abductor, while the anterior fibres alone cause flexion. The middle fibres abduct and the posterior fibres extend the glenohumeral joint. This fan-shaped muscle behaves like the glutei at the hip joint. The fibres recruited depend on the position of the arm and torso; those at the best mechanical advantage are recruited first. For the majority of daily activities the arm is abducted. This is initiated by supraspinatus to give deltoid the correct angle of pull to perform the power action required. Without this action of supraspinatus, contraction of the deltoid would result in the humerus rising in the glenoid cavity. Consider the action of abducting a straight upper limb and taking it to full elevation when standing. The centre of gravity of the upper limb is approximately at the elbow and the perpendicular distance to the fulcrum is at its greatest as the upper limb goes through 90°. At this point deltoid has to work hardest and it is also at its middle length range and at the strongest point on the active length:tension curve. Either side of this point the perpendicular distance from the elbow to the fulcrum decreases, as does the length of the movement arm forces that have to be overcome. Therefore, less strength is required from the muscle which is working in less favourable areas of the active length:tension curve and so is capable of producing less power.

Other powerful shoulder muscles are the pectoralis major and latissimus dorsi. These muscles together produce adduction. They are essential in activities that require stabilisation of the shoulder when the arm and the body are held close together. They also bring the arm and trunk forcibly towards each other in activities such as climbing. Strength in these muscles is necessary for activities such as crutch walking, where the body weight is taken through the upper limbs and the torso moves forwards and backwards.

When performing 'press ups', the scapula needs to be anchored and prevented from moving away from the chest wall in order to provide for the glenohumeral movement. The proximal fibres of serratus anterior work with the rhomboids as stabilisers while trapezius gener-

---

Task 2.7

Look at a colleague and see how the scapula, clavicle and glenohumeral joint move together in order to produce elevation of the arm.

The movement is complex; elevation through abduction is performed by abduction of the glenohumeral joint, but simultaneously there is a rotation of the scapula and clavicle. To gain full elevation there is a lateral rotation of the glenohumeral joint for the last 30°.

---

ates both power and stability. This allows subtle glenohumeral movement and the deltoid to generate powerful contractions.

The elbow joint

By comparison with the glenohumeral, the elbow joint is anatomically extremely stable. The convex ulna tightly hugs the lower end of the humerus and glides around the humerus, allowing flexion and extension. The flat radial head simply glides around the lower end of the humerus. The radius and the ulna unite at the superior radioulnar joint. Two very strong collateral ligaments hold the elbow joint together. From the ulna a very strong annular ligament hugs the rounded head of the radius, enabling it to rotate against the ulna. The capsule encompasses the elbow joint and the superior radioulnar joint.

Movements

The muscles acting across this joint are mainly the triceps posteriorly and the biceps and brachialis anteriorly, which produce extension and flexion respectively. The radial attachment of biceps also enables it to cause supination at the wrist.

Functional anatomy

In everyday life much of the activity at the elbow joint requires flexion or extension to be controlled against gravity. For example, biceps will work concentrically when flexing the elbow to raise a weight against gravity, isometrically to

maintain a given elbow position and eccentrically when controlling the rate of extension due to gravity.

The inferior radioulnar joint, just above the wrist, is very different to the superior radioulnar joint. Here the radius is allowed to rotate across the ulna by a very loose capsule. In the anatomical position, the forearm is held in supination; rotation or pronation is allowed through approximately 180°.

Wrist and hand

The wrist joint is normally defined as the radiocarpal joint since the radius alone articulates with the carpal bones. The ulna articulates with the carpal bones through a disc.

Movements

This joint allows for flexion, extension, radial and ulnar deviation. The flexors and extensors originate from the common flexor and extensor tendons on the medial and lateral humeral epicondyles, respectively. The muscles operating the wrist attach distally to the carpus and metacarpal bones. Running centrally across the wrist are the flexors and extensors of the fingers, flexor digitorum and extensor digitorum. Flexor carpi ulnaris and extensor carpi ulnaris have dual functions: working together they cause ulnar deviation at the wrist; independently they either flex or extend. Extensor carpi radialis longus and brevis, along with flexor carpi radialis, also have dual function: working synergistically they radially deviate the wrist, while independently they assist either extension or flexion of the wrist. Extensor digitorum with flexor digitorum profundus and superficialis are responsible for extension and flexion, respectively, of the wrist and the fingers.

The muscles of the thenar eminence are extremely important in assisting and generating force, as is the position of the thumb. The hypothenar eminence is much less developed but it is important in forming an opposition to the thumb. The interossei and lumbricals also work in assisting actions for the fingers.

Functional anatomy

The importance of the hand is that its anatomical and muscular construction enables it to be extremely flexible and yet it can become a rigid structure when required. The carpal bones can be made more rigid by muscular activity, as when pushing against a heavy door. Small and subtle movements also enable delicate actions such as cupping the hand and the delicate movements vital for everyday activity. The versatility of the hand, particularly the thumb, gives humans their unique ability to undertake a broad spectrum of activities ranging from precision activities to making a fist.

CONCLUSION

The body does not work segment by segment but as a unit. When standing, the skeleton is balanced by the coordination of muscles throughout the body in order to maintain the centre of gravity through the base of support (see Ch. 3). In relaxed standing there is some muscle activity though this is increased once actions are undertaken. Muscles act as prime movers to perform the activity and others act strongly to counter them, so maintaining posture and balance. If you stand on your right leg the peroneii, quadriceps hip abductors and trunk side flexors work hard on that side to balance the body over the smaller base of support. Once in position the muscles around the ankle co-contract to help maintain the balance.

Task 2.8

Consider the coordinated activity of opening a door, turning the handle and pulling the door towards you. What movements are occurring in the various joints; which muscles are active and how are they working? Start with the hand, work up the forearm to the elbow and finally the shoulder.

Consider the activity of eating an apple. Pick it up from the table and go through the motion of trying to eat, thinking of the movements of the arm and hand and the muscle activity necessary to produce them.

REFERENCES

Basmajian J V, Deluca C J 1979 Muscles alive, 5th edn. Williams and Wilkins, Baltimore

Binder-Macleod S A 1992 Force–frequency relation in skeletal muscle. In: Currier D P, Nelson R M (eds) Dynamics of human biologic tissues. F A Davies, Philadelphia

Bogduck N, Twomey L T 1991 Clinical anatomy of the lumbar spine, 2nd edn. Churchill Livingstone, Edinburgh

Broer M, Zernicke R F 1979 Efficiency of human movement, 4th edn. W B Saunders, Philadelphia

Chaffin D B, Anderson G B J 1990 Occupational biomechanics. John Wiley, New York

Clarkson P M, Newham D J 1995 Associations between muscle soreness, damage and fatigue. In: Gandevia S C, Enolta R M, McGomas A J, Stuart D G, Thomas C K (eds) Advances in experimental medicine and biology. Fatigue – neural and muscular mechanisms. Plenum Press, New York, pp 457–470

Gordon A M, Huxley A F, Julian F J 1966 The variation in isometric tension with sarcomere length in vertebrate muscle fibres. Journal of Physiology 184: 170–192

Gowitzke B A, Milner M 1980 Understanding the scientific bases of human movement, 2nd edn. Williams and Wilkins, Baltimore

Hennemann E, Clamann H P, Gillies J D, Skinner R D 1974 Rank order of motorneurons within a pool, law of combination. Journal of Neurophysiology 37: 1338–1349

Hodges PW, Richardson CA 1996 Inefficient muscular stabilisation of the lumbar spine associated with low back pain. Spine Vol 21: 2640–2650

Huxley A F, Simmons R M 1971 Proposed mechanism of force generation in striated muscle. Nature 233: 533–558

Jones D A, Round J M 1990 Skeletal muscle in health and disease. Manchester University Press, Manchester

Kapandji I A 1978 The physiology of the joints. Vol 2. Lower limb. Churchill Livingstone, Edinburgh

Komi P V 1986 The stretch shortening cycle and human power output. In: Jones N L, McCartney N, McComas A J (eds) Human muscle power. Human Kinetics, Champaign, Illinois

Lehmkuhl L D, Smith L K 1983 Brunnstrom's Clinical Kinesiology, 4th edn. F A Davies, Philadelphia

Lentell G L, Katzman L L, Walters M R 1990 The relationship between muscle function and ankle stability. Journal of Orthopaedic and Sports Physical Therapy 11: 605–610

Leveau B F, Bernhardt D B 1984 Developmental biomechanics. Effect of forces on the growth, development and maintenance of the human body. Physical Therapy 64: 1874–1881

Lieber R L 1992 Skeletal muscle structure and function. Williams and Wilkins, Baltimore

MacConaill M A, Basmajian J V 1977 Muscles and movements – a basis for human kinesiology, 2nd edn. R E Kreiger, New York

Nachemson A L F, Morris J M 1964 In vivo measurements of intradiscal pressure. Journal of Bone and Joint Surgery 46A: 1077–1092

Palastanga N, Field D, Soames R 1990 Anatomy and human movement. Butterworth Heinemann, Oxford
Singleton W T 1986 The body at work, 2nd edn. Cambridge University Press, New York

CHAPTER CONTENTS

Introduction   37
Basic concepts   38
Laws of motion   39

Force   39
Force systems   40
Force analysis   40
Types of force   43
Moment of force   44
Effects of force and moment of force   47

Centre of gravity and base of support   50
Body COG, line of gravity (LOG) and centre of
pressure (COP)   50
Base of support   52
Balance, equilibrium and stability   52

Work, power, energy and momentum   53
Forms of energy   54
Conservation of energy   54
Power   54

Movement analysis   55
Link-segment model and a free body diagram
(FBD)   56
Example of movement analysis   56
Moving up the limb   60

Deformation of materials   61
Stress and strain   61
Linear loading   61

Mechanical principles of fluids   64
Hydrostatics and hydrodynamics   64
Types of flow   66
Movement through a fluid   66

3

Biomechanics of human movement

R. W. M. van Deursen   T. Everett

OBJECTIVES

At the end of this chapter you will be able to:

1. **Describe the concept of force and its relevance for human movement**

2. **Discuss the general biomechanics of human movement**

3. **Apply your knowledge of biomechanics in specified situations, such as during gait and while immersed in water**

4. **Describe the graphical and mathematical analysis of force systems**

5. **Integrate the above knowledge to perform simple biomechanical movement analyses.**

INTRODUCTION

Biomechanics can be defined as the study of the structure and function of biological systems, such as the human musculoskeletal system, by application of (Newtonian) mechanics. The scope of biomechanics is both wide and deep but this chapter will highlight the aspects considered most relevant for the study of human movement. For a complete discussion of biomechanics there are basic textbooks (see 'Further reading' at the end of this chapter). The main focus of this chapter is centred on understanding forces and their effects. Principles of *kinematics* (the description of motion) and *kinetics* (the description of motion including the consideration of forces as the cause of motion) will also be discussed.

A first step in understanding human movement is knowledge of the anatomy and physiology of the human body, the musculoskeletal system in particular. However, anatomy books generally describe movement using the anatomical position as the starting point without considering the environment, as though the movement is occurring in a state of weightlessness. It is important to realise that movements cannot be considered out of context but occur in an infinite number of body configurations and within a mechanical environment. A biomechanical analysis is required to unravel these factors to determine which muscles (if any) are required to produce a given movement. In addition, such an analysis can quantify the amount of loading occurring on different anatomical structures. Although biomechanical analyses can be very powerful in providing information about movement, it should be noted that the environment within which the movement occurs is generally a lot richer than mechanics alone. Therefore, it is best to consider this field of study as a set of tools in a toolbox used to learn more about human movement.

Basic concepts

It is important that before any calculations can be attempted the basic elements of trigonometry are revised and some basic mathematical conventions are explained.

SI units

By convention the international system of units is used for the dimensions of biomechanical quantities. Table 3.1 gives the basic SIU (Le Système International d'Unites) and some conversions from imperial measurements.

Trigonometry

The most basic concept of trigonometry is that of the triangle with its three sides and three angles. The three angles of any triangle will always add up to 180°. If one of these angles is 90° (the right angled triangle) and the dimensions of the sides of the triangle are known, then the value of the

Table 3.1 SI units, their names and equivalents

Quantity	SI unit	Conversion
Mass	kilograms (kg)	1 kg = 9.807 N 1 kg = 2.2 lb 1 stone = 6.35 kg
Time	seconds (s)	
Length	metres (m)	1 m = approx. 39 inches 1 ft = 0.305 m
Angle	degrees (deg) radians (rad)	1 rad = 57.3 deg 1 deg = 0.0175 rad

angles can be calculated. If an angle and a side or two sides are known then it is possible to calculate all the remaining unknown parameters. This is possible by the use the *sine, cosine* and *tangent* rule. Figure 3.1 shows a right angled triangle where angle ABC is the right angle. Side b is known as the hypotenuse, side c as the base or adjacent and side a as the perpendicular or opposite. Mathematically the value of the angle CAB (φ) can be found using the formula:

$$sin\ \varphi = opposite/hypotenuse\ \text{or}\ sin\ \varphi = a/b$$

$$cos\ \varphi = adjacent/hypotenuse\ \text{or}\ cos\ \varphi = c/b$$

$$tan\ \varphi = opposite/adjacent\ \text{or}\ tan\ \varphi = a/c$$

It is also possible to calculate the lengths of the sides of the triangle by using Pythagoras' Theorem, which states that the square of the length of the hypotenuse is equal to the sum of the squares of the lengths of the other sides. In this case:

$$b^2 = a^2 + c^2 \quad \text{or} \quad b = \sqrt{(a^2 + c^2)}$$

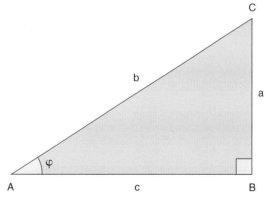

Figure 3.1 A right angled triangle is used for the definition of the sine, cosine and tangent of the angle φ.

Scalar and vector quantities

In biomechanics there are two types of quantities that are discussed. The first type are those that have magnitude only, such as mass, temperature, work and energy. These are called *scalar* quantities. The second type are those that have both magnitude and direction, such as force. These are called *vector* quantities. Scalar quantities can be added, subtracted, multiplied or divided without any problems. To manipulate vector quantities trigonometry will have to be used because those quantities may have varying directions.

Rotations

Figure 3.2 shows that rotations in biomechanical terms can occur in one of two directions: anti-clockwise as illustrated in (a) which is defined as positive rotation, and clockwise as illustrated in (b) which is defined as negative rotation. In this example the thigh is fixed and the leg is moving. The arrow indicates the direction of movement, and it is important that this direction arrow is added to any diagrammatic representation of movement.

Laws of motion

Although not the first to study movement, Sir Isaac Newton (1687) did provide a major breakthrough in the understanding of the causes of movement of objects. He explained this by addressing the relationship between force and one of its effects, namely motion. As a result of his studies Newton formulated three statements known as the laws of motion.

Newton's laws of motion

1. Law of inertia. Every body continues in a state of rest or uniform motion in a straight line except when it is compelled by external forces to change its state.
2. Law of acceleration. The rate of change of momentum of a body is proportional to the applied force and takes place in the direction in which the force acts.

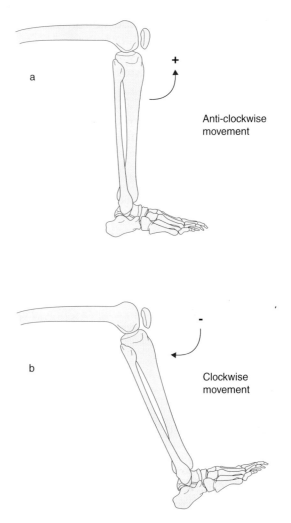

Figure 3.2 In describing the direction of a rotation, the convention is to call anti-clockwise rotation positive (a) and clockwise rotation negative (b).

3. Law of action/reaction. To every action there is an equal and opposite reaction.

These three laws still play a major role in the study of biomechanics and their implications will be considered and explained later in the chapter.

FORCE

Definition of force

A force is not a tangible object and should therefore be considered as a concept. It can be thought of as an entity that is generated by an action, for example a push or a pull, or imparted, as in a kick. The above examples will probably result in movement but the object to which the force is imparted may remain stationary while it deforms, as with the force imparted to a soft chair when somebody sits down. With this in mind a force can be defined as: *an influence that changes the state of rest or motion of a body or object.*

This definition is essentially what Newton described in the law of inertia, stating that a body/object which is at rest will remain at rest unless some external force is applied to it and a body/object which is moving at a constant speed in a straight line will continue to do so unless some external force is applied to it. Similarly, *inertia* of a body/object (or mass) can be defined as the resistance that a body/object offers to any changes in its motion. Inertia/mass is measured in kilograms (kg).

Description of a force

Force is a vector quantity and therefore has a magnitude and a direction. A force is represented graphically as an arrow with the following three descriptors:

- Magnitude: the longer the arrow the greater the magnitude
- Direction/line of action: the arrow points in the direction of the force
- Point of application: the origin of the arrow is located at the point of application.

Equation of force

Encapsulated in Newton's second law or the law of acceleration is the equation:

$$\text{Force} = \text{mass} \times \text{acceleration} \quad \text{or} \quad F = m \times a$$

where mass (m) is the quantity of matter that makes up a body/object measured in kilograms (kg) and the acceleration (a) may be the acceleration due to gravity, measured in m/s². The unit of force is the newton (N).

Force systems

It is unusual for forces to act singularly, since there is usually a combination of forces acting together. For convenience these forces can be described as *force systems* which are defined as two or more forces acting together. Force systems can be described as:

- Colinear (1-dimensional), where the forces are acting in the same plane and along the same line of action. They either point in the same or opposite directions. This is shown in Figure 3.3.
- Co-planar (2-dimensional), where the forces are acting in the same plane but not along the same line of action, as shown in Figure 3.4. *Special cases of co-planar force systems are:*
  - parallel forces, where the directions of the forces are parallel in the same or opposite directions (see Fig. 3.5a). Parallel forces in opposite directions may produce a force couple which is similar to handling a steering wheel.
  - orthogonal forces, where the directions of the forces are perpendicular to each other (see Fig. 3.5b).
  - concurrent forces, where two or more forces originate from the same point of application or their lines of action intersect at a common point (see Fig. 3.6).
- 3-dimensional force systems, where forces are acting in more than a single plane. Although this represents the situation most often encountered in everyday examples, this is more difficult to analyse. In this chapter examples will be used of 1- or 2-dimensional force systems only.

Force analysis

Because forces are vector quantities the analysis of force systems will involve trigonometry. Two basic techniques for manipulating vector quantities are important. These are summation and resolution of forces. *Summation* involves adding the force vectors to find the *resultant*, or the force that could replace the combined effect of all the forces acting on the body. Splitting a force into

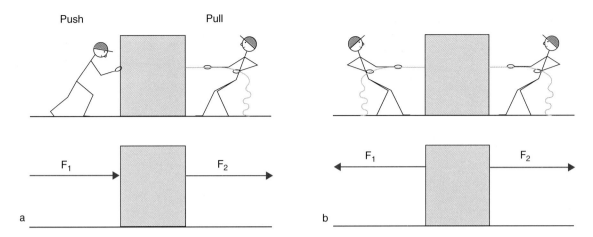

Figure 3.3 Two examples of colinear force systems: (a) two forces acting in the same direction along the same line of action and (b) two forces acting in the opposite direction along the same line of action.

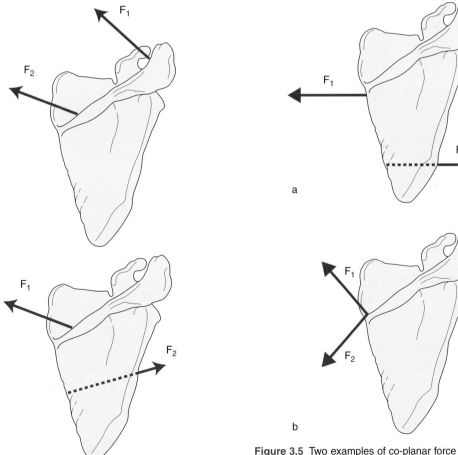

Figure 3.4 Two examples of co-planar force systems.

Figure 3.5 Two examples of co-planar force systems: (a) two forces acting in parallel and (b) two forces acting perpendicular to each other (orthogonal).

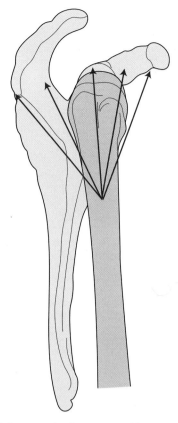

Figure 3.6 An example of a concurrent force system. The deltoid muscle is made up of multiple components that can act together.

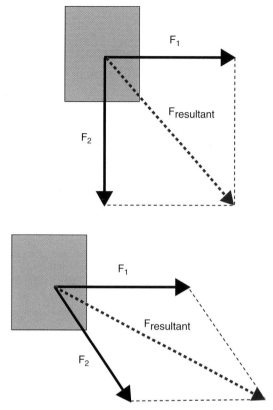

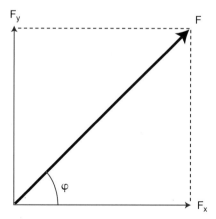

Figure 3.7 Two examples of obtaining the resultant force of a simple force system by means of the graphical method.

its components to establish its effects in two or three principal directions is called *resolution* of forces.

Simple force systems can be analysed using a graphical method. In a vector diagram each force vector is represented by an arrow drawn to scale. The resultant of two forces is determined by completing a parallelogram and joining the diagonally opposing corners (see Fig. 3.7). This diagonal is then measured and the magnitude determined by using the scale.

In cases of more complex force systems, the more useful method of force analysis is by means of trigonometry. Each force (F) is first split into its orthogonal (x and y) components (in three dimensions there is also a z-component), i.e. F_x and F_y illustrated in Figure 3.8. Referring back to the section on trigonometry earlier in this

Figure 3.8 Resolution of a force: the angled force (F) is resolved into two orthogonal components, F_x and F_y. The magnitude of the two components can be calculated by means of trigonometry.

chapter, F_x and F_y could be calculated using the following equations:

$$F_x = Force \times cos \; \varphi$$

$$F_y = Force \times sin \; \varphi$$

where F_x is the force component in the x direction and F_y is the force component in the y direction.

All the x-components are then added up if they point in the same direction or subtracted if they point in the opposite direction to obtain the resultant on the x-axis. The same is done with the y-components. The resultant force components on the x-axis and y-axis are then added up by means of the following equation:

$$F_{resultant} = \sqrt{(F_{x,\,resultant}^2 + F_{y,\,resultant}^2)}$$

Types of force

Force due to gravity

There is a force of attraction of the earth to any object on or near to its surface. The acceleration due to the gravitational pull of the earth is seen as the acceleration any mass has when it is allowed to freely fall to earth and has the value of 9.81 m/s². The weight of an object is the force exerted by the earth on the mass of the object or:

weight = mass × 9.81 (acceleration due to gravity).

Weight is expressed in newtons.

Ground reaction force

Newton's third law is demonstrated when considering the forces that are involved when standing on the ground. In this situation a force is applied by the feet to the ground which is equal to the weight of the person standing. This force is reflected back up into the feet through the same action line with the same magnitude. This is the *ground reaction force* and is illustrated in Figure 3.9.

Centripetal force

As stated earlier, a body/object which is moving at a constant speed in a straight line will continue

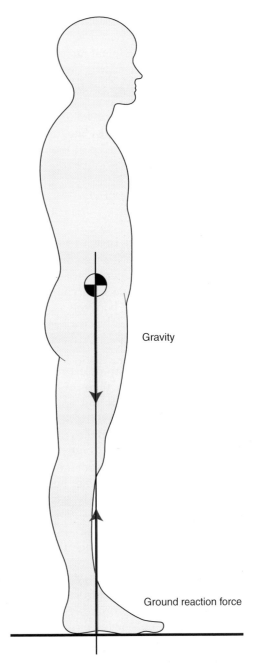

Gravity

Ground reaction force

Figure 3.9 The ground reaction force is the force of the floor acting on the body opposing the effect of gravity.

to do so unless some external force is applied to it. Therefore, if an object is to move in a circle, such as during a hammer throw, a force will have to be applied to make the object change direction continuously to maintain the circular movement. This force is called a *centripetal force*. In the hammer throw this centripetal force is produced by the thrower. The thrower will, however, experience a perception of being pulled by the hammer that is often called the *centrifugal force*. In a biomechanical analysis it is better to consider the centripetal force exerted by the thrower only. As soon as the thrower lets go of the hammer it will move in a straight line since the centripetal force is no longer operating.

Frictional forces

When two objects move, or tend to move, over each other they experience a resisting force. This force is referred to as *frictional force* and occurs if the objects are solid, fluid or a combination of both. Friction can occur between two surfaces moving over each other, between a wheel and the ground (rolling resistance), or between air/water and an object (drag).

If a force is applied to an object that does not move over a surface then there must be a frictional force (f) that is equal and opposite to the applied force (Newton's third law). As the applied force increases so will the resistance until it reaches a critical value (F_{max}). At this point the object will move. Until the object moves the friction is referred to as *static friction* but when the object is moving the friction is referred to as *dynamic* or *kinetic friction*.

The coefficient of friction (µ) is dependent upon the conditions under which the friction is occurring (static or dynamic), the condition of the surfaces of the material and the type and direction of the applying force. The frictional force can be calculated by multiplying the coefficient of friction (µ) and the force component perpendicular to the contact surface of the two objects (also called normal force).

In some instances frictional forces are useful as they allow controlled movement to take place (as in walking) or they may be a hindrance as they require energy to overcome them (as in some types of exercise). Friction can produce heat and wear and tear to the surfaces that are moving over each other.

Elastic forces

Elastic forces will be discussed in more detail in the section below about deformation of materials.

External and internal forces

Forces that act from outside the body, e.g. gravity, moving objects, ground reaction force, manual resistance by the therapist and wind or water resistance, are called *external forces*. Forces can also be generated inside the body by a muscle or be transmitted between body parts by, for instance, ligaments or bone on bone contact. These are examples of *internal forces*. It is important to realise that muscle forces that are under voluntary control are just one aspect of the force system acting on our body. Movement of the body depends on the resultant of the force system which includes external and internal forces and not only on muscle forces.

Pressure

Pressure is the manifestation of force when the surface area over which the force is acting is taken into consideration. Pressure can be defined as the force per unit area (in m^2) or $P = F/A$. The official unit of pressure is pascal (N/m^2) although the kPa (1000 Pa) is more useful for human application. It can be seen from the equation above that if a force remains the same and the surface area increases then the pressure exerted by the force will be less. Conversely, if the surface area is decreased whilst the force remains the same, greater pressure will be felt from the force. This is important when considering the pressure felt on the human body when lying in a bed. If the force is being channelled through a small surface area, like a bony point, then the pressure over that area would be much greater than if the force from the body was acting on a large surface area. In the latter case pressure sores would be less likely to occur.

Moment of force

When the result of an application of a force is a turning or rotary effect the force is said to be producing a *moment*. The twisting effect of a force, however, is often referred to as *torque*. There are no real differences between rotation and twisting so the words moment and torque cannot be considered separately. To calculate the magnitude of the moment of force the equation of moment/torque is used:

Moment = Force × moment arm or $M = F \times d$

In the above equation d stands for distance representing the moment arm. The *moment arm* is the shortest distance (perpendicular) from the line of action of a force to the axis of rotation. In Figure 3.10 the moment arm is shown for a weight on a see-saw (a) and the muscle moment arm is shown for the elbow flexor (b). A line is drawn parallel to the force line of action through the axis of rotation. The moment arm (d) is the

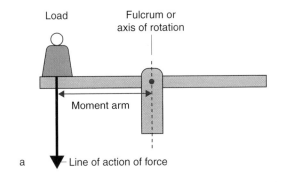

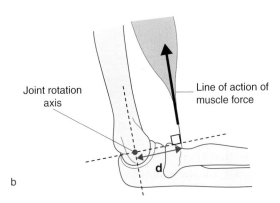

Figure 3.10 A typical lever within the physical world and the body are shown. In (a) the example is a weight on a see-saw and in (b) the muscle moment arm is shown for the elbow flexor. A line is drawn perpendicular to the force line of action and through the axis of rotation to determine the distance between the two.

distance between the two. The unit of moment/torque is the newton.metre or N.m.

Internal and external moments

When forces act from outside the body, for example gravity, ground reaction force, wind or water resistance, and produce rotatory effects they are called *external moments*. When the forces are acting inside the human body they produce *internal moments*. These are often muscle forces acting on the various segments of the body but they can also be forces acting from one segment to the next by means of the ligaments.

Task 3.1 Moment arms during strength testing

When testing the maximum muscle strength of the knee extensor, placement of the hand on the leg is important because of the effect on the moment arm of the resistance. If the left knee test produces a maximum resisted force of 300 N at a distance of 25 cm distal from the knee joint axis and the right knee test produces a maximum resisted force of 250 N at a distance of 30 cm distal from the knee joint axis, calculate which side is stronger.

Levers

When levers are considered, the moment of force is an important factor. A *lever* is defined as a rigid bar that rotates around a fixed point or fulcrum.

The rigid bar may be represented by a crowbar in the physical world or a bony segment inside the human body whilst the fulcrum may be the point about which the crowbar turns or it may be a joint.

Figure 3.10 represents typical levers within the physical world and the body. In Figure 3.10a, the resistance has to be met by a force on the other side of the lever to balance or lift the load. In Figure 3.11, the moment arms of a lever system are shown. The moment arm between the fulcrum and the load or resistance to be moved is called the load/resistance arm ($d_{resistance}$). The moment arm between the fulcrum and the effort or force is called the force/effort arm (d_{force}).

As can be seen from Figure 3.12 there are three distinct forms that the lever can take, the

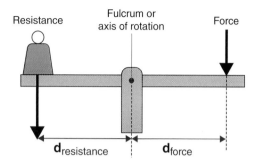

Figure 3.11 The moment arm is the distance between a force and the fulcrum. In this system, the resistance has to be met by a force on the other side of the lever to balance or lift the load. The moment arms for both are shown.

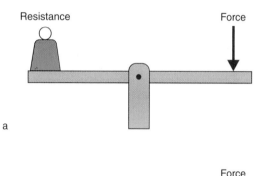

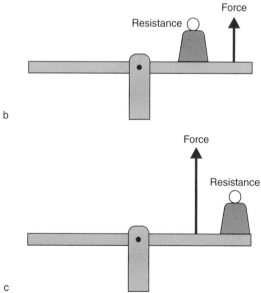

Figure 3.12 Depending on the position of the resistance, the force and the fulcrum relative to each other, levers are divided into (a) first order, (b) second order and (c) third order levers.

formation of which depends on the relative position of the fulcrum to the resistance and force. It is the form that the lever takes which decides its function. As is seen from everyday examples, a lever is often used to make work easier (as in the case of the crowbar). Figure 3.12a represents a lever where the fulcrum lies between the force and the resistance as in a see-saw. This type of lever is called a *first order lever*. In this example the moment arms are equidistant but they may vary. If the resistance lies between the fulcrum and the force (Fig. 3.12b) this is referred to as a *second order lever*. The lever is helpful for lifting a load, as less force is needed at the end to raise a load closer to the fulcrum (e.g. a crowbar or wheelbarrow). The final combination can be seen in Figure 3.12c where the force lies between the fulcrum and the resistance. This is called a *third order lever* and at first it appears quite difficult to see any advantage in this. However, this arrangement frequently occurs inside the body where the muscle insertion lies closer to the joint axis than does the load. The advantage for the muscle is that the distance and velocity of shortening during contraction is smaller. The tissue loading is obviously large.

Mechanical advantage

The reason why some levers help (*mechanical advantage*) and others do not has a mathematical explanation. The equation to calculate the mechanical advantage (MA) is given as:

$$MA = \text{force arm} / \text{load arm}$$

where force arm is the distance from the fulcrum to the force and the load arm is the distance from the fulcrum to the resistance (see Fig. 3.13).

From the example of the see-saw in equilibrium it can be seen that the MA will be 1. This means that there will be no advantage or disadvantage. If the example of the wheelbarrow is taken where the force arm is greater than the load arm then the MA is always going to be greater than 1. Any lever, therefore, with an MA of greater than 1 will have a true advantage. This advantage is sometimes called a force advantage which distinguishes it from a lever where the

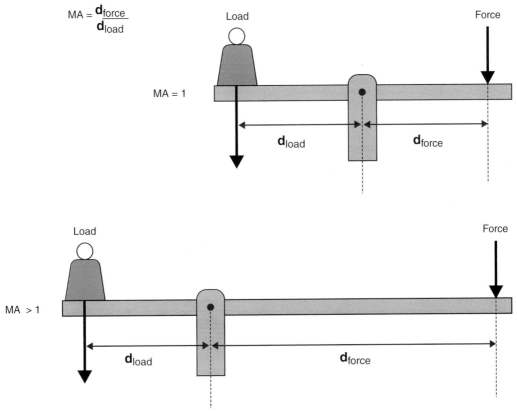

Figure 3.13 The mechanical advantage of levers can be calculated to determine whether the lever is beneficial in assisting to lift a load. A mechanical advantage greater than 1 indicates that the lever makes lifting easier. The terms d_{load} and d_{force} are the moment arms of the two forces acting on the lever.

load arm is always greater than the force arm, giving an MA of less than 1. This last lever has a speed advantage over the other two types of lever. This is because despite requiring a greater force to overcome the resistance, once done the load end of the lever will move with a greater velocity than the point at which the force is applied. Thus it has a speed advantage.

Task 3.2

Are there situations where a muscle in the body has an arrangement different to a third order lever? Consider the position of the fulcrum (joint), the resistance (for instance weight of the arm) and the force (point of application of the muscle force). What type of lever is operating and has it got a force or a speed advantage?

Effects of force and moment of force

It has already been said that a force can be described by its effects and there are two main effects, namely motion and deformation. Deformation will be described later in the chapter. Motion can be categorised as either linear or angular.

Linear motion

Linear motion is also referred to as translation. During a linear movement all the particles of the body describe equal and parallel paths. If the trajectory of the linear movement is a straight line it is called rectilinear movement and if the trajectory of the linear movement is curved it is called curvilinear movement.

Displacement is the shortest distance between two points as opposed to *distance* which may be travelled by a more circuitous route. This is shown in Figure 3.14.

Velocity can be defined as the rate of change of position (displacement) and is expressed in metres per second or m/s. *Acceleration/deceleration* is defined as the rate of change of velocity and is described in metres per second squared or m/s^2. Figure 3.15 shows the linear displacement, velocity and acceleration of a person running and then stopping. The total displacement during this period was almost 2 m (a). The velocity (b) was between 2 and 3 m/s at first and then

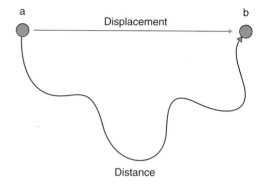

Figure 3.14 When moving from a to b the displacement between the two positions does not have to be the same as the distance travelled.

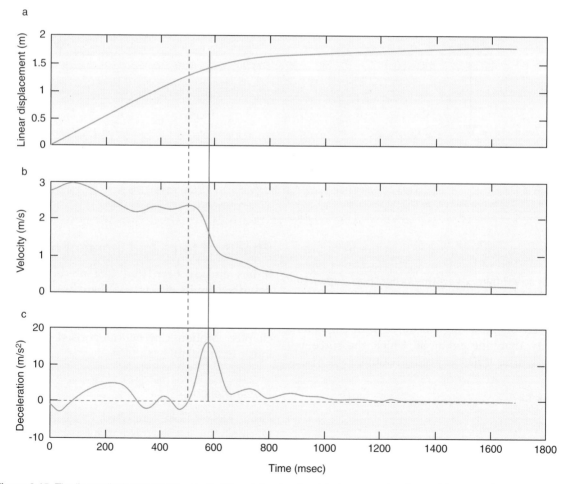

Figure 3.15 The linear displacement (a), velocity (b) and deceleration (c) of a person jogging and then stopping. In all graphs the point at which deceleration was started is indicated by the dotted vertical line. The solid vertical line indicates where the subject was decelerating the most, which is at the peak in the bottom graph.

rapidly declined as the person decelerated. Maximum deceleration (c) was over 15 m/s². The velocity gradually declined to zero after peak deceleration had occurred. It is obvious from this example that velocity and deceleration can vary from one moment to the next. The graph therefore represent the instantaneous velocity and deceleration as opposed to average velocity and deceleration for the whole time period.

Angular motion

Angular motion of a body is also known as rotation. The angular displacement (φ) is measured in degrees (one circle = 360°). In biomechanical calculations this is often expressed in radians (1 radian = 360/2π = 57.3°).

Angular velocity (ω) is defined as the rate of change of angle. It is measured in degrees per second or radians per second. *Angular acceleration* (α) is the rate of change of angular velocity and is expressed in degrees per second squared (°/s²) or radians per second squared (rad/s²). Figure 3.16 shows the angular movement of the right knee during the same activity of a person running and stopping displayed in the previous figure. The graphs begin at the point where deceleration started (dotted line in Fig. 3.15).

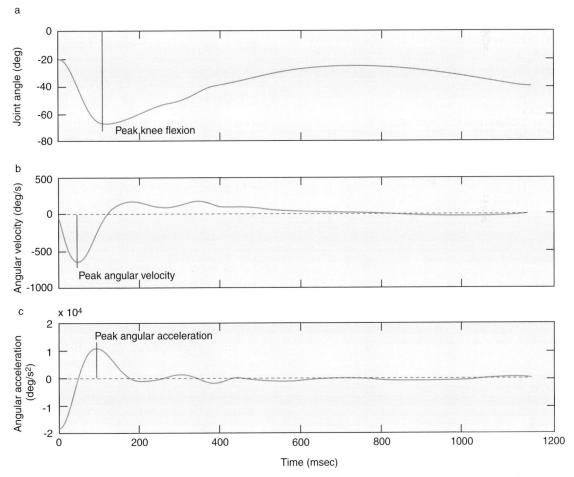

Figure 3.16 The knee angular displacement (a), velocity (b) and acceleration (c) of the same person jogging and then stopping as in Figure 3.15. A vertical line in each graph indicates the peak angular angle, velocity and acceleration. It is obvious that these peaks do not occur at the same point in time.

Peak knee flexion is close to 70° (a), peak knee angular velocity (towards knee flexion) is well over 500°/s (b), and peak angular acceleration (towards knee extension) is more than 10 000°/s^2 (c). Note that these peaks do not occur at the same instance.

Linear and angular motion combined

Human movement often involves a combination of linear and angular movement. For instance, during gait, rotation of the lower limbs is used to achieve curvilinear movement of the trunk represented by the dotted line in Figure 3.17. At the start of Figure 3.17 (left side), the first rotation occurs around the ankle (b) resulting in trunk linear movement (a). In the middle, the second rotation occurs around the hip resulting in curvilinear movement of the ankle (b'). The trunk continues to move forward because of the effect of the other leg. At the end of Figure 3.17, rotation occurs again around the ankle (b'').

Angular motion and moment of inertia

As discussed above, objects offer resistance to any changes in motion. For linear motion this was

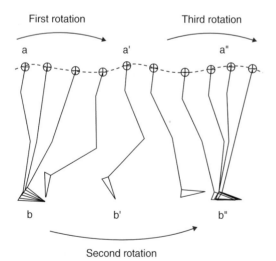

Figure 3.17 Gait involves rotation of the limbs to achieve curvilinear motion of the trunk (dotted line) through space. A single step is shown where a sequence of ankle (b), hip (a'), and ankle (b'') rotation provides for the forward progression of the body.

termed inertia. The tendency for an object to resist changes of angular motion is termed its *moment of inertia* or *I*. It can be represented by the equation:

$$I = m \times r^2$$

where *m* = mass of the object and *r* is the distance of the mass from the axis of rotation.

As the mass of the body increases so does its moment of inertia but as the mass distribution moves away from the axis of rotation, the radius increases and the moment of inertia increases in proportion to the square of that increased distance. The human body has different moments of inertia depending on the direction of rotation considered. Rotation about the longitudinal axis is easier to generate (Fig. 3.18a) than rotation about the frontal axis (Fig. 3.18b) because in the latter case mass of the body will be located at greater distances from the axis of rotation.

CENTRE OF GRAVITY AND BASE OF SUPPORT

Theoretically, mass is distributed throughout the segment and gravity (weight = mass × acceleration due to gravity) acts from every particle of mass of the segment. It would be almost impossible to perform any calculation if these were to be considered. So instead the *centre of mass* (COM) of the segment is used and is defined as the point about which the mass of an object is evenly distributed. The COM is closely associated with the *centre of gravity* (COG). The COG is sometimes explained as the point at which the force of gravity is said to act. The COM of an object is the geometrical centre of that object if it is symmetrical and regular (cube, cylinder or cone). The body segments do not fit exactly into these descriptions but can be approximated in this way. The percentage weight of the body segments and the position of the COM for each body segment can be seen in the Tables 3.2 and 3.3.

Body COG, line of gravity (LOG) and centre of pressure (COP)

The COG of the body as a whole can be thought of as the point about which the mass of all body

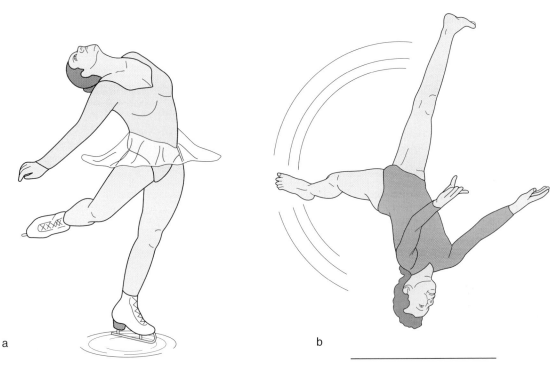

a   b

Figure 3.18 Rotation about one of the body axes is often performed in sports. In (a) a figure skater is spinning, which can reach high angular velocities. In (b) a gymnast is doing a straight somersault, which isn't very easy to achieve because of the larger moment of inertia involved.

Table 3.2 Mass of each body segment in percentage of total body mass

Segment	% of body mass
Trunk	49.7
Head and neck	8.1
Upper arm	2.8 each
Lower arm	1.6 each
Hand	0.6 each
Total arm	5.0 each
Upper leg	10.0 each
Lower leg	4.7 each
Foot	1.4 each
Total leg	16.1 each

Table 3.3 Location of the COM of each body segment in percentage of segment length (After Winter 1990)

Segment	Location
Trunk	50% between trochanter major and the glenohumeral joint
Head and neck	At the point of the ear canal
Upper arm	43.6% from proximal joint
Lower arm	43% from proximal joint
Hand	50% from proximal joint
Upper leg	43.3% from proximal joint
Lower leg	43.3% from proximal joint
Foot	50% between lateral malleolus and MTP5 joint

segments is evenly distributed. In the anatomical position it is thought to be at the level of the second sacral vertebra, inside the pelvis. However, as soon as the configuration of the body differs from the anatomical position, the COG will shift and can even be located outside the body. For instance, if both arms are elevated to a horizontal position, the COG moves forward and upward relative to its location in the anatomical position. This change of the COG location is an important consideration when discussing balance and equilibrium and the different human postures. See Chapter 13 for a full discussion on body posture and balance.

The *line of gravity* can be said to be the projection of the centre of gravity on the ground, represented by a line perpendicular to the ground through the COG. In Figure 3.19, the COG is represented by the target and the dotted line represents the line of gravity when the body is in the anatomical position. Although the position of the LOG is given relative to the different joints, it should be realised that there is a wide variation in posture between different people. The LOG is not very useful for biomechanical calculations.

The *centre of pressure* (COP) is the point of application of the ground reaction force. This force reflects Newton's third law, the law of action/reaction, in that the force exerted by the body onto the ground is reflected back at the centre of pressure. On average, during quiet standing, the ground reaction force and gravity pulling on the COG will be colinear forces but this is not necessarily the case during movements.

Base of support

Every object, unless it is floating in space, has to rest on a supporting surface. The surface area of the part which is involved in support of the object, inanimate or a human body, is known as the *base of support* (BOS). The shape and size of the base of support depends upon the posture that the body adopts (lying, sitting or standing, for example), the position of the feet and hands and the use of extra support (crutches or a chair, for example). When standing upright unsupported, the BOS is in between and underneath the feet (see Fig. 3.20).

Balance, equilibrium and stability

These terms are often interchanged in their use but they are all slightly different paradigms. If the line of gravity is within the base of support then the body is said to be in *balance*. When all the resultant forces and moments acting on a body are equal to zero then *equilibrium* is said to occur. If the body is stationary when all the forces add up to zero then the body is said to be in *static*

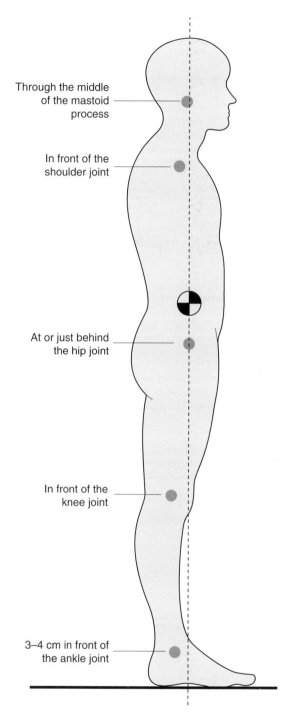

Through the middle of the mastoid process

In front of the shoulder joint

At or just behind the hip joint

In front of the knee joint

3–4 cm in front of the ankle joint

Figure 3.19 A line projected through the centre of gravity onto the floor is called the line of gravity. In the picture this line is shown on a person standing ideally upright. Some anatomical landmarks give a better indication of where the line is located.

equilibrium. If, on the other hand, the body moves with a constant linear velocity it is said to be in *dynamic equilibrium.* If, after a displacement by a force of short duration, the body tends to return to its original starting position then it is said to be *stable.*

Types of stability

If an object tends to return to its original starting position after a force of short duration is applied or if the object is placed such that an effort to disturb it would require its COG to be raised, then the object is said to be *stable* (in other words if the LOG remains well within the BOS when the object is tilted).

In the situation where an object tends to continue its displacement under the influence of gravity after a force of short duration is applied then it is said to be unstable. When the relationship of the LOG to the base and the height of the COG are the same after displacement (rolling of a tube, for example) then the stability is said to be neutral. The stability of a body depends upon:

● The surface area of the BOS
● The location of the LOG within the BOS
● The height of the COG above the BOS
● The mass of the body.

Base of support, stability limit and centre of pressure

In Figure 3.20, the BOS in quiet standing, with the feet parallel and slightly apart, is drawn around the outer edges of the feet and the area in between. In theory, a person should be able to move their line of gravity to the edge of the BOS and still be stable. This is, however, very difficult to do because it would require a lot of muscle force, particularly at the ankle joint, to maintain stability. There is, therefore, a limited area within the BOS within which a person can move their line of gravity safely. This area is called the *stability limit* (see Fig. 3.20). The centre of pressure (COP) was defined as the point of application of the ground reaction force. During quiet standing the COP lies well within the BOS and the stability

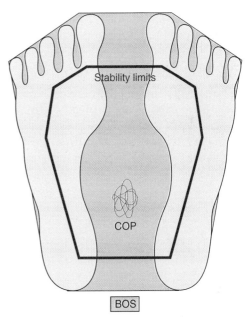

Figure 3.20 During quiet upright standing, the contact area with the floor underneath the feet and the area in between the feet is the base of support (BOS: dark red area in the graph). Because people cannot easily move their line of gravity to the outer edges of the BOS, the stability limit has been defined as the area within which people can move their line of gravity without losing balance. The centre of pressure (COP) of the ground reaction force is located well within those two areas. Because a person will always sway a bit, the COP oscillates with a certain amplitude.

limit. The COP is usually located a few centimetres in front of the ankle joint and moves with an amplitude of approximately 1 cm because a person sways when standing (see Fig. 3.20).

WORK, POWER, ENERGY AND MOMENTUM

When a force moves an object in a specified direction the extent to which it can be moved is the amount of *work* it can perform. The unit of work is the joule (J). The capacity of the force to do this work is the *energy.* It is also measured in joules (J). The rate at which this work is done is called the *power* and is measured in watts (W).

Work can either be linear or rotational and can be calculated by using the following equations:

Linear work = Force × distance of linear
displacement

Rotational work = Moment × angular displacement

Forms of energy

There are many forms that energy can take. *Metabolic energy* is the energy obtained from food by means of the metabolic process. *Heat energy* is the energy that a system can derive from a heat source. *Mechanical energy* is a measure of the ability to do work.

Forms of mechanical energy

Potential (gravitational) energy is defined as the capacity of a body to do work due to the location of an object in a gravitational field above a certain baseline. The equation for calculating this energy is shown below:

$$E_p = \text{mass} \times \text{gravity} \times \text{height}$$

where E_p is potential energy, mass is the mass of the body or object, gravity is the acceleration due to gravity and height is the position of the body above the baseline.

Kinetic energy is the capacity of an object to perform work due to its motion. It can be calculated using the equations below:

Linear kinetic energy: $E_k = \frac{1}{2} m \times v^2$

where m is mass and v is velocity.

Rotational kinetic energy: $E_r = \frac{1}{2} I \times \omega^2$

where I is moment of inertia and ω is angular velocity.

Elastic (strain) energy is the capacity a body has to do work after being deformed from its original shape. It is calculated by using the equation below:

$$E_s = k \times x$$

where k is the constant of spring stiffness and x is the change in length.

Conservation of energy

The total sum of energy is assumed always to be constant. One form of energy can be transformed into another but the total amount of energy is never lost.

Power

The rate at which work is performed is termed the *power* of the system. Power is the product of force and distance in a specified time. This can be calculated by using the equations below.

For linear motion:

Power = Force × distance/time

or

Power = Force × velocity

For rotational motion:

Power = Moment × angular displacement/time

or

Power = Moment × angular velocity

Muscle work

Muscle can only contract by using metabolic energy. The physiology of muscle work is described in Chapter 13.

Muscle work can be calculated using the following equations. If the muscle force and the distance between muscle origin and insertion are known:

Work = Muscle force × muscle length change

If the net joint moment (see section on movement analysis later in this chapter) and joint rotations are known:

Work = Net joint moment × joint angular displacement

During a concentric contraction the muscle force and the muscle length change are in the same direction. The above equation will then result in a positive outcome and therefore results in positive work. During an eccentric contraction the muscle force and the muscle length change are in the opposite direction. The above equation will then result in a negative outcome and therefore results in negative work. During an isometric contraction there is no length change of the muscle and therefore, in biomechanical terms, there is no work done.

Muscle power

The rate of doing muscle work is termed *muscle power*. Muscle power can be calculated using the following equations. If the muscle force and the distance between muscle origin and insertion are known:

Power = Force × velocity of contraction

If the net joint moment and joint rotations are known:

Power = Net joint moment × joint angular velocity

During concentric contractions, power is generated (positive power). During eccentric contractions, power is absorbed (negative power).

Momentum and impulse

Momentum can be defined as the quantity of motion possessed by an object, measured by the product of its mass and the velocity of its COM. A linear momentum is relevant when an object moves linearly and angular momentum is relevant when an object rotates.

The summation of a force over time is called the *impulse*. It is also described as the area under the force-curve (see Fig. 3.21) and can be interpreted as the change of momentum. Momentum and impulse have the same dimension, namely newton.second (N.s).

Momentum and impulse are useful quantities when a force applied over time does not result in a change of position as happens during gait. The ground reaction force applied to the foot during the stance phase of gait is substantial but the foot remains in the same position relative to the floor. Without a distance or velocity over which this force is applied, work or power generated by this ground reaction force would be zero. The impulse of the ground reaction force in that case is more revealing.

These quantities are also useful to explain what happens during collisions (kicking a ball, rugby tackle). The sum of the momentum of colliding objects remains constant, being known as conservation of momentum.

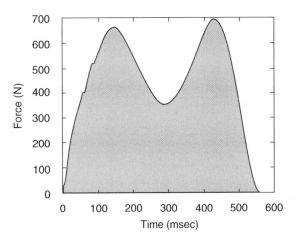

Figure 3.21 This is a typical graph of the vertical ground reaction force under one foot during gait. The double hump shape arises from the heel strike and push off phases. Because the foot does not move during the stance phase, this force would not result in any work. Therefore, the impulse (area under the curve in red) is a better indication of the impact the foot has on the ground or vice versa.

MOVEMENT ANALYSIS

The majority of human movements are quite complex because body segments move relative to each other and relative to the environment. This makes it difficult to predict what combination of muscle actions is required to generate a particular movement. A quantitative movement analysis can clarify which muscles should be active during a posture or movement in the context of several external forces acting on the body. For this purpose *inverse dynamics* is an often-used technique. The word inverse indicates that the causes of movement (forces and moments) are calculated from the outcome (movement as it is measured). The aim of such an analysis is to determine the forces and moments at the different joints. In particular net joint forces and net joint moments are calculated. A net joint force is the resultant force of all the forces acting on the different anatomical structures at the joint interface between two body segments. In equivalent terms, a net joint moment is the resultant moment. Muscles generate the main components of a net joint moment and therefore these net joint moments can be used as an indication of which muscles contribute to an activity. A limitation of the method is that it does not clearly predict the coactivation of muscles. Once net joint forces and moments are known and given certain assumptions, it is possible to estimate what loading muscle tendons, joint surfaces and passive joint structures undergo during an activity.

Link-segment model and a free body diagram (FBD)

Movement analysis by means of the inverse dynamics approach involves a number of steps. First of all a link-segment model is used to represent the body in biomechanical terms. In a two-dimensional link-segment model the segments of the body can be represented by a bar or a line and the joints by a hinge. A free body diagram is a graphical representation of the whole or part of the body. To be able to do any calculations three different types of information are necessary. These are anthropometric information on the segments (e.g. segment mass and length), kinematic information (linear and angular segmental movement), and some information about the external forces acting on the body (e.g. ground reaction force). Each segment is analysed separately using a free body diagram and the equilibrium equations of force and moment. The analysis is usually started at the distal segment. The results (net joint forces and moments) from that distal segment can then be used in the analysis of the next segment in the link. The calculation therefore progresses in steps from one segment to the next.

Example of movement analysis

To illustrate this process of movement analysis, we will use an example of the lower limb during gait. The phase of the gait cycle to be analysed is at the end of mid-stance just before the push off phase (see Fig. 3.22). At that point in time the foot is normally flat on the ground and not yet moving.

To analyse the right leg, we need to start by constructing a link-segment model of the right

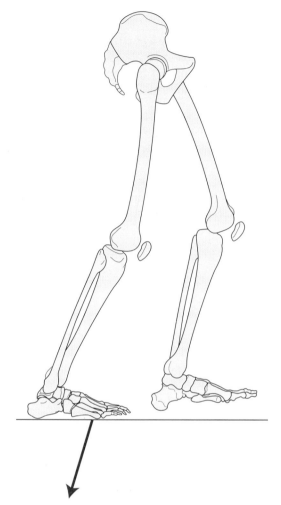

Figure 3.22 This is the phase during gait that is used in the example of movement analysis. The right foot is starting the push off but heel off has not yet occurred. The other leg is in terminal swing phase and heel strike will occur soon. The vector shows the force applied by the foot on the ground (magnitude, direction and point of application).

lower limb (see Fig. 3.23). Of each segment we need to know the mass, the length, the location of the centre of mass and the moment of inertia about the centre of mass. This information is available in the literature (Winter 1990). In our example, information about the ground reaction force (magnitude, direction and point of application) is available from measurement.

The biomechanical calculations are performed in steps.

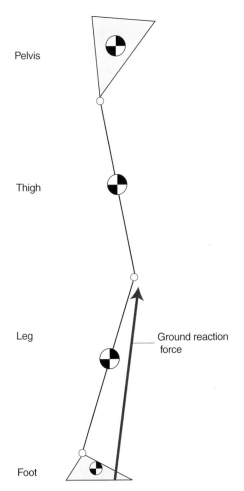

Pelvis

Thigh

Leg

Ground reaction force

Foot

Figure 3.23 A link-segment model describes the relation of the body segments relative to each other in mechanical terms, using bars to represent the segments and hinges to represent the joints. The targets indicate the positions of the centre of mass of each segment. The vector shows the magnitude, direction and point of application of the ground reaction force acting on the foot.

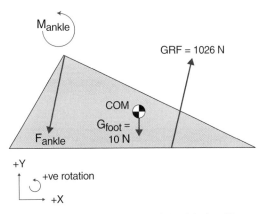

Figure 3.24 A free body diagram of the right foot. Vectors indicate forces and moments acting on the foot during the late stance phase of gait.

Step 1 – creating a free body diagram

Calculations are started at the foot since sufficient information about the external forces is available, therefore a free body diagram of the right foot is constructed (see Fig. 3.24). The free body is analysed as a separate entity. The environment and neighbouring parts of the body are represented in the FBD by arrows indicating the forces and moments that are applied by these factors to the free body.

In our example the relevant forces and moments to be included in the FBD are the ground reaction force (GRF), the effect of gravity on the centre of mass of the foot (G_{foot}), the net joint force at the ankle (F_{ankle}), and the net joint moment at the ankle (M_{ankle}). The latter two factors represent the net linear and rotational effects of the rest of the body on the foot acting at the ankle joint. These factors are unknown but will be solved by calculation. The net joint force and net joint moment are entered in the FBD as arrows in the locations where they act (ankle). The directions of the forces and moments are not always easy to predict. It is not essential to make an accurate prediction so long as the equilibrium equations are written on the basis of the FBD. The results of the calculations will then tell you whether the direction of the arrow was correct or not. A negative result indicates that the force or moment is pointing in the direction opposite to the one drawn.

Step 2 – type of equilibrium

The next step is to consider whether the foot is accelerating/decelerating (dynamic equilibrium) or not (static equilibrium). In our example the foot at that particular instant is not moving or starting to move. Therefore, all the forces acting on the foot should add up to zero since there is no linear acceleration/deceleration and all the moments should also add up to zero since there is no angular acceleration/deceleration (static equilibrium).

Step 3 – the equilibrium equations and finding the force

With the above information the equilibrium equations of force and moment for this free body diagram can be written and solved. The net joint force is solved first, followed by the net joint moment. Before the forces can be summed they need to be resolved into their orthogonal components. For instance, the ground reaction force can be resolved (see Fig. 3.25) into a vertical component pointing upward (positive direction) and a horizontal component pointing to the right (positive direction). The net ankle force can be resolved into a vertical component pointing down (negative direction) and a horizontal component pointing to the left (negative direction).

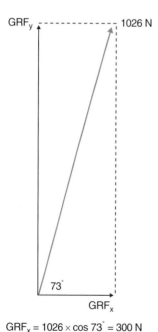

$GRF_x = 1026 \times \cos 73° = 300$ N
$GRF_y = 1026 \times \sin 73° = 981$ N

Figure 3.25 The ground reaction force (GRF) is an angled force and therefore must be resolved into its orthogonal components to be able to do further calculations. The magnitude of these force components is calculated by means of trigonometry (see section on trigonometry earlier in the chapter).

The effect of gravity is always pointing vertically down so that it does not have to be resolved.

Step 4 – the horizontal force

The horizontal forces in this FBD are the horizontal components GRF_x and $F_{ankle,x}$ These should add up to zero as stated earlier. This results in an equation that can readily be solved.

Horizontal forces:

$$GRF_x - F_{ankle,x} = 0$$

$$300 - F_{ankle,x} = 0$$

$$F_{ankle,x} = 300 \text{ N}$$

The result is a positive number, therefore the direction of the arrow, pointing in the negative direction, in the FBD was correct.

Step 5 – the vertical force

In the vertical direction there are three forces to consider: the vertical component of the GRF_y and the $F_{ankle,y}$ and the effect of gravity on the foot (G_{foot}). They should also add to zero because there is no foot movement, resulting in an equation that can readily be solved.

Vertical forces:

$$GRF_y - F_{ankle,y} - G_{foot} = 0$$

$$981 - F_{ankle,y} - 10 = 0$$

$$F_{ankle,y} = 971 \text{ N}$$

The total net ankle force can now be calculated by summing the horizontal and vertical components: $F_{ankle,x}$ and $F_{ankle,y}$.

Net ankle force:

$$F_{ankle} = \sqrt{(F_{ankle,x}^2 + F_{ankle,y}^2)}$$

$$F_{ankle} = \sqrt{(300^2 + 971^2)} = 1016 \text{ N}$$

Step 6 – the ankle moment

Now that all the unknown forces for this FBD (Fig. 3.24) have been solved, the net ankle moment

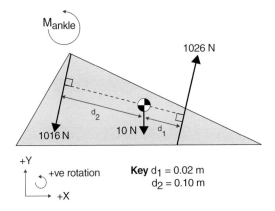

Figure 3.26 Once all the forces acting on the foot have been calculated, the rotatory effects of these forces also need to be considered. The same free body diagram used in Figure 3.24 is shown, but the moment arms of the GRF (d_1) and ankle force (d_2) are entered as well.

can also be solved. Note that by convention the moments of force are calculated about the COM of the free body and not about the ankle joint. In that case gravity does not have a moment of force about the COM. Therefore, the moment of force of the GRF and of the net ankle force and the net joint moment are to be included in the equation. The moment of force can be calculated by multiplying the force by the moment arm, i.e. the perpendicular distance between the axis of rotation (fulcrum) and the line of action of the force (Fig. 3.26).

Another aspect to consider is in which direction each force would rotate the free body if acting alone. In this FBD the GRF would result in an anti-clockwise (positive) rotation around the COM if it was the only force acting on the foot. The net ankle force would result in an anti-clockwise (positive) rotation. These will therefore be entered in the moment equation as positive. The net joint moment has been drawn as an anti-clockwise moment (see Fig. 3.26) so this is also entered into the same equation as positive. All these factors should add up to zero because the foot is not rotating, i.e. there is no angular acceleration.

Net ankle moment:

$$(GRF \times d_1) + (F_{ankle} \times d_2) + M_{ankle} = 0$$

$$(1026 \times 0.02) + (1016 \times 0.10) + M_{ankle} = 0$$

$$M_{ankle} = -122 \text{ N.m}$$

Step 7 – the internal moment

The result of this calculation of the net joint moment is negative. Therefore, the moment should be drawn as a clockwise moment, which means that it is an internal plantar flexing moment. This internal moment is mainly generated by the plantar flexors of the ankle. The triceps surae is the major contributor because of its large physiological cross sectional area (PCSA) and because of its large moment arm compared to the other flexors. Therefore it is not unreasonable to assume that this muscle almost entirely generates the ankle moment calculated in our example.

This assumption that one muscle produces the net joint moment makes it possible to calculate the force that will occur within the tendo calcaneus. A muscle moment is the product of the force within the muscle and the distance between the line of action of the muscle and the axis of rotation of the ankle joint (see Fig. 3.27). This distance or moment arm for the Achilles tendon can be estimated at 5 cm.

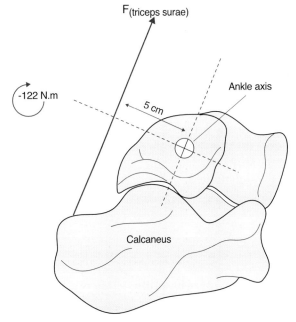

Figure 3.27 The net ankle moment calculated in the example is mainly provided by the triceps surae muscle. The moment arm of the muscle determines what muscle force is required to generate this moment. In this example the muscle moment arm is estimated to be 5 cm. $F_{(triceps)}$ represents the force generated by the triceps surae muscle.

The muscle force is therefore calculated as follows:

Net ankle moment generated by the triceps surae:

$$M_{ankle} = Force_{(triceps)} \times distance_{(Achilles\ tendon)}$$

$$-122\ N.m = Force_{(triceps)} \times -0.05\ m$$

$$-122\ N.m/-0.05\ m = Force_{(triceps)}$$

$$Force_{(triceps)} = 2440\ N$$

Step 8 – muscles, forces and their effects

The calculated force acting on the Achilles tendon is quite high but not out of the ordinary. In fact, the tensile loading in this example is equivalent to approximately three times the body weight of an average person. In more strenuous activities such as jumping this loading is expected to be much higher still.

The force of the triceps surae muscle is much larger than the net ankle force that was calculated earlier (F_{ankle} = –1016 N) and is pointing in the opposite direction. The net ankle force is the resultant force of all the different structures producing forces at the ankle joint. The muscle is just one of these structures. In this example the other structures are therefore generating the remainder of the forces so that the resultant force equals the net ankle force that was calculated. Because all forces in this example are parallel, the force of the other structures ($F_{(bone-on-bone)}$ in Fig. 3.28) can be easily determined.

Bone-on-bone forces:

$$F_{ankle} = F_{(triceps)} - F_{(bone-on-bone)}$$

$$-1016 = 2440 - F_{(bone-on-bone)}$$

$$F_{(bone-on-bone)} = 2440 + 1016 = 3456\ N$$

It is assumed that the main structure to contribute to this force is the force of the tibia on the talus, although the ligaments cannot be ignored. The bone-on-bone force results in a compression of the ankle cartilage. This load is the largest of all the values that were calculated. It is interest-

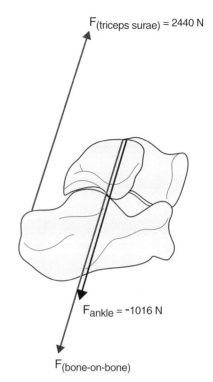

Figure 3.28 The triceps surae applies a large force in the direction opposite to the net joint force that was calculated. Therefore, there needs to be a third force that balances the force system. This would have to be the force that the bones of the lower leg apply to the foot. The resultant of the $F_{(triceps)}$ and the $F_{(bone-on-bone)}$ is the net ankle force (F_{ankle}).

ing to note that the activity of the triceps surae muscle was the major contributor to this cartilage loading. Body weight contributed to the cartilage loading to a much lesser extent. This is mainly due to the direction of pull of the muscle, which is almost parallel to the tibia, and to the 'small' moment arm of the muscle. The Achilles tendon has one of the largest moment arms of the muscles of the limbs. The result of this example, therefore, illustrates in general that joint loading is mostly due to muscle contractions.

Moving up the limb

The calculations so far have provided us with insight into which muscle group needs to be active to provide the appropriate moment at the ankle joint and has given us an idea of the magnitude of the tissue loading at the ankle joint during the particular phase of the gait cycle studied in this example. The same type of calculation can be carried out for the knee joint. For this purpose an FBD of the lower leg is required. The unknowns are the net joint force and net joint moment at the knee. The net ankle force and moment have already been solved for the FBD of the foot. These can be used for the FBD of the lower leg as well because according to Newton's third law of motion 'to every action there is an equal and opposite reaction'. In other words, the force (or moment) applied to the foot by the lower leg is equal but opposite to the force (or moment) applied by the foot to the lower leg. Once the net knee force and moment have been solved the analysis can be progressed to the hip joint. This will not be elaborated on in this chapter.

Note that the calculation for the example provided could be done in different ways but the proposed method allows analysis of more complex situations as well. It is the process that is demonstrated and not so much the calculation of the example.

DEFORMATION OF MATERIALS

So far this chapter has considered the effects of force on an object if the object moves or has the propensity to move. There are conditions when the object to which the force is being applied does not perform linear or angular motion. If sufficient force is applied then the object will undergo deformation. The type and extent of deformation will depend on the magnitude, direction and duration of the applied force and the composition of the object itself.

Stress and strain

The application of a force to an object is termed *loading*. The standardised measurement of loading is termed *stress*. The intensity of the applied stress is a result of the applied force divided by the surface area over which the force acts. This is expressed in N.m^{-2} (pascals). The equation is:

σ = Force/cross sectional area

Once the stress has been applied the object will undergo a *deformation* which can be defined as the change in shape or dimensions produced by the applied force. Not all materials will deform in the same way or to the same extent. Some materials will offer greater resistance to being deformed. This resistance is known as the materials' *stiffness*. The measure of deformation undergone by the object due to the stress that has been placed on it is termed the *strain*; it has no units and it is denoted by the letter epsilon (ε) and is expressed by the equation:

$\varepsilon = \Delta L / L_0$

where ΔL is change in dimension and L_0 is original dimension.

Figure 3.29 gives an number of examples of the types of stress that can act on an object. For every stress there is a corresponding strain. The relationship between the two parameters is unique to every material.

Linear loading

There are three types of linear stress that can be applied to the object. These are described below:

1. *Linear tension* occurs when two equal loads are applied to an object in such a way that they act along the same action line but in opposite directions, the resultant deformation being a lengthening and some narrowing (Fig. 3.30a).
2. *Linear compression* occurs when two equal loads are applied to an object such that they act along the same action line towards each other, i.e. squeezing. The resultant deformation will therefore be shortening with some widening (Fig. 3.30b).
3. *Shear* occurs when two parallel and equal loads are applied in opposite directions but not on the same line of action (Fig. 3.30c).

It can also be seen from Figure 3.30 that the calculation of the linear compression and tension strain is relatively straightforward. When considering the shear stress and strain there is not a change in length but there is an angular deformation. If, as illustrated in Figure 3.30c, the block is acted upon by a stress and the top of the block moves a

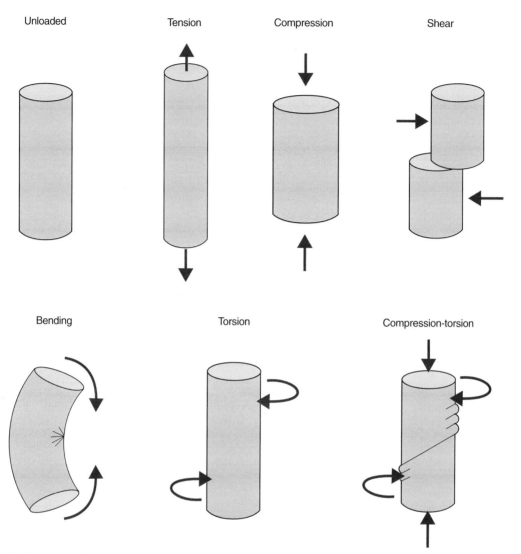

Figure 3.29 Examples of linear and rotational types of tissue loading.

distance d relative from the bottom of the block, then there is an angle Θ produced, as shown. This angle is the angle of shear strain and can be calculated by dividing the displacement by the height.

Young's modulus

The relationship of the changing stress and strain results is a constant of proportionality for each individual material. This constant is called *Young's modulus* and is represented by the equation:

Young's modulus = $\Delta\sigma/\Delta\varepsilon$

where $\Delta\sigma$ is the change in linear stress and $\Delta\varepsilon$ is the change in linear strain.

The constant of proportionality for shear stress is the *shear modulus* and is represented by the equation:

Shear modulus = $\Delta\sigma/\Delta\Theta$

where $\Delta\sigma$ is the change in shear stress and $\Delta\Theta$ is the change in shear strain.

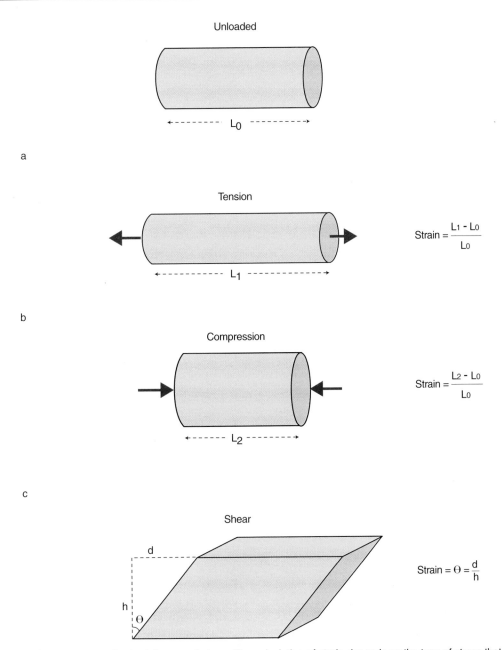

Unloaded

L_0

a

Tension

$$\text{Strain} = \frac{L_1 - L_0}{L_0}$$

L_1

b

Compression

$$\text{Strain} = \frac{L_2 - L_0}{L_0}$$

L_2

c

Shear

$$\text{Strain} = \Theta = \frac{d}{h}$$

d

h

Θ

Figure 3.30 Strain occurs under the influence of stress. The calculation of strain depends on the type of stress that is active. The examples provided are for the linear stresses of (a) tension, (b) compression and (c) shear.

Stress-strain curves

One of the more useful relationships between the stress placed on an object and the corresponding strain is seen when a graph is plotted with strain on the x-axis and stress on the y-axis. A general *stress/strain* curve is illustrated in Figure 3.31 below. The relationship found for any material is dependent only on the type of loading and the

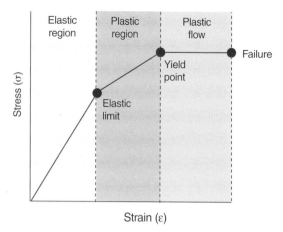

Figure 3.31 A typical stress-strain curve that applies to many types of materials. Generally, materials have an elastic region and a plastic region until failure. The elastic limit and the yield point are shown in the graph, marking the transition from one region to the next.

mechanical properties of the material. It is interesting to note that the relationship will stay the same for any object made from the same material irrespective of its size or shape. By experimentation the relationships between stress and strain for different materials have been found and all display variations of a basic pattern.

As can be seen from the diagram there are three distinct regions separated by the vertical dashed lines. The first region is the linear section of the graph as seen between the start and the elastic limit. This is referred to as the elastic region. It is in this region that the material under stress obeys Hooke's Law. This means that for every incremental unit of stress there is a corresponding incremental increase in strain, i.e. there is a linear relationship between the two. It is within the elastic region that, if the stress is released, the material will return to its original position. Therefore, there is no permanent deformation occurring and the deformation (and material) is referred to as elastic. This section of the graph is represented mathematically by Young's modulus.

Once the stress has increased past the elastic limit the graphical representation is seen to occur in the plastic region (up to the yield point). If the stress does not exceed the yield point then the

material will still exhibit some elastic properties but will not return to its original position. Some permanent deformation has taken place. The material is said to have undergone *plastic change*.

If the stress is maintained at the yield point the material will undergo *plastic flow* where the strain continues with no increase in stress until failure occurs and the material will fracture. The amount of stress that a material can absorb prior to failure is called its *ductility* and will vary for different materials.

Some materials will exhibit the property of *creep*, which is the ability to increase their deformation under a constant load. This is dependent on time. The behaviour of biological materials under stress will be discussed in Chapter 7.

MECHANICAL PRINCIPLES OF FLUIDS

Hydrostatics and hydrodynamics

Hydrostatics is the study of the effects of force and pressure on a fluid at rest whereas hydrodynamics is the study of fluid in motion (flow).

To understand hydrostatics we must look firstly at some of the physical properties of liquids. In this section only water will be described, as it is water that is generally used in the treatment of patients. Water itself can take the form of any of the three states of matter, being solid below temperatures of 0°C and gaseous above 100°C. Hydrotherapy pools are normally heated to temperatures of between 33° and 38°C and thus the water is always a liquid.

The structure of a liquid is such that it has different properties to solid objects. At a basic level the atomic structure of a liquid can be said to have weaker cohesive bonds (attractive forces between the same type of molecules) than a solid. This means that the motion of these molecules is much greater than in solids, so much so that a liquid is unable to maintain its own shape and therefore has to take the shape of the receptacle in which it is placed. A liquid also has the property of retaining its volume, showing a molecular repulsive force when it is being compressed. It is this repulsive force that produces the almost continuous flow of the liquid when an outside force is applied to it, hence the term fluid.

The cohesive force is responsible for giving water its property of *surface tension*. This is the 'film like' covering on the surface of the water which is caused by the stronger cohesive forces of the water to water molecules than the weaker adhesive forces (the attractive forces between different molecules) of the water to air molecules. The force of surface tension for a hydrotherapy pool is so weak that it can be ignored. The adhesive forces between the water and whatever is placed in it, part of the body or an oar, for example, are also very weak, being greater than moving through the air but insignificant when compared to the frictional forces experienced on land.

Pressure

When a force is applied to a fluid in a confined container it experiences pressure. Earlier in the chapter pressure was described as the force per unit area and this was the pressure on a plane surface. In fluids, however, the pressure is said to be acting at a point and this point can be thought of as a small plane surface (Bell 1998). Even without an additional force, hydrostatic pressure is felt within the fluid in all directions as the randomly moving molecules collide into each other, the container and any object immersed in it. Pascal's law states that this force is equal in all directions and is independent of gravity. Pressure within the fluid is also the result of the weight of the fluid above a given point and it is equal to the vertical distance from the point to the surface, multiplied by the weight density of the fluid. So it can be seen that the deeper an object is in the fluid the greater pressure it will experience. Hydrostatic pressure is usually measured in pascals which equals 1 N.m^{-2}.

Density

Along with depth, pressure in a fluid will change when the density of the fluid changes. Density is defined as the mass of the fluid divided by its volume. This then gives us the fluid's mass density (ρ) expressed in kg.m^{-3}. If we multiply the fluid's mass by the acceleration due to gravity and divide it by its volume then we have the fluid's weight density.

Relative density/specific gravity

This is the density of a material (solid or liquid) relative to that of pure water at 4°C. As the relative density of water is, by definition, 1 then the relative densities of other materials will determine whether that material will float or sink in water. A relative density less than 1 will mean that the material will float and with a relative density greater than 1 it will sink. The relative density of the human body is in the region of 0.86–0.97 (Bell 1998). This number will vary depending on the proportion of the different body tissues and the amount of air within the lungs.

Buoyancy

It has already been said that the pressure on a body within the water is equal on all aspects of that body and this pressure increases with the depth of the water. The point forces will be greater on the deeper aspects of the object, thus there will be a resultant upward force on that body. This resultant upward force is the upthrust experienced in the water and is termed the force of *buoyancy*.

The amount of force a body will experience is governed by Archimedes' principle which states that any body which is wholly or partially immersed in a fluid will experience an upward thrust equal to the weight of fluid displaced. The force of buoyancy can be said to be acting through the *centre of buoyancy*, which is the centre of gravity of the displaced fluid. Therefore, the centre of buoyancy does not have to coincide with the centre of gravity of the body in the water.

Stability

The stability of a body on dry land is subject to the relationship of the centre of gravity to the base on which it rests. In fluids, however, the relationship of the centre of gravity to the centre

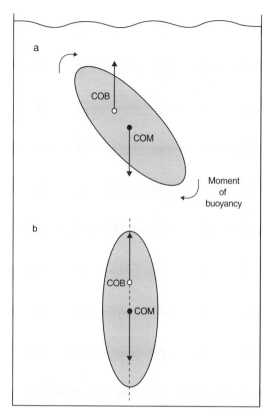

Figure 3.32 A moment of buoyancy occurs when the force due to gravity and due to buoyancy is not colinear (a). The object will rotate until colinearity has been achieved (b). In this example the centre of buoyancy and the centre of mass never coincide.

of buoyancy is the predominant factor controlling stability. If a body is placed in water it will rotate until the centre of buoyancy and the centre of gravity are coincident. This point is referred to as the *metacentre*. This is illustrated in Figure 3.32.

Moment of buoyancy

If the centres of buoyancy and gravity do not lie in the same vertical line then the body, as explained above, will not be in equilibrium and will rotate. The cause of this rotation is the *moment of buoyancy*. The moment of buoyancy is the same as any turning effect of a force on dry land in that it causes the body to rotate until it is compelled to stop by another force, or in this example, because the forces of buoyancy and gravity are colinear.

The moment of buoyancy is calculated, as on dry land, by multiplying the force (buoyancy) by the perpendicular distance from the fulcrum. As can be seen from Figure 3.33, the nearer the body segment is to the water's surface the greater the perpendicular distance from the knee axis of rotation and hence the greater is the moment of buoyancy, thus facilitating knee extension.

Types of flow

When a fluid flows from a point of higher to lower pressure the fluid molecules form themselves into layers or laminae. The layers at the centre of the flow move faster than those nearer the edge of the fluid, whilst those at the very edge may even be stationary. If these layers run smoothly along without any disturbance then the flow is said to be *laminar* or *streamlined*.

The fluid will flow in a streamlined way until it reaches a critical velocity. At this velocity the laminae break up and the flow is said to be *turbulent*. Turbulence is created because shear stress between the different laminae depends on the viscosity of the fluid and the rate of change of velocity in the direction of flow and perpendicular to the flow. Thus, with the increase in the flow rate, the laminar pattern will break up and the molecules will no longer travel in layers but take on an irregular pattern of motion. Once turbulent flow has been established the back current or *eddy currents* may become exaggerated and cause areas of reduced pressure downstream (the wake) of these eddy currents.

Movement through a fluid

If a streamlined object moves through the fluid then the fluid offers little resistance to its flow. There is very little turbulence caused by the movement of the object and thus the frictional resistance is low. If the object is non-streamlined then there will be a much greater resistance to its progress. The type of resistance it will meet will depend on the shape of the object. As can be seen from Figure 3.34a a streamlined object produces little disturbance in the fluid. Figure 3.34b shows the formation of eddy currents and an area of reduced

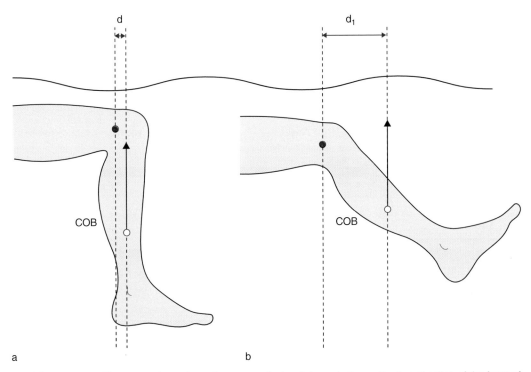

Figure 3.33 The moment of buoyancy depends on the perpendicular distance between the line of action of the force of buoyancy and the knee axis of rotation. In (a) the moment of buoyancy will be smaller than in (b) because of the greater distance (moment arm).

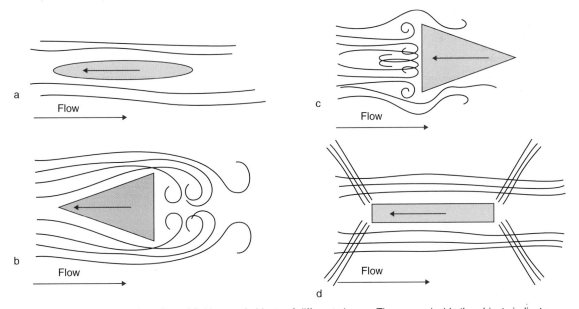

Figure 3.34 Four examples of the flow of fluid around objects of different shapes. The arrows inside the objects indicate movement of the objects from right to left. The fluid is moving in the opposite direction as indicated. In (a) there is a streamlined object that does not disturb the flow in laminae. In (b) the object results in turbulence with an area of reduced pressure and eddy currents in its wake. In (c) there are turbulence and eddy currents in front of the object. In (d) waves form at the front and the back of the object.

pressure, which together form a *wake*. Figure 3.34c shows the formation of eddy currents with the turbulent flow in front of the object, which provides a much greater resistance to movement. As seen from Figure 3.34d, there is also the formation of waves, one travelling out in front of the object and one travelling out from behind. Both these waves will require energy to overcome their resistance. The resistance to movement is increased even further if the fluid in which the movement is taking place is already turbulent.

Task 3.3
With a group of colleagues walk around in a circle in single file in a swimming pool. After a few seconds change the direction you are all walking (from clockwise to anti-clockwise). What happens? Try this again but this time vary the depth and speed of your walk and the frequency of your direction change. What differences do you find?

REFERENCES

Bell F 1998 Principles of mechanics and biomechanics. Stanley Thomas, Cheltenham

Winter D 1990 Biomechanics and motor control of human movement. John Wiley, New York

FURTHER READING

Craik R L, Oatis C A (eds) 1995 Gait analysis: theory and application. Mosby Year Book, St Louis

Enoka R M 1994 Neuromechanical basis of kinesiology. Human Kinetics, Champaign, Illinois

Hollis M 1989 Practical exercise therapy. Blackwell Scientific, Oxford

Zatsiorsky V M 1998 Kinematics of human motion. Human Kinetics, Champaign, Illinois

CHAPTER CONTENTS

Introduction   69

Overview of movement and postural control   70

Organisation of the spinal cord for movement control   70

Muscle receptors – their role in muscle control   72
Role of the muscle spindle in voluntary motor activity   72
The golgi tendon organ   73

Brain stem and basal ganglia level of control of posture and movement   76

Cerebral cortex (cortical) control of movement   77

Cerebellar control of motor function   79
Functions of the cerebellum in motor control   79

Sensory feedback control of motor function   82

4

The neural control of human movement

J. L. Crow   B. M. Haas

OBJECTIVES

When you have completed this chapter you should be able to:

1. **Describe the roles of the different levels of the central nervous system in the neural control of movement**

2. **Explain the various interconnections between the different levels of the central nervous system and the periphery**

3. **Understand how information from the periphery can alter or shape a movement response**

4. **Demonstrate knowledge of the overall control of the body with specific reference to rapid movements**

5. **Consider the close relationship between postural control and active movements.**

INTRODUCTION

Human movement is a complex affair. Normal movements are often automatic in nature and only come under volitional control when circumstances change or as a consequence of new experiences. The unique functional ability of humans is possible through the quality of movement produced from normal coordinated patterns of movement. Such patterns are produced on a background of normal sensory information and feedback, normal tone, reciprocal innervation, normal balance and postural reactions (Edwards 1996).

The control of movement has traditionally been considered to be hierarchical with the highest, cortical level of control organising voluntary, skilled movement. However, in reality there is no separation between voluntary movements and the background of postural control that maintains the body in an upright position with the aid of automatic reflexes and responses. Therefore, parallel systems of control, with integration of all levels rather than just a serial hierarchy, may be a more appropriate description. All levels of control, from the spinal cord up to the cerebral cortex, are necessary and integrated to provide the base of axial stability for more normal distal mobility and skilled or refined coordinated limb movements (Kidd et al 1992).

In addition, the environmental context and the movement task itself may influence how the nervous system organises movement. Expansion of the many movement control theories which have been proposed are reviewed by Plant (1998) and by Shumway-Cook & Woollacott (1995). This chapter will therefore consider only the specific role of the nervous system in normal movement control. Such an understanding is essential for the assessment and treatment of disorders of movement resulting from musculoskeletal injury and damage to the nervous system. The neural control of posture and movement, whether voluntary or automatic, will be considered briefly as an overall system and then subdivided into centres (levels) of control within the central nervous system (CNS).

A basic knowledge of neuroanatomy and neurophysiology is assumed in those reading this chapter and these subjects will not be covered directly. Rather, the applied neurophysiology of the control of movement will be discussed. Therefore, readers may find it useful to recap their knowledge of the basic neurophysiology with particular reference to the role of the muscle spindle, the stretch reflex, action potentials and inhibition and excitation of nerve impulses, prior to studying this chapter.

The development of motor control is well described elsewhere and provides a useful background to the study of normal child growth and development. This section will, therefore, restrict itself to the control of posture and movement of the normal adult.

OVERVIEW OF MOVEMENT AND POSTURAL CONTROL

For any normal motor function to occur an input of sensory information is required. Sensory information is integrated at all levels of the nervous system and causes appropriate motor responses, i.e.:

- Spinal cord: simple reflexes (automatic, stereotyped reflex movement); the peripheral execution level of movement.
- Brain stem and basal ganglia: more complicated responses (postural and balance reactions), able to affect the spinal cord to produce or change automatic movement.
- Cerebrum: most complicated responses controlled (variable and adaptable skilled voluntary movement based on stored programmes of learned movements). The motor, sensory and associated areas begin the chain of commands for most movements, though this may be initiated or modified at lower levels.
- Cerebellum: planning, timing and predictive function to produce coordinated skilled and rapid movements.

Figure 4.1 illustrates this movement control system with the interconnections between the main levels of the central nervous system suggesting a concurrent parallel organisation (Kidd et al 1992).

ORGANISATION OF THE SPINAL CORD FOR MOVEMENT CONTROL

The grey matter of the spinal cord is the integrative area for the cord reflexes and other automatic motor functions. As the region for the peripheral execution of movements, it also contains the circuitry necessary for more sophisticated movements and postural adjustments. Sensory signals enter the cord through the sensory nerve roots and then travel to two separate destinations:

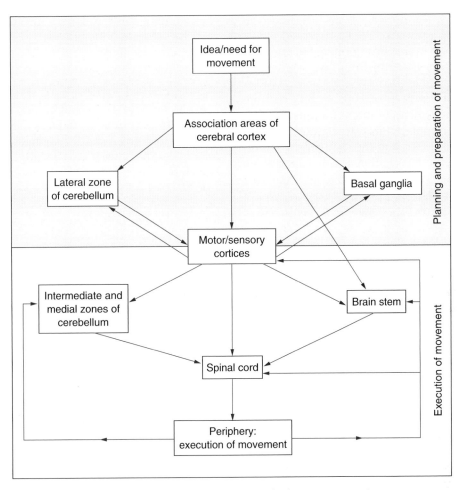

Figure 4.1 A schematic representation of the main control processes of voluntary movement.

• Same or nearby segments of the cord where they terminate in the grey matter and elicit local segmental responses (excitatory; inhibitory; reflexes, etc.).

• Higher centres of the CNS, i.e. higher in the cord, and brain stem cortices where they provide conscious (and unconscious, i.e. cerebellum) sensory information and experiences.

Each segment of the cord has several million neurones in the grey matter that include sensory relay neurones, anterior motor neurones and interneurones.

Interneurones are small and highly excitable with many interconnections, either with each other or with the anterior motor neurones. They

have an integrative/processing function within the spinal cord as few incoming sensory signals to the spinal cord or signals from the brain terminate directly on an anterior motor neurone. This is essential for the control of motor function. One specific type of interneurone is called the Renshaw cell, located in the anterior horn of the spinal cord. Collaterals from one motor neurone can pass to adjacent Renshaw cells which then transmit inhibitory signals to nearby motor neurones. So stimulation of one motor neurone can also inhibit the surrounding motor neurones. This is termed *recurrent* or *lateral inhibition*. This allows the motor system to focus or sharpen its signal by allowing good transmission of the primary signal and suppressing the tendency for the signal to spread to other neurones (Rothwell 1994).

In addition to interneurones there are also pro-priospinal fibres that run from one segment of the cord to another, so providing pathways for multisegmental reflexes, i.e. those reflexes that coordinate movement in different limbs simultaneously. Segmental circuits can activate networks of anterior horn cells and thus trigger the stimulation of specific muscle fibres. This can activate circuits (called central pattern generators) that control locomotion and possibly also a number of other repetitive motor activities (Marieb 1998).

MUSCLE RECEPTORS – THEIR ROLE IN MUSCLE CONTROL

For control of motor function, muscles need to be activated by excitation of the motor neurones. There is also a need for continuous feedback from each muscle to the central nervous system giving the status of that muscle, i.e. length, instantaneous tension and rate of change of length and tension. Muscle spindles detect changes and rate of change in the length of a muscle whereas golgi tendon organs detect degree and rate of change of tension. Signals from these sensory receptors operate at an almost subconscious level, transmitting information into the spinal cord, cerebellum and cerebral cortex where they assist in the control of muscle contraction.

The muscle spindle has both a static and a dynamic response. The primary and secondary endings respond to the length of the receptor, so impulses transmitted are proportional to the degree of stretch and continue to be transmitted as long as the receptor remains stretched. If the spindle receptors shorten, the firing rate decreases. Only the primary endings respond to sudden changes of length by increasing their firing rate and only whilst the length is actually increasing. Once the length stops increasing, the discharge returns to its original level, though the static response may still be active. If the spindle receptors shorten, then the firing rate decreases.

Control of the static and dynamic response is by the gamma motor neurone. Normally, the muscle spindle emits sensory nerve impulses continuously with the rate increasing as the spindle is stretched (lengthened) or decreasing as the spindle shortens.

The stretch or myotactic reflex can therefore be considered as:

- *Dynamic*, i.e. an instantaneous, strong reflex elicited from primary endings only, with the function to oppose sudden changes in length of muscle as the muscle contraction opposes the stretch.
- *Static*, i.e. a weaker reflex elicited from primary and secondary endings which continues for a prolonged period with the function to continue to cause muscle contraction as long as the muscle is maintained at excessive length.

The stretch reflex also has the ability to prevent some types of oscillation and jerkiness of body movements even if the input is jerky, i.e. a damping function (Palastanga et al 1994).

Role of the muscle spindle in voluntary motor activity

When the motor cortex or other areas of the brain transmit signals to the alpha motor neurones, the gamma motor neurones are nearly always stimulated simultaneously, i.e. a co-activation of the alpha and gamma systems so that intra- and extrafusal muscle fibres (usually) contract at the same time. This stops the muscle spindle opposing the muscle contraction and maintains a proper damping and load responsiveness of the spindle regardless of change in muscle length. If the alpha and gamma systems are stimulated simultaneously and the intra- and extrafusal fibres contract equally, then the degree of stimulation of the muscle spindle will not change. If the extrafusal fibres contract less because they are working against a great load, the mismatch will cause a stretch on the spindle and the resultant stretch reflex will provide extra excitation of the extrafusal fibres to overcome the load (Fig. 4.2).

The gamma efferent system is excited/controlled by the bulboreticular facilitatory region of the brain stem with influences from impulses transmitted to that region from the cerebellum, basal ganglia and cerebral cortex. The bulboreticu-

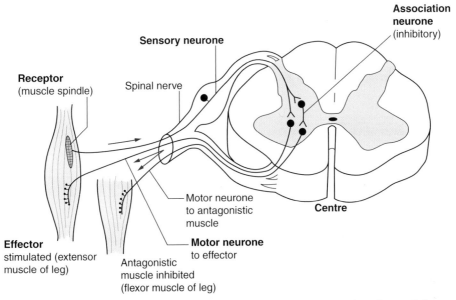

Figure 4.2 Reflex reaction to stimulation of the muscle (spindle stretch reflex). (Adapted from Tortora & Anagnostakos 1987; reprinted by permission of HarperCollins Publishers, Inc.)

lar facilitatory area is concerned with anti-gravity muscle contractions (anti-gravity muscles have a higher density of muscle spindles). Therefore, the gamma system has an important role in controlling muscle contraction in positioning different parts of the body and for damping the movement of the different parts (Guyton 1991). However, the monosynaptic spinal stretch reflex may not always be able to produce a contraction of sufficient force and is therefore followed by a long loop stretch reflex (functional stretch reflex) involving the cerebral cortex (Mathews 1991).

The golgi tendon organ

The golgi tendon organ, as a sensory receptor in the muscle tendon, detects relative muscle tension. Therefore, it is able to provide the CNS with instantaneous information of the degree of tension on each small segment of each muscle. The golgi tendon organ is stimulated by increased tension. When the increase in tension is too great, the tendon reflex response is evoked in the same muscle and this response is entirely inhibitory. The brain dictates a set point of tension, beyond which automatic inhibition of

muscle contraction prevents any further change. Alternatively, if the tension decrease is too low, then the golgi tendon organ reacts to return the tension to a more normal level. This leads to a loss of inhibition so allowing the A-alpha motor neurone to be more active and increase the muscle tension.

Information from the golgi tendon organ has both a direct and an indirect effect. Signals travel to local areas of the spinal cord and excite a single inhibitory interneurone that directly inhibits the A-alpha motor neurone to that individual muscle only. Information is then also spread to all the higher centres through indirect means (Guyton 1991).

The golgi tendon organ is similar to the muscle spindle in that it has a static and a dynamic response. The static response provides a low level of steady state firing proportional to the muscle tension. The dynamic response allows rapid/intense firing when muscle tension suddenly increases.

If the golgi tendon organ is stimulated by an increased tension, the signals transmitted cause an inverse stretch reflex effect in the respective muscle, which is entirely inhibitory (Fig. 4.3).

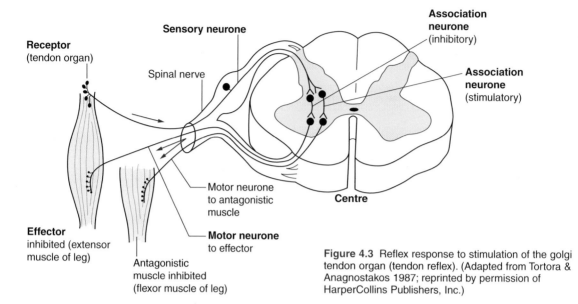

Figure 4.3 Reflex response to stimulation of the golgi tendon organ (tendon reflex). (Adapted from Tortora & Anagnostakos 1987; reprinted by permission of HarperCollins Publishers, Inc.)

This serves as a negative feedback to prevent development of too much tension. If the tension is extreme, the golgi tendon organ tendon reflex effect is to cause sudden relaxation of the entire muscle, a lengthening reaction. This protective mechanism prevents muscle tears or tendon avulsions.

With the golgi tendon organ being in series with the muscle fibres it is stimulated by both passive and active stretch. A passive stretch has a slow response as the more elastic fibres take up most of the stretch first. It actually takes a strong active contraction of the muscle to produce the relaxation of autogenic inhibition (Ganong 1995).

Table 4.1 summarises and compares the roles of the golgi tendon organ and the muscle spindle.

With the stretch reflex, as the supplied muscle is excited, the antagonistic muscle is simultaneously inhibited to allow movement to occur (Figs 4.2 and 4.4). This phenomenon is called reciprocal inhibition (postsynaptic) with the neural mechanism termed reciprocal innervation or a flexor reflex. With the inverse stretch reflex, the direct effect to the muscle supplied is one of inhibition and relaxation with additional information being sent to the motor neurones supplying the antagonist muscle causing excitation in that muscle group (Fig. 4.3).

Table 4.1 Comparison of the roles of golgi tendon organs and muscle spindles

Golgi tendon organ	Muscle spindle
Detects relative muscle length	Detects relative muscle tension
In series with the muscle fibres	In parallel with the muscle fibres
Tendon reflex is a feedback mechanism to control muscle tension	Stretch reflex is a feedback mechanism to control muscle length
Has dynamic and static responses	Has dynamic and static responses
During active concentric movement	
Increase in tension in the tendons	Decrease in muscle length
During passive movement	
Increase in tension in the tendons	Increase in muscle length

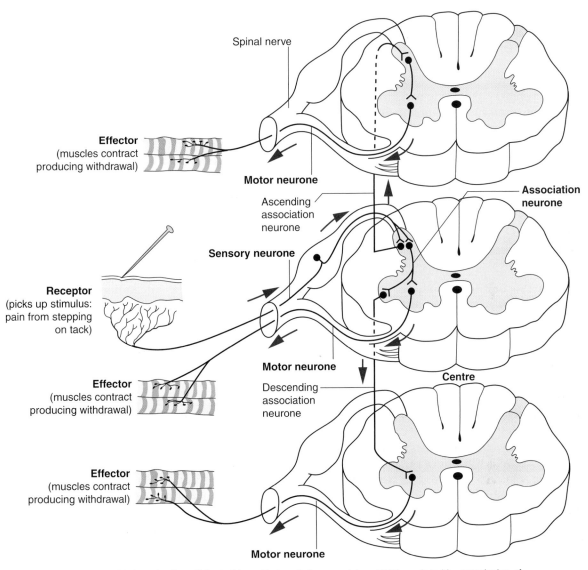

Figure 4.4 The flexor withdrawal reflex. (Adapted from Tortora & Anagnostakos 1987; reprinted by permission of HarperCollins Publishers, Inc.)

Task 4.1

Answer the following challenges before moving on to the next part of the chapter. You will need to refer to the earlier parts of this chapter and also to other books related to this subject.

Paraplegics with complete lesions of the spinal cord often demonstrate uncontrollable movements below the level of the lesion. How can you explain this when the neural connections from that part of the body to the brain are no longer intact?

With proprioceptive neuromuscular facilitation techniques the importance of fully elongating a muscle before maximal concentric contraction is emphasised. Using your knowledge of the neural control of movement can you suggest the reasons for this?

BRAIN STEM AND BASAL GANGLIA LEVEL OF CONTROL OF POSTURE AND MOVEMENT

The principal role of the brain stem in control of motor function is to provide background contractions of the trunk, neck and proximal parts of limb musculature so providing support for the body against gravity. The relative degree of contraction of these individual anti-gravity muscles is determined by equilibrium mechanisms, with reactions being controlled by the vestibular apparatus, which is directly related to the brain stem region.

The brain stem connects the spinal cord to the cerebral cortex. It comprises the midbrain (mesencephalon), pons and medulla oblongata. The central core of this region is often referred to as the reticular formation. This region of the central nervous system comprises all the major pathways connecting the brain to the spinal cord in a very compact, restricted space. It is also the exit point of the cranial nerves from the central nervous system.

The central core of the brain stem region is the reticular formation. This is the collection of neurones (nerve fibres, etc. that form the ascending and descending pathways), the connections with the cerebellum and other parts of the brain, collateral fibres and the origin of some pathways. Therefore, the area functions as a relay station processing sensory information and organising motor output (Gordon 1990). The reticular formation influenced through the reticular activating system also controls alertness.

It is through the integration of the information reaching the reticular formation that axial postural control and gross movements are controlled. Input to the reticular formation is from many sources, including the spinoreticular pathways, collaterals from spinothalamic pathways, vestibular nuclei, cerebellum, basal ganglia, cerebral cortex and hypothalamus. The smaller neurones make multiple connections within the area whereas the larger neurones are passing through, being mainly motor in function.

The vestibular nuclei are very important for the functional control of eye movements, equilibrium, the support of the body against gravity and the gross stereotyped movements of the body. The direct connections to the vestibular apparatus of the inner ear and cerebellum, as well as the cerebral cortex, enable the use of preprogrammed, background attitudinal reactions to maintain equilibrium and posture. Working with the pontine portion of the reticular formation, the vestibular nuclei are intrinsically excitable; however, this is held in check by inhibitory signals from the basal ganglia (Guyton 1991).

Overall, the motor related functions of the brain stem are to support the body against gravity, generate gross, stereotyped movements of the body and maintain equilibrium. Therefore, it is predominately concerned with the muscular control of the axial and proximal limbs (trunk and girdle movements). This is not in isolation but assisted by the integration of information from the cerebellum, basal ganglia and cortical regions.

The brain stem influences motor control directly through the descending pathways of the spinal cord and indirectly through ascending pathways to higher centres where their role is controlling overall activity of the brain and so of alertness (Gordon 1990). The descending pathways, which help control axial and girdle movements, can be divided into medial and lateral motor systems.

The medial system descends in the anteromedial columns of the spinal cord and projects directly (through interneurones) to medial motor neurones of the anterior horn, influencing groups of proximal limb muscles and axial body regions, often bilaterally. It is important for organising and controlling whole body movements that require groups of muscles working together. The vestibulospinal pathways are specifically related to the position and movement of the head, making them important in the organisation of postural movements in balance control. The reticulospinal pathways influence postural movements and locomotion through pontine portions that are inhibitory (Guyton 1991), so facilitating the support of the body against gravity by exciting the anti-gravity muscles. The tectospinal pathways link the midbrain with the cervical and upper thoracic spinal cord and are important for organising and orientating movements of the head and neck.

The lateral system descends in the dorsolateral columns of the spinal cord and directly or indirectly innervates the motor neurones to the distal muscles of the limb, i.e. it is for more discrete muscle actions that are concerned with the individual, agile and skilled movements of the extremities (Kidd et al 1992). The brain stem is probably involved in the circuits that produce the central pattern generators that coordinate locomotion. The impulse for walking may come from higher cortical centres but these central pattern generators are able to provide the motor pattern for walking (Grillner et al 1995).

The basal ganglia region forms part of the internal structure of the cerebral hemispheres. It comprises five subcortical nuclei (the putamen; caudate nucleus; globus pallidus; subthalamic nucleus and substantia nigra) which seem to serve as side loops to the cerebral cortex as they receive their input from the cerebral cortex and project almost exclusively back to the cerebral cortex. The basal ganglia are involved in all types of movements but have a predominant role in the provision for internal cues for the smooth running of learned movements and in the maintenance of the preparedness for movement (Morris and Iansek 1996). It is believed that the basal ganglia play an essential role in the selective initiation of most activities of the body or selective suppression of unwanted movements. A number of distinct feedback loops have been described including the putamen circuit (the direct pathway), which is responsible for the facilitation of movement, and the caudate circuit (the indirect pathway), which is more involved in the inhibition of unwanted movements. Thus the interplay of inhibitory or excitatory neurotransmitters within this region explains the clinical features that emerge in disorders of the basal ganglia (Rothwell 1994). Figure 4.5 shows a hypothetical model of the direct pathway. Excitation of the striatum from areas of the cerebral cortex inhibits the globus pallidus (internal part) and thus reduces the inhibitory influences of this area upon the thalamus. This in turn disinhibits the thalamus to excite areas of the cere-

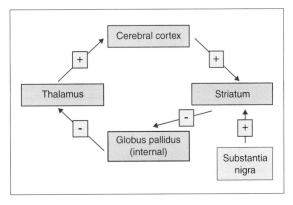

Figure 4.5 Hypothetical model of the direct pathway in the basal ganglia.

bral cortex for the initiation of movement. The normal functioning of this loop is reliant upon excitatory neurotransmitter impulses from the substantia nigra.

CEREBRAL CORTEX (CORTICAL) CONTROL OF MOVEMENT

Posture and equilibrium are controlled subconsciously by the brain stem and spinal cord; however, the cerebral cortex is the main centre for the control of voluntary movement. It works with the information it receives from the cerebellum, basal ganglia and other centres in the CNS to bring movements under voluntary control.

The cerebral cortex provides the advanced intellectual functions of humans, having a memory store and recall abilities along with other higher cognitive functions. The cerebral cortex is, therefore, able to perceive, understand and integrate all the various sensations. However, its primary movement function is in the planning and execution of many complex motor activities, especially the highly skilled manipulative movements of the hand (Gilman & Newman 1987).

The motor cortex occupies the posterior half of the frontal lobes. It is a broad area of the cerebral cortex concerned with integrating the sensations from the association areas with the control of movements and posture. It is closely related to other motor areas including the primary motor area and the premotor or motor association area.

The primary motor area contains very large pyramidal cells that send fibres directly to the spinal cord and anterior horn cells via the corticospinal pathways. In contrast, the premotor area has only a few fibres connecting directly with the spinal cord. It mainly sends signals into the primary motor cortex to elicit multiple groups of muscles; i.e. signals generated here cause more complex muscle actions usually involving groups of muscles that perform specific tasks, rather than individual muscles. This area connects to the cerebellum and basal ganglia which both transmit signals back, via the thalamus, to the motor cortex. Projection fibres from the visual and auditory areas of the brain allow visual and auditory information to be integrated at cortical level to influence the activity of the primary motor area. The premotor area is activated when a new motor programme is established or when the motor programme is changed on the basis of sensory information received, i.e. exploring a new environment. The supplementary motor area is thought to be the site where external inputs and commands are matched with internal needs and drives to facilitate formulation (programming) of a strategy of voluntary movement. So altogether the motor cortex and related areas of basal ganglia, thalamus and cerebellum constitute a complex overall system for voluntary control of muscle activity (Afifi & Bergman 1986).

The primary motor area has a topographical representation of the body on the surface of the cerebral cortex. This demonstrates the connections of the cerebral cortex to the different areas of the body with the size of the representation being proportional to the degree of innervation in that area. The hands are exaggerated in form as the refined skilled movements produced by the hand require more innervation to achieve that level of control (Palastanga et al 1994).

For voluntary movement to occur, information has to reach the motor cortex, mainly from the somatic sensory systems plus auditory and visual pathways. The sensory information is processed with information from the basal ganglia and cerebellum to determine an appropriate course of action. As can be seen there are many two-way pathways between the various centres of the CNS.

The organisation of the motor cortex is in vertical columns which act as functional units. Information enters a column from many sources and is amplified as necessary to produce appropriate muscle contraction. Each functional unit is responsible for directing a group of muscles acting on a single joint. So movements, not individual muscles, are represented in the motor cortex. Individual muscles are represented repeatedly, in different combinations, amongst the columns. Neurones of the motor cortex, having axons in the corticospinal pathways, function chiefly in the control of the distal muscles of the limb. They function to:

- change their firing rate in advance of limb movements
- fire at a frequency that is proportional to the force to be exerted in a movement and not in relation to the direction of the movement (Gilman 1992).

Each time the corticospinal pathway transmits information to the spinal cord the same information is received by the basal ganglia, brain stem and cerebellum. Nerve signals from the motor cortex cause a muscle group to contract. The signal then returns from the activated region of the body to the same neurones that caused the contraction, providing a general positive feedback enhancement if the movement was successful and recording it for future use.

At any segment of the spinal cord multiple motor pathways enter/terminate in the cord from the brain stem or higher centres. Generally, the corticospinal and rubrospinal pathways lie in the dorsal portions of the lateral columns of the spinal cord and terminate on the interneurones when concerned with the trunk, leg and arm areas of the cord. However, at the cervical enlargement where the hands and fingers are represented, the motor neurone supplying the hands and fingers lies almost entirely in the lateral portions of the anterior horns. In this region a large number of corticospinal and rubrospinal fibres terminate directly onto the anterior horn cells, i.e. a direct route from the brain in keeping with a high representation for fine control of the hand, fingers and thumb in the primary motor cortex (Ganong 1995).

The spinal cord can provide specific reflex patterns of movement in response to sensory nerve stimulation that are also important when the anterior horn cells are excited by signals from the brain. The stretch reflex is functional all the time helping to dampen the motor movements initiated from the brain. For example, when brain signals excite agonist muscles it is not necessary to inhibit the antagonistic muscles at the same time because reciprocal innervation will occur through the flexor reflex (Fig. 4.4).

CEREBELLAR CONTROL OF MOTOR FUNCTION

The cerebellum is vital for the control of very rapid muscular activities such as running, talking, playing sport or playing a musical instrument. Loss of the cerebellum leads to inco-ordination of these movements such that the actions are still available but no longer rapid or coordinated. This is due to the loss of the planning function.

The cerebellum monitors and makes corrective adjustments in the motor activities elicited by other parts of the brain. It is able to do this as it continuously receives information from the motor control areas of the cerebrum on the desired motor programme and from the periphery to determine the status of the body parts. With these feedback systems the cerebellum compares the actual instantaneous status of each part of the body, as depicted by peripheral information, with the status that is intended by the motor system. Corrective signals can then be transmitted if necessary to alter levels of activation (Gordon 1990).

Although the cerebellum is anatomically divided into three lobes (anterior, posterior and flocculonodular lobes), functionally the anterior and posterior lobes which control movement are divided longitudinally into a medial zone, or the vermis, and the intermediate and lateral zones from the cerebellar hemispheres (Fig. 4.6). The medial zone controls motor function of the axial body (neck, trunk and limb girdles), whereas the intermediate zone is concerned with control of the distal portions of the upper and lower limbs.

The lateral zone operates more remotely to provide overall planning of sequential motor movement such as timing and coordination (Ghez & Fahn 1985).

Extensive input and output systems operate to and from the cerebellum. Input pathways to the cerebellum from the cerebral cortex, carrying both motor and sensory information, pass through various brain stem nuclei before reaching the deep nuclei of the cerebellum. Likewise, output from the three zones of the cerebellum exit via the deep nuclei with the fibres from the lateral zone passing to the cerebral cortex to help coordinate voluntary motor activity initiated there. Fibres from the intermediate zone usually pass to the thalamus then on to the basal ganglia, cerebral cortex or brain stem regions to coordinate reciprocal movements. Those from the medial zone pass to the brain stem region to function in close association with the equilibrium apparatus to control postural attitudes of the body. Output from the deep nuclei of the cerebellum is continually under the influence of both excitatory and inhibitory influences, excitatory from the afferent fibres that enter the cerebellum and inhibitory from the functional unit of the cerebellar cortex, the Purkinje cell. A balance between the two effects is relatively constant with a continuous level of stimulation from both sources. However, when rapid movements are required, the timing of the two effects on the deep nuclei is such that excitation appears before inhibition. A rapid excitatory signal is initiated to modify the motor programme followed by an inhibitory signal, which is negative feedback having the effect of damping the movement and preventing overshooting. The cerebellum has a purely input and output system with no reverberating pathways (Gordon 1990, Guyton 1991).

Functions of the cerebellum in motor control

The cerebellum does not initiate motor activities but plays an important role in planning, mediating, correcting, coordinating and predicting motor activities, especially for rapid movements. The medial zone of the cerebellum represents the

Anatomical divisions of the cerebellum

Superior/inferior view

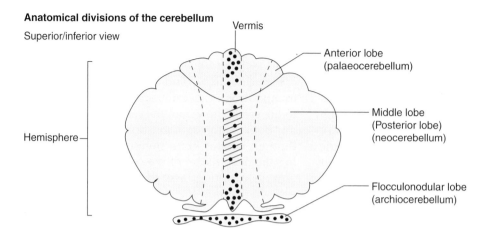

Functional representation of the areas of the cerebellum

Topographical representation

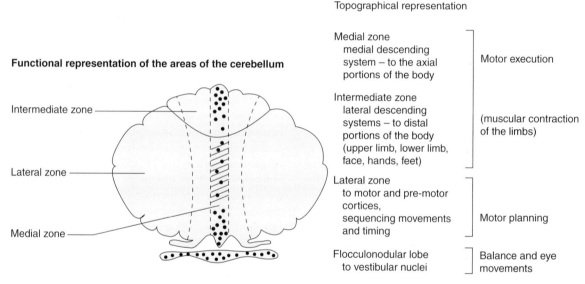

Figure 4.6 Anatomical divisions, functional divisions and representation areas of the cerebellum. (Adapted from Ghez & Fahn 1985.)

axial and girdle parts of the body with a predictive function for the control of posture and equilibrium. The intermediate zones control the distal parts of the limbs that produce the more refined and highly skilled movements in a smooth, co-ordinated and controlled manner. The lateral zones, with no topographical representation, oversee the overall control of the entire body with the function of planning and correct timing of sequential movements.

The medial zone of the cerebellum with the flocculonodular lobe works with the spinal cord and brain stem regions to control postural and equilibrium movements and provides a predictive function for rapid movement. Information from the muscle spindles is used to enhance and prolong the spinal cord stretch reflex. Thus, postural attitudes and adjustments of axial and limb girdle parts of the body are controlled with the help of the vestibular apparatus. During rapid movements the continuous feedback of the body's status by the cerebellum provides up to date and predictive information on body positions to other parts of the motor system. It is thought that the rapidly conducted information from the vestibular apparatus is used within a feedback control circuit to provide this instantaneous correction of postural motor signals in preparation for or anticipation of the body's needs (Ghez 1991).

Working with the basal ganglia and thalamus, the intermediate zones of the cerebellum help to control voluntary movement by utilising feedback circuits from the periphery and the brain. The distal parts of the limbs are controlled by information from the motor cortex and from the periphery and this information is integrated in the cerebellum. This provides smooth, coordinated movements of agonists and antagonistic muscle groups, allowing the performance of accurate, purposeful intricate movements that are especially required in the distal part of the limbs. This is achieved by comparing the intentions of the higher centres of the motor cortex with the performance of respective parts of the body. In general, the motor cortex sends more information than is needed so the cerebellum has to inhibit the motor cortex at an appropriate time after the muscles have begun to move. This provides both a damping function and control of ballistic (rapid) movements with a specific intention. The cerebellum assesses the rate of movement and calculates the length of time required to reach the point of intention. Inhibitory signals are then transmitted to the motor cortex to inhibit the agonist and excite the antagonist muscle groups and apply the brakes so that the movement stops on target. There is no time for feedback control of such highly skilled movements, therefore they have to be previously planned or learned. The damping function prevents overshooting and pendular movements. This point of reversal of excitation depends on the rate of movement plus previously learned knowledge of the movement. Consequently, voluntary movements, despite their name, are not purely voluntary but are also controlled at a subconscious level. Likewise, ballistic movements need the excitation from the cerebellum to get the speed of

a movement and then inhibition to stop the movement. The lateral zone of the cerebellum is concerned with the overall control of movement of the entire body by having a planning and timing function working with the premotor, sensory and association areas of the cerebral cortex. Planning the sequence of movements is necessary for a smooth and orderly transition of one movement to the next. The lateral zones draw on the cerebellum's predictive ability to recognise the pattern of action, how far different parts of the body will move in a given time and, so, the next movement. A timing function is then needed to predict and control the transition from one movement sequence to the next in a coordinated and accurate manner. This is possible because a two-way traffic between the sensory and premotor areas of the cerebral cortex and the lateral zones of the cerebellum exists. Thus, the deep nuclei of the cerebellum, through the lateral zones, are already involved in the activity pattern of the next movement at the same time as the present movement occurs (Guyton 1991).

In addition, extra motor predictive functions from other senses (auditory and visual) are alerted to environmental factors so providing additional situational detail. Such information is important in interpreting spatiotemporal relationships and recognising the specificity of the movement, i.e. how rapidly the body is approaching an object or an object is approaching the body. This is essential in avoiding collisions.

Overall, the cerebellum serves as an error correcting device for goal directed movements. It receives information on the body's position and movements in progress, then computes and delivers appropriate signals to the brain stem effector centres to correct posture and smooth out movements. The cerebellum is important in the process of learning and acquisition of motor skills.

Task 4.2

Ataxia is a disorder of movement control resulting in slow, uncoordinated motor actions. Some patients with this problem only show these clinical features when their eyes are closed. Can you explain why?

SENSORY FEEDBACK CONTROL OF MOTOR FUNCTION

Once a movement is learned, a sensory engram is established in the sensory cortex and used as a guide for the motor system of the brain to reproduce the same pattern of movement. If the engram and pattern of movement do not match, then the additional motor signals automatically activate appropriate muscles for the correct performance of the task. The sensory engram is projected according to a time sequence and the motor control system automatically follows from one point to the next, so it is not a controlling system but rather a following process. If the motor system fails to follow the pattern, this is fed back to the sensory cortex and corrective signals are transmitted to the appropriate muscles.

The establishment of rapid motor patterns that are too quick for sensory feedback is based on motor engrams. Rapid movements such as typing are initially learned slowly so there is time for sensory feedback to guide a movement through each step. Successive performance of a skilled activity results in an engram for the activity being laid down in the motor control areas as well as the sensory system. The motor engram causes a precise set of muscles to go through a specific sequence of movements to perform a task. The pattern can then be performed without sensory feedback, but the sensory system still determines if the act was performed correctly. In addition, a variety of patterns are stored to allow for the variety of movement necessary in different situations (Guyton 1991).

In summary, the control of movement is a complex process involving more and higher levels of the CNS as the movement becomes more complicated. Learning a new movement can be a slow process and takes time and practice, but once established the learned movement and variations on that theme become more automatic, adapting to the minor alterations necessary for a potentially changing environment. As a totally integrated system, with many direct and indirect feedback circuits, information is constantly being gathered on the status of the body parts for the present and for the future. This is frequently compared with past movement activities to see if a stored posture and movement pattern is already available. An efficient system can then utilise previous experiences with less effort demanded of the CNS, enabling attention to be given to other aspects of a task.

Task 4.3

Here are two final challenges. As before, you should use the information in this chapter plus other sources of information on neurology to work out the answers. If you are able to complete these final two tasks, then you will have a reasonable grasp of the basic relationship between neurological control and human movement. If you find the tasks difficult, it would be advisable to undertake some more reading.

Draw a flow chart that details the hierarchical levels of control of movement in the central nervous system. Add to this the alternative parallel routes connecting the different levels of control. Now consider in turn the result of damage to each of the levels of control. Would normal movement still be possible?

Why do postural attitudes adopted following musculoskeletal injury continue long after the injury is resolved?

REFERENCES

Afifi A K, Bergman R A 1986 Basic neuroscience: a structural and functional approach, 2nd edn. Urban & Schwarzenberg, Baltimore

Edwards S 1996 Neurological physiotherapy. Churchill Livingstone, Edinburgh

Ganong W F 1995 Review of medical physiology, 17th international edn. Appleton & Lange, Connecticut

Ghez C 1991 The cerebellum. In: Kandel E R, Schwartz J H, Jessell T M (eds) Principles of neural science, 3rd edn. Elsevier, New York

Ghez C, Fahn S 1985 The cerebellum. In: Kandel E R, Schwartz J H (eds) Principles of neural science, 2nd edn. Elsevier North Holland, New York

Gilman S 1992 Manter and Gatz's essentials of clinical neuroanatomy and neurophysiology, 8th edn. F A Davis, Philadelphia

Gilman S, Newman S W 1987 Manter and Gatz's essentials of clinical neuroanatomy and neurophysiology, 7th edn. F A Davis, Philadelphia

Gordon J 1990 Disorders of motor control. In: Ada L,

Canning C (eds) Key issues in neurological physiotherapy. Butterworth Heinemann, London

Grillner S, Deliagina T, Ekeberg O 1995 Neural networks that coordinate locomotion and body orientation in lamprey. Trends in Neurosciences 18(6): 270–279

Guyton A C 1991 Basic neuroscience – anatomy and physiology. W B Saunders, Philadelphia

Kidd G, Lawes N, Musa I 1992 Understanding neuromuscular plasticity. Edward Arnold, London

Marieb E N 1998 Human anatomy and physiology. Longman, California

Mathews P B C 1991 The human stretch reflex and the motor cortex. Trends in Neurosciences 14(3): 87–91

Morris M E, Iansek R 1996 Characteristics of motor disturbance in Parkinson's disease and strategies for movement rehabilitation. Human Movement Science 15: 649–669

Palastanga N, Field D, Soames R 1994 Anatomy and human movement, 2nd edn. Butterworth Heinemann, London

Plant R 1998 Theoretical basis of treatment concepts. In: Stokes M 1998 Neurological physiotherapy. Mosby, London

Rothwell J 1994 Control of human voluntary movement. Chapman and Hall, London

Shumway-Cook A, Woollacott M H 1995 Motor control – theory and practical applications. Williams & Wilkins, Baltimore

Tortora G J, Anagnostakos N P 1987 Principles of anatomy and physiology, 6th edn. Harper Collins, New York

CHAPTER CONTENTS

Introduction   85

Range of movement   88

Facilitation and restriction/limitation of
movement   90
Normal facilitation   90
Normal limitation/restriction   90
Abnormal limitation   91

Types of joint movement   93

Passive movements   94
Relaxed passive movements   94
Auto-relaxed passive movements   95
Mechanical relaxed passive movements   96

Stretching   96
Stretching of biological material   96
Therapeutic stretching   99

Accessory movements   100

Manipulation   101

Active movement   102

Conclusion   103

5

Joint mobility

T. Everett

OBJECTIVES

At the end of this chapter you should be able to:

1. **Describe the structure and function of joints**

2. **Discuss ranges of joint movement**

3. **Describe how movement is produced at joints**

4. **Discuss factors that influence normal facilitation and restriction of joint range**

5. **Discuss the causes of abnormal restriction of joint range**

6. **Classify joint movement**

7. **Discuss the rationale of the use of movement to increase joint mobility.**

INTRODUCTION

Biomechanically the body can be considered as composed of segments divided between the axial and appendicular skeleton. There are many models which describe this segmental arrangement; the one that is used in this book divides the body into eight segments. The head and neck, and trunk, make up the two segments of the axial skeleton. The other six segments comprise the appendicular skeleton and are equally divided between the upper and lower limbs; the upper limb consists of arm, forearm, and wrist and hand, whilst the lower limb consists of the thigh, leg, and foot and ankle. All movements, including locomotion, involve the motion of these bony segments, be they in the appendicular or axial skeleton. Junctions between these segments are provided by the joints (juncture, articulations or arthroses) which are themselves classified into three groups: fibrous or fixed (synarthroses), cartilaginous (amphiarthroses) or synovial (diarthroses), the last being the only freely moveable joints (Williams 1995). It is at these joints that the motion actually takes place. Movements of the segments are produced by forces, mainly the internal forces provided by muscles, but also the force of gravity, which is modified by the internal muscle forces acting in opposition. This combination of the bones that form the core of the segments and the muscles that produce the force that provides movement is described as the musculoskeletal system. It is vital that this musculoskeletal system is intact for functional movement to occur. The role of the muscles producing the movement is covered in Chapters 2 and 14 of this text, but the vital components of this system, the synovial joints, will be described below.

The major characteristics of a synovial joint include the surface of opposing bones being in contact, but not in continuity, and covered in hyaline cartilage. These bony ends are joined together via ligaments and the whole joint complex, which may or may not include the ligaments, is surrounded by an extensive synovial lined fibrous joint capsule. The viscous synovial fluid secreted by this synovial membrane not only provides the articular cartilage with nutrition but acts with it to decrease the coefficient of friction within the joint to a level that is low enough to reduce the possibility of joint surface destruction. Intracapsular structures are usually covered by synovium. Intra-articular discs or menisci may be found within the synovial joint helping congruity and acting as shock absorbers. Labra and fat pads may also be found within the joints, having the function of increasing joint surface area (and possibly stability) and shock absorption respectively.

There are a large number of different types of synovial joints, classified according to their shape, for example plane, saddle, hinge, pivot, ball and socket, condylar or ellipsoid (Palastanga et al 1998), but movement at all of these joints can

be considered as either physiological or accessory. A *physiological movement* is the movement that the joint performs under voluntary control of the muscles or is performed passively by an external force but still within the available range of the joint. Maitland (1986) defines *accessory movements* as those movements of the joints that a person cannot perform actively, but that can be performed on that person by an external force. It is an integral part of the physiological movement that cannot be isolated and performed actively by muscular effort.

Although there may seem to be a large number of directions in which joints may move, a system of description has been devised to make the visual analysis of movement more simple. From the anatomical position (standing upright with the upper limbs at the side and palms and head facing forward), movements can be described as occurring in three planes and around three axes. The frontal plane splits the body into front and back halves, the sagittal plane splits the body into right and left halves and the transverse plane splits the body into top and bottom halves.

Movements within these planes take place around three axes. The axes can be described as being perpendicular to the plane of movement. Therefore, there are two horizontal axes and one vertical axis. The sagittal axis is at 90° to the frontal plane and therefore allows movements within that frontal plane. These movements consist of abduction, adduction, deviation and lateral flexion. The frontal axis allows movements of the segments within the sagittal plane and consists of the movements of flexion and extension. Both frontal and sagittal are horizontal axes. The vertical axis is at 90° to the horizontal plane and movements around this axis give rotatory motion.

The actual movements performed can be described in terms of the degrees of freedom the joint allows. A uniaxial joint will possess only one degree of freedom, i.e. rotation about only one axis. An example of this is flexion and extension at the elbow. A biaxial joint has two degrees of freedom, such as the radiocarpal joint which has flexion and extension at the wrist about one axis and ulnar and radial deviation about the other axis. The movement available at a multiaxial joint can be des-

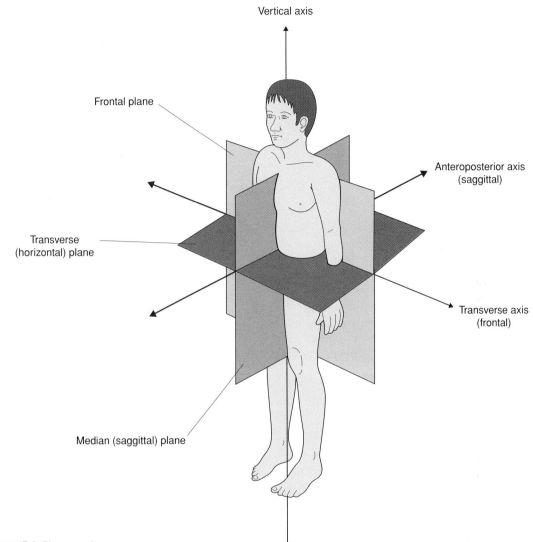

Vertical axis

Frontal plane

Anteroposterior axis
(saggittal)

Transverse
(horizontal) plane

Transverse axis
(frontal)

Median (saggittal) plane

Figure 5.1 Planes and axes.

cribed as having three degrees of freedom. This type of movement can be described at the shoulder where flexion, extension, abduction, adduction and internal and external rotation all take place.

Task 5.1

Movements of the body segments are described in terms of their planes and axes. For each of the major joints of the body describe the planes in which the segments move followed by the axes that they move around.

The above system of movement analysis is only truly applicable if the movement takes place within the anatomical position and does not cross planes and axes. This, however, is not really the case. The shape of most joints is rather complex and they have axes that permit movement in more than one direction. Most movements are also functional in nature and therefore do not take place from the anatomical position. This makes the analysis system rather artificial.

An alternative system for describing movement is the Cartesian coordinate system which

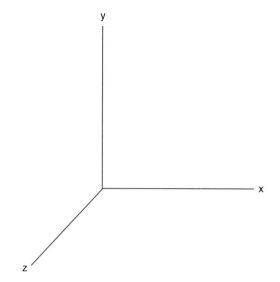

Figure 5.2 The Cartesian coordinate system.

allows any permutation of movement to be described in the three planes. It has, as shown in Figure 5.2, three coordinates in the directions of:

- anteroposterior – the x coordinate
- mediolateral – the z coordinate
- superior-inferior – the y coordinate.

RANGE OF MOVEMENT

With the combination of uniaxial, biaxial and multiaxial joints, the body may adopt a multitude of functional positions. When analysing these positions or movements the components are broken down to each individual joint with the range of movement (ROM) of that joint being described. This movement may not be the maximum movement that the joint is capable of achieving, i.e. its full range of movement (FROM) but only a functional component of it.

Movements of the joints are dependent on many factors and the description of these factors is largely dependent on the discipline by which the movement is being studied. One such discipline is arthrokinematics. This is the intimate mechanics of the joints and is dependent, for its description, largely on the shape of the joint surfaces. Most of the synovial joints are complex in their formation, having more than one axis

within the joint. These joints, being ovoid in different axes of the same joint, have the ability to bring about these different movements. This means that, although joints have roughly reciprocally-shaped surfaces, the maximum congruity of the articular surfaces occurs at specific positions within the range of movement and does not necessarily equate with the end of range of the physiological movement. This position of maximum congruity is called the *close pack* position and is the position of greatest joint stability. At this close pack position not only is there most joint surface contact, but the ligaments are often taut. *Loose pack* position, on the other hand, is where the apposition of the joint surface is the least; muscle, ligaments and capsule are usually lax and the joint is in its least stable position (Hall 1995).

Physiological movements are rarely pure but usually contain different combinations of physiological or accessory movements. These may be a combination of physiological movements, such as side flexion of the cervical spine which, if examined closely, will be seen to involve both side flexion and rotation in combination. By studying the arthrokinematics of the joint it can be shown that there is a combination of accessory type movements occurring in the physiological joint movement. These accessory movements are considered to be of three types: spin, roll and glide. A roll refers to one surface rolling over another as a ball rolling over a surface. An example of roll is seen when the femoral condyle rolls over a fixed tibial plateau during knee extension. Gliding, on the other hand, is a pure translatory movement, one fixed point sliding over the other joint surface. A glide usually takes place in an anteroposterior or mediolateral direction and this type of movement is again seen when the femur slides forward on a fixed tibia at the knee joint. Spin is like a top spinning, a pure rotatory motion. These movements are illustrated in Figure 5.3 below. Accessory movements enable the range of movement to be increased at the joint and also maximise the congruency of the joint surfaces to improve stability (Norkin and Levangie 1992). Descriptions of these movements and their combinations for specific joints can be found in many anatomical texts.

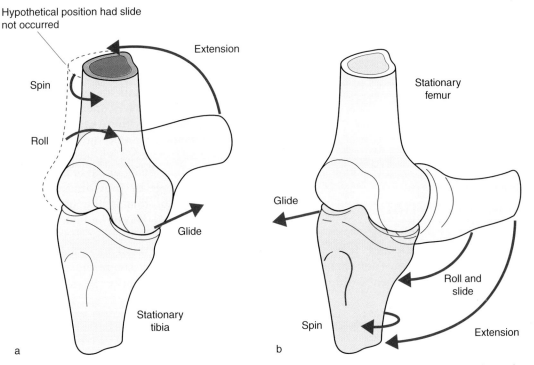

Figure 5.3 Diagrammatic representation of roll, spin and glide at the knee. (a) With stationary tibia (b) with stationary femur.

So it can be seen that movement at joints is not the straightforward unidimensional process that it may at first appear. Movement is caused by a force acting on the bony segment, which in turn produces the movement at the joint. This force may be an internal force, the concentric or eccentric work of the muscle, or an external force, the force of gravity, for example.

When the joint is moved by the force of muscle contraction, either concentrically or eccentrically, the range of joint movement may be described in terms of the excursion of the muscle. This excursion consists of the full range of the muscle, i.e. the inner, middle and outer range, each being roughly a third of the full range of movement. The inner range is where the muscle is at its shortest, middle range is the middle third of the muscle excursion and the outer range is where the muscle is at its longest. This is graphically illustrated in Figure 5.4.

The actual range through which the joint moves, either actively or passively, is measured in degrees of a circle. Range of movement is

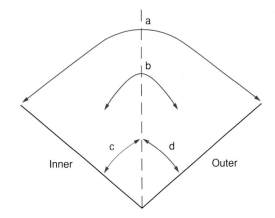

Figure 5.4 Diagrammatic representation of ranges of movement.

usually measured by goniometry. This gives an accepted objective measurement that may be used when analysing joint motion as a part of movement analysis or used as an objective marker when assessing patients. Chapter 8 will give a fuller description of the process of goniometry.

Task 5.2

Work in small groups and choose some simple activities. One person perform the activity whilst the others observe the movement very closely. Try to estimate the range of movement of each joint and identify the muscles that are working to produce the movement. Describe the range of movement of the muscle and the type of muscle contraction throughout the activity.

FACILITATION AND RESTRICTION/LIMITATION OF MOVEMENT

Anatomical, physiological and arthrokinaesiological factors combine to give normal facilitation to, and restriction of, movement within a joint.

Normal facilitation

ROM is facilitated by the following:

- bony shape
- hyaline cartilage
- capsule supporting synovial membrane
- additional structures
- elastic ligaments
- intact neuro- and musculoskeletal system.

The reciprocal convex and concave shapes of the joint surfaces combined with the accessory movements of roll, spin and glide provide a greater surface area over which the two bone ends can move. Hyaline cartilage, present on the articulating surfaces of the bone ends, has the dual function of providing a smooth surface over which the bone ends can glide and affording the joint protection from wear and tear. Both the functions of the hyaline cartilage are enhanced by the presence of synovial fluid within the joint. The fluid layer over the two joint surfaces will reduce the amount of friction between the bone ends when movements occur and act as a form of shock absorber to reduce the trauma of constant impact, particularly in weight bearing joints. Synovial fluid produced by the synovial membrane also provides the joint with some of its nutrition. Most of the capsule surrounding joints

is lax, thus permitting a large range of movement by the joint. Many joints have additional structures within the joint; examples of these are the menisci in the knee or the glenoidal labrum within the shoulder. Both these structures, and others like them, can act as a mechanism for increasing joint surfaces, increasing congruity or affecting stability within the joint. Occasionally, the ligaments surrounding the joints contain yellow elastic fibres in addition to the usual collagen, enabling the ligament to allow the joint an increase in range by providing more flexibility. An example of this is the ligamentum flava which connects adjacent laminae of the spine. It permits separation of these laminae in flexion and ensures that the end range is not reached abruptly. It also assists in returning the spine to the erect position after flexion has occurred (Williams 1995).

Normal limitation/restriction

Normal limitation of range of movement is brought about by:

- articular surface contact
- limit of ligament extensibility
- limit of tendon and muscle extensibility
- apposition of soft tissue.

The two main factors that limit joint mobility are the shape of the joints and the type of structures that run over them. Articular surface contact could mean that the joint is in the close pack position, as in the elbow, where the joint is actually prevented from extending beyond approximately 180° by the olecranon of the ulna impinging onto the humerus. Flexion of the elbow, on the other hand, is limited by the bulk of the biceps brachii pressing against the forearm, this being an example of soft tissue apposition.

Most ligaments and all tendons are primarily composed of white fibrous collagen. One of the properties of collagen is that it is fairly inelastic and stretching achieved by deformation requires strong forces. Therefore, within normal activities, if the ligaments or tendons are at their maximum length, no more movement is possible at that joint. This is illustrated by McMahon et al (1998) who point out that the inferior band of the inferior glenohumeral ligament is the primary restraint to anterior stability post shoulder dislocation. When considering normal movement Branch et al (1995) point out that the anterior and posterior components of the glenohumeral capsuloligamentous complex limit the external and internal rotation of the glenohumeral joint respectively.

It must be remembered, as O'Brien et al (1995) describe, that differing positions of joints enable different structures to limit movement. This point is taken a stage further by Warner et al (1999) who show that glenohumeral compression through muscle contraction provides stability against inferior translation of the humeral head and this effect is more important than intercapsular pressure or ligament tension. This agrees with Wuelker et al (1998) who found that the rotator cuff force significantly contributes to stabilisation of the glenohumeral joint during arm motion.

The structure of muscle, on the other hand, offers the opportunity of more stretch as it crosses the joint and thus affords greater mobility but it still has a limit of extensibility. The limitation that muscle offers to joint mobility is seen particularly when the muscle stretches over two joints, such as the hamstrings stretching over the hip and knee. If the hip is flexed then the amount of knee extension is limited as the muscle is already near its maximum possible length. If the hip is extended then the hamstrings are no longer near the limit of their potential length and will therefore allow for a greater range of knee extension.

It is important that the therapist becomes aware of the normal limitations and can recognise these both by visual analysis and recognising how the joint feels at the end of passive range. This is referred to as the 'end-feel' of the joint and will be different according to the circumstance of the particular joint. For example, the feel of a bony end block, as in the elbow extension, is quite different from that of soft tissue apposition, as in full flexion of the elbow. There is also the 'springy' end-feel of normal tendon, ligamentous and other joint structures. It is only by recognising the normal end-feel of joints that the therapist will become skilled at recognising pathological joint changes.

Task 5.3

Work with a partner and move the major joints of the body passively to their physiological limits. Identify (by end-feel if possible) what is preventing further movement and remember what the end-range feels like. Move to a different partner and perform the same passive movements. See if you can detect any differences and similarities. Discuss your findings with your colleagues.

Abnormal limitation

Although both normal facilitation and limitation are important factors to consider when discussing joint range, joint range becomes an issue when there is an abnormal limitation in that range. Abnormal limitation of joint range is usually brought about by either injury or disease to its structure, surface or surrounding soft tissue, i.e. the muscles producing the movement or their functioning.

The above factors can be summarised as:

- destruction of bone and cartilage
- bone fracture
- foreign body in joint
- tearing or displacement of intracapsular structures
- adhesions/scar tissue
- muscle atrophy or hypertrophy
- muscle tear, rupture or denervation
- pain
- psychological factors
- oedema
- neurological impairment

Destruction of bone and cartilage. Any disease that destroys the articular cartilage, such as osteoarthritis or rheumatoid arthritis, will impair the functioning of the joint and thus the movement will be limited. This may be for two reasons. Either the destroyed surface will physically prevent the movement, or the pain produced when the two exposed surfaces grind together may produce a reduction in range or a deterioration in the quality of the movement. Either singly or together these may actually prevent movement altogether.

Fracture. A fracture near to or within the joint will also prevent movement via mechanical obstruction or pain. The same applies to a foreign body within the joint complex.

Tearing or displacement of intracapsular structures. Field et al (1997) demonstrate that recurrent anterior unidirectional shoulder instability is most commonly associated with an avulsion of the glenoidal attachment of the labroligamentous complex (Bankart lesion). This would limit the range of movement available.

Soft tissue lesions. If there has been an injury to the soft tissue surrounding or within the joint, then repair to that tissue usually takes place by the formation of fibrous or scar tissue which does not have the same extensibility as the tissue it is replacing. Fibrous adhesions may also form and these would bind structures together and hence movement would be restricted.

Injury or immobilisation. If immobilisation of soft tissue occurs there are biomechanical, biochemical and physiological changes that occur within 1 week. These changes are magnified in the presence of trauma or oedema (Cyr and Ross 1998). These structural changes are a result of stress deprivation causing structural changes in the matrix of the tissue due to the remodelling of tissue to its new resting length while being held immobile (Hardy and Woodall 1998). The net result of this will be a decrease in the range of movement. If muscle tissue is held in a shortened position there appears to be absorption of the sarcomeres, causing a change in length. This shortening in length is termed adaptive shortening and will limit joint movement.

Muscular changes and pathology. The joint itself may be intact, but if the muscles that produce the movement have a dysfunction then the net result is a decrease in ROM. If the muscle is atrophied to a large degree then it would not create sufficient force to move the joint through its full range. Conversely, if there was a large amount of muscle hypertrophy, ROM would also be decreased due to the increased amount of soft tissue apposition.

Neurological impairment. The muscle itself may be intact, but its neural control may be impaired. This could range from total denervation, causing flaccidity of the muscle, to lack of higher centre control, which may cause spasticity. Local spinal reflexes may also have the effect of limiting movement by causing the muscle to be in spasm.

Pain. The body's response to pain is usually to keep the part still and avoid movement. This may be only short term, but if the pain becomes chronic then adaptive shortening may occur. The pain may disappear, but the pattern that the brain has adopted due to the memory of pain that occurred on movement may continue. Other psychological problems such as depression, lack of motivation or self-confidence may also be responsible for the subject not moving. This may also be transient and cause no physical limitation of movement, but if the condition persists then adaptive shortening may occur.

Hypermobility. It is important to remember that what has so far been discussed describes a decrease in movement (hypomobility), but the opposite may also occur. This is termed hypermobility where the range of movement exceeds that of the expected physiological range. This could be due to pathological change either at the joint, or elsewhere within the musculoskeletal or neuromuscular systems. It may, however, be a natural phenomenon caused mainly by laxity of ligaments or a congenital joint deformity, but it can also result from a deliberate attempt by stretching to increase the joint range well beyond that which is functionally acceptable, as in a gymnast or ballet dancer for example. As Lewit (1993) states, this may be an advantage to these sportspeople but with increased mobility there may be a decrease in stability with the disadvantage of possible problems in the future. There is also the possibility of subluxation of the joint occurring during movement, which could result in neurological damage. If the joint is hypermobile there is also the possibility that the joint will articulate on bone that is not designed for this function and therefore there is a great risk of increasing the possibility of degenerative changes occurring at the joint surfaces.

Task 5.4

In groups, look at the major joints of the body and assess visually the differences in the range of movement between each person. Can you discover what is limiting the movement for each joint? Can you find anyone with hypermobility? Are there any differences between males and females in ROM or hypermobility?

Treatment

Before treatment can be given for any decrease in the range of movement it is obvious from the above that the cause of the decrease will have to be known. It has been shown that the cause may be in the joint structure (surface or intracapsular), the structures surrounding or running over the joint (ligaments or tendons), or the neuromuscular system that produces the movements. So, to establish the pathological changes that have occurred, it is vital that the therapist performs a full and detailed assessment. Once the pathology is known, the therapist can choose a method of treatment whose physiological effects alter the pathological changes that have occurred to limit joint movement.

Once the assessment has been made it is important to know the physiological effects of the possible treatment options and match them with the effects they will have on the pathological changes. This is the rationale of the treatment.

Limitation of movement, from whatever cause, impairs function of the joint and the muscles producing the movement. Measures that increase the range of movement must also include methods that strengthen the muscles in their new, lengthened position. The degree of ROM gained must be able to be controlled, and the stability of the joint maintained, or further injury may result.

It is important that the details of the anatomy and arthrokinaesiology are understood as well as the pathology of the joint, as these have an effect on the rationale of the treatment choice when there is a pathological reduction on joint range.

Many studies have looked at actual joint ranges of physiological ROM and presented tables of values (Norkin and White 1995). It is accepted, however, that each ROM is specific to each individual and discrepancies may even exist when comparing both sides of an individual. Two of the factors that have an effect on the ROM obtained are age and gender. Younger children appear to have a greater amount of hip flexion, abduction and lateral rotation, and a greater amount of ankle dorsiflexion, than an adult. Elbow movements are also shown to be greater than those of an adult, whilst there is found to be less hip extension, knee extension and ankle plantarflexion. Older age groups seem to have a generalised appendicular and axial joint decrease. Gender appears to have different effects on different joints depending on what movement that joint is performing (Norkin and White 1995).

There are many physiotherapy modalities to increase the ROM. The most obvious is the use of movement itself. The main classifications of the therapeutic movements are described below.

TYPES OF JOINT MOVEMENT

Movement is one of the main methods that therapists use to increase joint range. The therapist will use the different ways in which the joint moves as a basis for these different methods. There are two main types of movement:

- passive movement
- active movement.

Passive movement is defined as those movements produced entirely by an external force, i.e. no voluntary muscle work. These can be subdivided into:

- relaxed passive movements
- stretching
- accessory movements
- manipulations.

Active movements are those movements within the unrestricted range of a joint produced by an active contraction of the muscles crossing the joint. These can be subdivided into:

- active assisted exercise
- free active exercise.

PASSIVE MOVEMENTS

Relaxed passive movements

These are movements that are performed within the unrestricted range by an external force and involve no muscle work of the particular joint, or joints, at which the movement takes place.

These movements can be performed in three ways:

- *Manual relaxed passive movements* are movements that are performed by another person, usually the physiotherapist, within the unrestricted range.
- *Auto-relaxed passive movements* are performed within the unrestricted range by the person herself, i.e. with her unaffected limbs.
- *Mechanical relaxed passive movements* are performed by a machine but still occur within the unrestricted range.

Relaxed passive movement has been a core skill of the physiotherapist for many years and is still widely used today. As with many of the traditional skills, little evidence of its clinical effectiveness has been published (Basmajian and Wolf 1990) but the following is the accepted rationale for its use.

Indications

These movements are indicated when the patient is unable to perform an active full range movement. The reason for this inability may include: unconsciousness, weak or denervated muscle, spinal injury, pain, neurological disease or enforced rest.

Effects

- maintain ROM
- prevent contractures
- maintain integrity of soft tissue and muscle elasticity
- increase venous circulation
- increase synovial fluid production and therefore joint cartilage nutrition
- increase kinaesthetic awareness
- maintain functional movement patterns
- reduce pain.

Maintaining ROM and preventing contractures. If muscle is not moved through its full range then it will adapt to the demands being placed upon it. The actin and myosin protein filaments (the contractile element) will be reabsorbed and thus the area for cross bridge formation will be decreased. This will cause muscle weakness and the inability to perform the movement. The muscles will adopt the new position and will be shortened, i.e. they will have adaptive shortening. The non-contractile elements within the muscle, the connective tissue, will add to this effect by increasing the collagen turnover rate, which is the balance of collagen production and destruction (Basmajian and Wolf 1990). If more collagen is produced, it increases the stiffness of the muscle and decreases its propensity to stretch. If no movement takes place then the muscle will adapt to the new position and thus contractures will occur.

Other soft tissues, such as ligaments and tendons, will also be similarly affected. As they have a greater proportion of collagen, the increase and change in consistency will also lead to stiffness and eventually to contractures.

Maintaining integrity of soft tissue and muscle elasticity. By placing stresses on these tissues the collagen turnover rate is normalised and the elasticity of the tissues is maintained. As Cyr and Ross (1998) conclude, early controlled motion is vital to prevent the negative effects of immobilisation and maintain normal viscoelasticity and homeostasis of connective tissue. Passive movements will not, however, increase the strength of the muscle as this requires the greater physiological demand of active and resisted work.

Increase venous circulation. If a limb, particularly the lower limb, is not moved, venous congestion may occur. This is because the muscle pump does not work to aid venous return. Pooling occurs and is increased through dilation of the vessels caused by the physical pressure of the blood on the veins and the possible lack of sympathetic tone. This decrease in flow can lead to an increased risk of deep vein thrombosis. Passive movements will act as a prophylaxis to prevent stagnation. This is achieved by physically compressing the veins and one way flow is achieved via the valves within the veins themselves. Lymph is also encouraged to move. Compression of the tissues increases the hydrostatic pressure and thus encourages tissue perfusion and fluid reabsorption. This may be useful in reducing oedema.

Joint cartilage nutrition. If the synovial fluid is swept over the articular cartilage it will provide nutrition and help prevent the deterioration of the surface. Production and absorption of the synovial fluid by the synovial membrane is stimulated by movement of the joint. This is quite an important effect and is lost if the joint is immobile for any length of time. If the immobility is due to injury then movement is of greater importance as one of the consequences of injury is inflammation and repair by fibrosis, which in itself will increase the risk of adhesions forming within the joint. Thus, with passive movement, this risk will be decreased.

Kinaesthetic awareness. To perform coordinated, energy efficient and safe movement it is important for the central nervous system to receive information about the position and movement of the joints and soft tissue. This information is supplied by sensory nerve endings in the many structures in and surrounding the joints. This is kinaesthetic awareness and it may be lost if there is a long period of immobilisation. The kinaesthetic pathways may be maintained when performing passive movements by stimulating the nerve endings within the joint complex.

Maintain functional patterns. The brain is said to recognise gross movement patterns, so if these patterns are not able to occur then there is the possibility of the memory of the pattern being lost. Passive movement in these patterns will decrease this risk.

Reduce pain. Rhythmical movements are said to reduce pain by causing a relaxation effect within the muscles (Gardiner 1981). This may partly be achieved by removing waste products and chemical irritants from the area through increased circulation. Stimulation of the joint mechanoreceptors may also subserve the sensations from the pain nerve ending and thus decrease their effect (see accessory movements, p. 100, for further explanation).

Contraindications

- Immediately post injury as this may increase the inflammatory process.
- Early fractures where movement may cause disruption of the fracture site.
- Where pain may be beyond the patients' tolerance.
- Muscle or ligament incomplete tears where further damage may occur.
- Where the circulation may be compromised.

Principles of application

Passive movements may either be performed in the anatomical planes or in functional patterns. The choice and type of movement will depend on the findings of the assessment and the aims of the treatment. The same basic principles of application need to be considered whichever movement is chosen. These include:

- The segment should be comfortable, supported and localised to the specific joints.
- The patient should be comfortable, warm and supported.
- Hand holds should support the segment and protect the joint.
- The motion should be smooth and rhythmical.
- Speed and duration should be appropriate for the desired effects.
- Range should be the maximum available without stretching or causing pain.
- Segments should be positioned so that muscles that stretch over two or more joints are not restricting joint range (after Hollis 1989).

Auto-relaxed passive movements

Although the rationale is the same, the method of application must be modified. Patients who have to perform their own passive movements are usually those with a long-term problem. People with spinal injuries, for example, must retain their joint range and muscle length if they are to perform the functions necessary for daily living (Bromley 1998).

Mechanical relaxed passive movements

Unlike manual or auto-passive movements which, by their nature, have to be carried out intermittently, mechanical passive movements may be carried out continuously. Mechanical devices for producing continuous passive movement (CPM) were first used by Salter in 1970 (McCarthy et al 1993). Although their designs and protocols of use may differ, they all have essentially the same function.

The rationale is the same as for any relaxed passive movement but the benefits of continuous movement are particularly evident following surgery (Kisner and Colby 1990). Basso and Knapp (1987) found that CPM decreased joint effusions and wound oedema whilst increasing range of movement and decreasing pain in post-operative knee patients.

STRETCHING

Stretching differs from relaxed passive movement in that it takes the movement beyond the available range. This available range may be limited due to disease or injury. Stretching may also take the joint beyond the normal physiological range. Whereas relaxed passive movements are designed to maintain length of soft tissue and hence joint range, stretching should result in a change in length of the soft tissue structures crossing over the joint, with the consequent increase in joint range. Passive stretching is not the only method of increasing joint range via the soft tissues. This can also be attained via active stretching which will be discussed later (p. 103).

Stretching of biological material

Most biological materials are viscoelastic. This means that they exhibit both viscous and elastic properties. Viscosity is the property of a fluid that is a measure of the resistance to flow. Elasticity is the property of a solid. Therefore, viscoelastic materials posses both solid and liquid properties, which means that stress is not the only function of strain. There is also a strain rate. This differs from most of the purely elastic materials discussed in Chapter 3 where there was no time dependency, i.e., how quickly the stress was applied to the material. This time dependency is described in the equation below:

$$E = de/dt$$

where E is the strain rate and t is the time.

As was discussed in Chapter 3, a useful way of describing the relationship between stress and strain is to plot a graph of the stress versus strain and discuss the resulting curves.

Loading and unloading paths

For elastic materials strain energy is stored within the substance as potential energy. When the load is released it is this energy that returns the material to its original stress. This is represented graphically in Figure 5.5.

For viscoelastic materials some of the strain energy is stored as potential and some is dissipated as heat. Therefore, once the applied load is removed there is not enough stored energy to regain the normal configuration. This is shown in Figure 5.6.

Within the enclosed area shown in the graph is the hysteresis loop which represents the energy dissipated as heat when the material is stretched and the stress released, allowing a return to the non-stressed condition. Therefore continual loading and unloading will produce heat. The

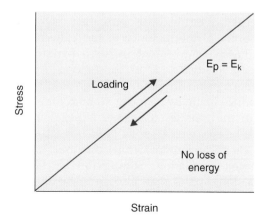

Figure 5.5 Loading and unloading paths (where *Ek = Ep*).

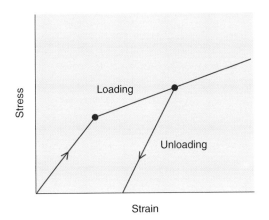

Figure 5.6 Elastic materials exhibiting hysteresis.

amount of hysteresis (heat produced) is dependent on the strain rate. This loss of energy does not allow the material to return to its original state, hence permanent deformation has taken place.

When considering biological tissues it is important to know the micro and macro structure of the tissue concerned. Not many biological tissues are pure, as most are a composite of materials. This may mean that they have fibres in an aqueous matrix (which therefore makes them viscoelastic) or that they have a combination of different fibres or both. Orientation of the composite fibres is also of importance. If the fibres are arranged in parallel and the stress is applied in the direction of the fibres then the material will be strong and possibly

stiff (a measure of the resistance to stress). If there is irregular orientation of the fibres then there will be less strength, but what strength there is will be multidirectional.

The stress/strain curve for a 'general' biological tissue can be seen in Figure 5.7. Although not presenting the graph of any particular tissue, it shows the characteristics that are common to most biological tissues.

The *toe region* of the graph represents the straightening of the wavy collagen (see p. 98). It represents no change in the structure of the tissue under stress. The *elastic range* is the area under the graph that obeys Hooke's Law in that the tissue will return to its original length once the tension is released. The *elastic limit* is that point beyond which the tissue does not return to its original length when the stress is removed. *Plastic range* refers to that area in which the tissue will undergo permanent deformation and will not return to its original position. The strength of the tissue at this point is referred to as its *yield strength*, whereas the *ultimate strength* is the greatest load the tissue can sustain before strain occurs without further stress. There is a point, which is usually greater than the ultimate strength, where *necking* occurs. Necking is where considerable weakening occurs and strain continues to increase even if the stress or loading is greatly reduced or even removed. At the point of *failure* of the tissue it has reached its *breaking strength*, i.e. the load at the time the tissue fails and rupture occurs.

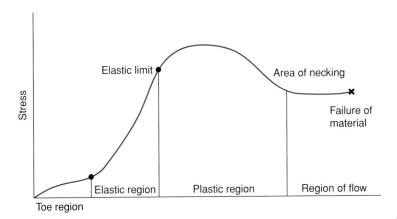

Figure 5.7 Typical stress/strain curve for biological material.

Another property of tissue that is important when considering stretching is its *stiffness* which is a measure of the resistance offered by the tissue to deformation. The stiffness of a tissue is often rate and speed dependent. The *ductility* of the tissue is its capacity to absorb plastic deformation before failure occurs. If the tissue has an increase in strain with a constant stress then this increase in length is referred to as *creep*. This phenomenon is often used in serial splinting where the tissue is held in a cast under constant load and over time the tissue undergoes further lengthening. The *resilience* of material is its ability to recover quickly from its deformation whereas *damping* refers to the slow return to shape (Soderberg 1997).

Bone

Bone is non-homogenous, thus it will vary in its response to stress. It is a composite of compact and cancellous bone and during loading compact bone is seen to be stiff, with a high ultimate strength and a large modulus of elasticity (see Ch. 3, on deformation of materials). It can resist rapidly applied loads better than loads that are applied slowly. Cancellous bone, on the other hand, is more compliant, hence it has greater shock absorbing capacity. These properties are shown in Figure 5.8, where the different amounts of stress that are needed to produce the same amount of strain and ultimate failure are shown for loads in the longitudinal and transverse directions. The graphs of fast and slow loading also illustrate the time dependent response of the bone to stress (Fig. 5.8).

Soft tissue

Most soft tissue found in the musculoskeletal system is a composite material of mainly collagen, elastin and the aqueous ground substance. The collagen is composed of crimped fibrils which are aggregated into fibres, and its prime function is to withstand axial tension.

On stretching the crimps straighten out, and the collagen then stores the potential energy that returns the fibril to the original position. As the

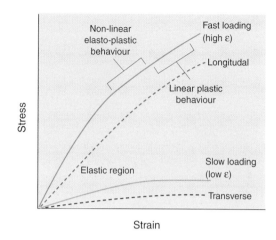

Figure 5.8 Strain rate dependent stress/strain curves for cortical bone under longitudinal stress (continuous line) and direction dependent stress (dotted line).

collagen is surrounded by fluid (gel like ground substance), it also possesses fluid properties of creep and hysteresis.

Elastin is highly elastic even at high stress strains, i.e. it possesses a low modulus of elasticity, whereas that for collagen is high. The importance of these properties is illustrated in Figure 5.9 which shows the stress/strain curves for the ligamentum flava (70% elastin) and the anterior cruciate ligament (90% collagen).

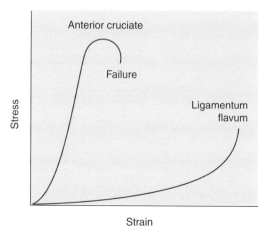

Figure 5.9 Stress/strain curves for anterior cruciate ligament and ligamentum flavum.

Tendons. Fibrous connective tissue is mainly composed of collagen and ground substance, functioning primarily as a passive transmitter of the force produced by muscle contraction. Compared to muscle the tendon is stiffer, has higher tensile strength and can endure larger stresses. The tendon can support a large stress with only a small strain and thus makes muscle contraction more efficient as not much of the muscle action is wasted on movement of the tendon. This facilitates greater apposition of the bones. The properties of a tendon are dependent on the type and proportion of its fibres, as shown in Figure 5.10. The resultant strain of a tendon is also time dependent and the tissue exhibits a hysteresis loop showing that deformation of the tendon will be permanent. This can be seen from Figure 5.11. Tendons have a low shear modulus therefore they can act as pulleys to redirect high forces.

Ligaments. Most ligaments contain a greater proportion of elastin than tendons, therefore there is higher flexibility and lower strength and stiffness than tendons. Sometimes, however, ligaments have greater strength if resistance is applied quickly.

Muscle. Muscles vary in their reaction to stress, depending on which muscle is being studied and the age of that muscle (see Ch. 15). The structure of the muscle with its attendant tendon also has a role in the strain that occurs when stress is applied to the muscle-tendon-bone complex (Soderberg 1997).

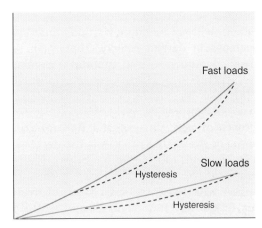

Figure 5.11 Stress/strain curve showing rate dependency and hysteresis for the tendon.

Muscle, however, is an active tissue and the force produced within the muscle is due to its contraction. *Active tension* is developed in the muscle as a result of cross bridge formation and *passive tension* is developed as a result of the stress placed upon the connective tissue elements of the muscle when it is stretched past its resting length. Active tension is decreased, however, as the cross bridges are pulled apart. Therefore as muscle lengthens, passive tension increases.

Cartilage. Cartilage has a high fluid content, therefore it has greater viscoelastic properties and becomes very variable in its properties.

Therapeutic stretching

Therapeutic stretching of soft tissue is a passive movement and is an important physiotherapeutic skill that can be carried out for a variety of reasons. The usual indications for performing stretching are to regain range of movement or to facilitate an increase in the available range of movement.

Changes in collagen that affect the stress/strain response

Immobilisation. During immobilisation there will be a decrease in the collagen turnover rate with a consequent weak bonding between the new, non-stressed, fibres. There will also be adhesion formation, with the consequent greater cross

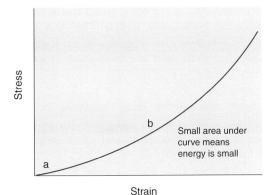

Figure 5.10 Stress/strain curve for a typical tendon. (a) Low strain (elastic fibres dominate and crimping straightens), (b) stiffer (viscoelastic matrix takes over).

linking between disorganised fibres, and ground substance will not retain its viscous properties.

Decrease in normal activity. There will be a decrease in the size and amount of collagen fibres, leading to weakened tissues and possibly an increase in elastin with the consequent increase in compliance.

Effects of age. One of the natural consequences of the ageing process is the decrease in tensile strength and elastic modulus of all soft tissues. This may lead to a decrease in the rate of adaption with the increased chance of overuse injury, fatigue and trauma (Cribb and Scott 1995).

Effects of drugs. Corticosteroids cause a long-term decrease in tensile strength.

All the above effects must be taken into consideration when stretching is performed.

As has been described, stretching of collagen, therefore, is due mainly to plastic deformation as the material is fairly inelastic. Connective tissue will reorganise itself in response to a sustained stretch provided the stress is not too great or applied for too long (Basmajian and Wolf 1990). Therefore, any stretch that does occur will be fairly permanent. It can be seen, then, that care must be taken not to reach the necking phase as this would compromise the integrity of the tissue and could thus lead to a diminishing of the function of the tissue being stretched. This could lead to a decrease in stability and a greater risk of further injury to the joint.

To summarise, the effects of stretching:

- increase joint ROM
- increase soft tissue length
- relieve muscle spasm
- increase tissue compliance in preparation for an athletic event (Vujnovich and Dawson 1994).

Performing a stretch

Passive stretching can, like passive movements, be performed as manual, auto- or mechanical stretching.

In manual (or auto) stretching the therapist (or patient) produces the sustained stretch at the end of range with the patient relaxed. It is generally accepted that the stretch should be held for at least 15 seconds and repeated several times. When stretching a muscle tendon complex it is important that the muscle has an opportunity for the sarcomeres to 'give' before the tendon can be stretched. Sarcomere give occurs when the force applied to the muscle is sufficient to separate the actin and myosin filaments so that the non-elastic components of the complex can be stretched.

Mechanical stretching involves a low stress being applied by a machine over a prolonged period.

The above text refers to *static stretching*, which is defined as a slow sustained stretch at the end of range. This should be held, as stated, for up to 15 seconds, but it is possible that a patient will be unable to tolerate a stretch held for this long and therefore the duration may have to be built up from a few seconds. This type of passive stretching is in contrast to *ballistic stretching*, which is defined as small end of range bounces. Despite having been used for many years the ballistic method of stretching has been shown to increase the risk of injury and should not be performed (Vujnovich and Dawson 1994).

ACCESSORY MOVEMENTS

As described earlier, Maitland (1986) defines accessory movements as those movements of the joints which a person cannot perform actively, but that can be performed on that person by an external force. Although these movements form an integral part of the normal physiological movement, and occur throughout the ROM, they cannot be physically isolated by the patient himself. However, if the accessory movement was being performed by the physiotherapist, the patient would be able to stop the movement from taking place.

These movements take the form of glides (medially, laterally, longitudinally), compressions, distractions or rotations.

Anatomists group accessory movements into two categories: type one are those that cannot be performed unless resistance is provided to the active movement; and type two are the movements that can be produced only when the subject's muscles are relaxed (Williams 1995).

The latter are the type that are used for therapeutic purposes. Accessory movements are used to increase the range of movements at joints and also to decrease any pain that is present. The mechanism for decreasing pain depends, of course, on the cause of that pain. If the pain is caused by the decrease in ROM then the rationale of treatment will be the same as that for increasing the range. If not, then the usual effect of small amplitude movements, applied rhythmically to the joints, is to have an inhibitory effect on the afferent impulse traffic from articular receptors, blocking the pain (Grieve 1988).

Twomey (1992) suggests that articular cartilage facilitates the ROM of joints. If there is joint immobility the articular cartilage will degenerate more quickly, as it requires movement and loading to ensure adequate nutrition. This nutrition is facilitated by the synovial fluid which is swept over the joint surface. As the stimulation of the synovial membrane decreases, the amount of synovial fluid produced is decreased, becoming thicker with decreased osmolarity. Accessory movements assist in the maintenance of synovial production and, by the small oscillatory movements they make, produce the washing effect of the synovial fluid over the joint surfaces.

Twomey (1992) also suggests that movement is important for the nutrition of all collagenous tissue as well as the prevention of adaptive shortening. Small amplitude movements at the end of range will elongate connective tissue, ligaments, joint capsule and other periarticular fascia via the processes described in the section dealing with stretching (p. 96). End-range movements will also break down any intra-articular adhesions that have been formed (Grieve 1988).

If joint stiffness is caused by fibrocartilaginous blocks and subsequent connective tissue shortening, Threlkeld (1992) claims that the relative positions of the joint surfaces can be altered to restore normal accessory movement and restore displaced material.

MANIPULATION

Joint manipulations differ from all other types of therapeutic movement because the patient has no control over the procedure. These movements are potentially dangerous and should therefore only be performed by skilled professionals with much experience in the mobilisation of joints. Manipulations are small amplitude forceful movements that take the joint past the available physiological range. As Maitland (1986) states, manipulations are performed very quickly before the subject has time to prevent the movement from taking place. Lewit (1993) describes manipulation as a technique for treating end-range blocking of joints. Displaced intra-articular material may be one reason for the restriction of movement. Joint misalignment may be another. This blocking, or restriction of movement, he claims, has two effects: one is the restriction of the subject's functional movement; the other is the effect on the accessory movement or joint play. Restrictions caused by meniscal or other material within the joint are termed loose bodies.

Lack of movement of a joint may lead to adaptive shortening of the soft tissue structures surrounding it; capsule, ligaments, tendons or muscles, for example. This secondary consequence will in itself cause a restriction of movement and possibly pain when movement is attempted. Thus, a vicious circle is set up. The initial immobility may be as a consequence of pain. If the pain is caused by trauma to the joint, then the problem may be compounded by the presence of adhesions within and around the joint that are the natural consequence of the inflammatory process.

Shortened soft tissue structures may also be manipulated to physically break the structures.

Effects

The primary effect of manipulating the joint is to restore its mobility. A secondary effect may be to decrease pain, if the pain was a direct result of abnormal tension on structures due to incorrect functioning of the joint.

These effects are brought about in a variety of ways. As the joint is manipulated the surfaces are caused to gap, creating space. The movement of the surfaces, together with the greater space created, possibly causes any physical obstruction between the joint surfaces to be moved clear. Joint surfaces may then be realigned, causing the correct afferent information to be sent to the spinal cord. Fibrous adhesions, caused as the result of the inflammatory exudate, the organisation of the synovial fluid or the adaptive shortening of any soft tissue structure, will be physically torn. This takes the structure through the plastic phase and very rapidly past the breaking point. The hopeful consequence of this procedure is to free the joint to perform its full functional excursion.

Contraindications for the above technique are the same as those for relaxed passive movements.

ACTIVE MOVEMENT

Active movement can be thought of as movements of the joint within the unrestricted range that are produced by the muscles that pass over that joint. The movements may be active assisted or free active. Therapeutically, these movements are performed as exercise.

Active assisted exercise is exercise carried out when the prime movers of that joint are not strong enough to perform the full ROM of the joint. The forces that need to be overcome are friction, gravity and the effects of the mechanical disadvantage of lever length. Assistance may be given by any external force but it is important that the external force provides assistance only, and that the movement is simply augmented and does not become a passive movement. The external force has to be applied in the direction of the muscular action but not necessarily at the same point. External assistance may be:

- manual assistance
- mechanical assistance
- auto-assistance.

Manual assisted exercise is the assistance to the subject's muscular effort by the therapist. The therapist is able to change the assistance as the muscles progress through their ROM, compensating for such factors as angle of pull and length tension relationships. The amount of assistance may also be changed as the muscle strength increases.

Mechanical assistance may be provided by a variety of apparatus. Isokinetic equipment has

the facility for active assisted movement provided the trigger forces are set low enough. The most useful mechanical assistance is that of sling suspension, where the assistance is given in two ways. Firstly, the resisting force of friction is reduced by physically lifting the segment clear of its resting surface, which also helps to counteract the force of gravity by supporting the segment. Secondly, depending on the point of fixation of the sling suspension, gravity may be used to assist the movement, provided the desired movement occurs on the downward arc of the curve produced by the segment within the sling suspension.

Auto-assisted exercise may be performed by the subject herself using the same principles as those of manual assistance. More common, however, is for the assistance to be a combined form of auto- and mechanical assistance. This is seen in the use of bicycle pedals for lower limb mobility or pulleys for upper limb mobility.

Free active exercise differs from assisted exercise in that the movement is carried out by the subject herself, with no assistance or resistance to the movement, except that of the force of gravity. There are many ways that free active movements can be performed. These include:

- Rhythmical: this uses momentum to help perform the movement taking place in one plane but in opposite directions.
- Pendular: these are movements performed in an arc and are useful for improving mobility as, on the down curve of the arc, the movement is assisted by gravity.
- Single or patterned: depending on the aims of the intended movement, the choice of single or patterned movements is made. As a general rule, single movements are used to demonstrate or restore actions, whereas patterned movements are used for functional activities. The use of biceps brachii to flex the elbow as a pure movement is an example of a single movement. Reaching out to pick up an object (food) and taking it to the mouth also involves flexion of the elbow but this movement also contains other joint movements in a functional pattern (the feeding pattern).

These movements may also be classed as to their effect:

- Localised: designed to produce a local or specific effect; mobilising a particular joint or strengthening a particular muscle.
- General: gives a widespread effect over many joints or muscles; running, for example (Gardiner 1981).

Exercise affects all the systems of the body and is covered elsewhere in this and many other textbooks. What must be remembered, however, is that the effects produced cannot be isolated to one particular system or even one effect within that system. Exercise, for example, will maintain muscle length and joint range but it may also alter the strength (aerobic and anaerobic capacity) of that muscle and have a more widespread effect on the cardiovascular system.

One of the major local effects of exercise is the increased rate of protein synthesis, thus producing more actin and myosin as a response and facilitating an increase in muscle length. Connective tissue also responds to increased exercise by becoming stronger in order to cope with the increase in function that is required of that muscle (Basmajian and Wolf 1990).

If active exercise is performed regularly and through the available physiological range, it has all the effects of passive exercise that were previously explained, including maintaining joint range, increasing joint nutrition and decreasing pain. Active movement has the advantage of strengthening muscles to some extent, thus providing stability for the joint with its increased range. Another advantage of performing active movements is that, if they are performed in a rhythmical manner, they may promote relaxation of the muscles surrounding the joint. If this happens then the joint range may well be increased, especially if the restriction was due to muscle spasm.

CONCLUSION

Movement occurring at joints depends upon a variety of anatomical and biomechanical factors which can facilitate and/or limit the range of movement available. How movements are classified and described will depend on which discipline is being studied. For this text, movements are classified as either active or passive, with subdivisions of each. Restriction of movement, caused by pathological changes, can be successfully managed by the therapist using different forms of movement. This is achieved once the rationale of the chosen method is known and correctly applied to the fully assessed patient.

The preceding descriptions by no means represent an exhaustive survey into the therapeutic modalities to improve joint range and muscle length. They are, however, representative of the basic principles of the techniques that are used based on normal joint movement.

REFERENCES

Basmajian J, Wolf S 1990 Therapeutic exercise, 5th edn. Williams and Wilkins, Baltimore

Basso D, Knapp L 1987 Comparison of two continuous passive motion protocols for patients with total knee implants. Physical Therapy 67: 360–363

Branch T P, Lawton R L, Iobst C A, Hutton W C 1995 The role of glenohumeral capsular ligaments in internal and external rotation of the humerus. American Journal of Sports Medicine 23(5): 632–637

Bromley I 1998 Tetraplegia and paraplegia; a guide for physiotherapists, 5th edn. Churchill Livingstone, Edinburgh

Cribb A M, Scott J E 1995 Tendon response to tensile stress: an ultrastructural investigation of collagen: proteoglycan interactions in stressed tendon. Journal of Anatomy 187 (part 2): 423–428

Cyr L M, Ross R G 1998 How controlled stress affects healing tissues. Journal of Hand Therapy 11(2): 125–130

Field L D, Bokor D J, Savoie F H 1997 Humeral and glenoid detachment of the anterior inferior glenohumeral ligament: a cause of anterior shoulder instability. Journal of Shoulder and Elbow Surgery 6(1): 6–10

Gardiner M D 1981 The principles of exercise therapy, 4th edn. Bell and Hyman, London

Grieve G 1988 Contraindications to spinal manipulations and allied treatment. Physiotherapy 75(8): 445–453

Hall S 1995 Basic biomechanics, 2nd edn. Mosby, St. Louis

Hardy M, Woodall W 1998 Therapeutic effects of heat, cold and stretch on connective tissue. Journal of Hand Therapy 11(2): 148–156

Hollis M 1989 Practical exercise therapy, 3rd edn. Blackwell Science, Oxford

Kisner C, Colby L 1990 Therapeutic exercise, foundations and techniques, 2nd edn. F A Davies, Philadelphia

Lewit K 1993 Manipulative therapy in rehabilitation of the locomotor system, 2nd edn. Butterworth-Heinemann, Oxford

McCarthy M, Yates C, Anderson M, Yates-McCarthy J 1993 The effects of immediate continuous passive movement on pain during the inflammatory phase of soft tissue healing following anterior cruciate ligament reconstruction. Journal of Sport and Physical Therapy 17(2): 96–101

McMahon P J, Tibone J E, Cawley P W et al 1998 The anterior band of the inferior glenohumeral ligament: biomechanical properties from tensile testing in the position of apprehension. Journal of Shoulder and Elbow Surgery 7(5): 467–471

Maitland G 1986 Vertebral manipulation, 5th edn. Butterworths, London

Norkin C, Levangie P 1992 Joint structure and function: a comprehensive analysis, 2nd edn. F A Davies, Philadelphia

Norkin C, White J 1995 Measurement of joint motion: a guide to goniometry, 2nd edn. F A Davies, Philadelphia

O'Brien S J, Schwarts R S, Warren R F, Torzilli P A 1995 Capsular restraints to anterior-posterior motion of the abducted shoulder: a biomechanical study. Journal of Shoulder and Elbow Surgery 4(4): 298–308

Palastanga N, Field D, Soames R 1998 Anatomy and human movement: structure and function, 3rd edn. Butterworth-Heinemann, Oxford

Soderberg G L 1997 Kinesiology – application to pathological motion, 2nd edn. Williams and Wilkins, Baltimore

Threlkeld J 1992 The effects of manual therapy on connective tissue. Physical Therapy 72(12): 61–70

Twomey L 1992 A rationale for the treatment of back pain and joint pain by manual therapy. Physical Therapy 72(12): 53–60

Vujnovich J, Dawson N 1994 The effect of therapeutic muscle stretch on neural processing. Journal of Sport and Physical Therapy 20(3): 145–153

Warner J J, Deng X H, Warren R F, Torzilli P A 1999 Static capsuloligamentous restraints to superior-inferior translation of the glenohumeral joint. American Journal of Sports Medicine 20(6): 675–685

Watkins J 1996 An introduction to mechanics of human movement. Petroc Press, Plymouth, pp 74–75

Williams P (ed) 1995 Gray's anatomy, 38th edn. Churchill Livingstone, Edinburgh

Wuelker N, Korell M, Thren K 1998 Dynamic glenohumeral joint stability. Journal of Shoulder and Elbow Surgery 7(1): 43–52

CHAPTER CONTENTS

Introduction 105

Strength 107
Contraction force 107
Power 107
Development, ageing and gender 107
Body types (somatotypes) 108
Measurements of strength 109

Endurance 110
Peripheral fatigue 110
Central fatigue 110
Limitations and ageing 111
Measurement of endurance 111

Muscle training 111
General principles of training 111
Warm-up 113

Strength training 113
Types of muscle activity 113
What is the best type of exercise to increase strength and performance? 115
Specificity 115
Intensity, repetition and frequency 116
Types of strength training programmes 116
Changes during strength training 116

Training for power 117

Training for endurance 117
Changes during endurance training 119

Circuit training 118

Therapeutic exercise 118
Assessment and measurement 118
Selecting and using an exercise programme 119
Preparation for treatment 120
Body positioning 120
The choice of activity 120
Patterns of movement 122
Irradiation, overflow and cross transfer 122
Trick movements 122
Muscle imbalance 123
Starting and finishing positions 123
Teaching and learning 124
Review and progression 124
Early re-education of movement 124
Later stage treatment 126
General maintenance 126
An unsatisfactory training programme 126

6

Strength, power and endurance

D. J. Newham

OBJECTIVES

At the end of this chapter you should be able to:

1. **Define and explain the concepts of work, strength, force and power**

2. **Discuss the effects of various factors on the above concepts**

3. **Discuss the measurement of the above**

4. **Describe fatigue and the other limits to the above concepts**

5. **Explain the factors involved in muscle training for strength, power and endurance**

6. **Discuss the parameters involved in muscle training with the different aspects of muscle functioning**

7. **Discuss the physiological effects of the training on the three aspects of muscle function**

8. **Describe the factors involved in therapeutic exercise**

9. **Develop and justify an exercise programme for the three concepts of muscle function.**

INTRODUCTION

The aim of this chapter is to give an understanding of the factors affecting force generation and how they are utilised in training programmes for both clinical and athletic purposes. Factors influencing strength, power and endurance are discussed, along with how they may be affected by training. The chapter builds on existing knowledge of the structure and function of skeletal muscle.

We require our muscles for two main purposes: to maintain a given posture (when they generally adopt a static role) and to move our bodies in a coordinated fashion and enable effective functional performance.

The concepts for force, strength, work and power are fundamental to an understanding of muscular action but are often used incorrectly. As they each have precise and different meanings it is important to clarify them.

Force cannot be seen but its effects can be measured. It can be defined as that which changes, or tends to change, the state of rest or motion of matter. For example, when a critical amount of force is applied to a stationary object, it will start to move. The application of an increased force will result in faster movement in the absence of any opposing resistive force such as friction. Application of a force less than the critical amount will not result in movement, but can still be measured with the appropriate technology. The unit of measurement of force is the newton (N) which is the force required to accelerate a mass of one kg at one metre/sec/sec.

Strength is the ability to generate force and is obviously central to muscle performance. A critical amount of strength is required to perform any function: if the strength of an individual is below this level, that function cannot be performed. Strength is measured in newtons or torque. The latter is the effectiveness of a force to produce rotation about an axis, e.g. a joint, and is measured in newton meters (N.m).

Work is the product of the force exerted and the distance through which it acts. The unit of measurement is the joule (J). It is important to note that work is only done when movement occurs; therefore, someone exerting considerable muscle strength and force by pushing against an immovable object is not doing any work, since there is no external movement.

Power is the rate of doing work, i.e. work divided by time, and is measured in watts (W). As velocity is distance divided by time, power can also be calculated by multiplying force by velocity.

The interactions between these different terms is illustrated by considering two individuals who each weigh 70 kg, but who have muscles of very different strengths. When standing still, no work is being done as there is no movement but each is exerting the same force of about 700 N (70 kg × force of gravity (9.81 m/s/s)). This force will represent a lower proportion of the maximal strength for the stronger person. If they are unable to exert a force of 700 N they will be unable to stand.

If each one covers a distance of 10 m, they have moved and therefore work will have been done. The work done is 7000 J (70 kg × 10 m) and will be the same for each person. In life there is a requirement for speed and therefore the rate of doing work, i.e. power, is important. If the 7000 J of work described above is performed by one person in 2 s, then the power output (7000 J/2 s) will be 3500 W. If the other person takes longer to perform the same work then his power output will be less. Covering the 10 m distance in 4 s will result in a power output of 1750 W.

It can therefore be seen that the key components of muscle function are strength and velocity. Endurance, the ability to continue activity and withstand fatigue, is also essential. These factors will be considered in further detail along with the causes and effects of improved performance with training. Strength and endurance must be considered separately as either primary or secondary muscle problems may affect either one alone or both together.

Task 6.1

Make sure you understand the definitions of force, work and power. Think of some examples of normal activities and work out which definitions do, and do not, apply.

STRENGTH

Intuitively we think that bigger muscles are stronger than smaller ones. It has also been shown experimentally that the strength of a muscle is proportional to its cross-sectional area (CSA) and independent of its length (Jones & Round 1990). In other words, the number of sarcomeres in parallel determines the strength of a muscle.

Contraction force

Most activities of daily life do not require a person of normal strength to make maximal contractions. However, each action requires a certain amount of absolute strength, i.e. lifting a bag of shopping or raising the body weight from sitting to standing. For a weak person these activities will require contractions at a greater proportion of their maximal strength than for a stronger person. The weaker person will therefore fatigue more rapidly.

Since a given amount of strength is necessary for a particular function, it will be easier to perform for a stronger person than a weak one since the former is producing a force which is a smaller proportion of his maximal. Strength below the critical value for that function will result in an inability to perform it and may have such profound functional consequences as being unable to rise from a chair or toilet seat.

For activities involving moving the body, its mass is of great importance. A person with weak thigh muscles is further disadvantaged by being overweight; losing a few kilograms of body mass may be the difference between being able or unable to stand from sitting, even in the absence of any increase in strength.

Power

As previously mentioned, we frequently want our muscles to produce power and bring about movement rather than simply generate force. The determinants of power are force and velocity and so an alteration in either will affect power output.

Muscle velocity (speed of contraction and relaxation) is largely influenced by the distribution of fibre types within a muscle. It is little affected by reduced activity or muscle injuries but may be changed by some neurological and primary muscle diseases. Fibre typing is also relatively constant whilst the muscle remains normally innervated and is only marginally influenced by training.

Therefore, power output is most likely to be affected by changes in muscle strength.

Development, ageing and gender

Reliable measurements of strength can be made in children from about the age of 5 years. From this age until puberty, when a growth spurt occurs, there is a steady increase in size and muscle strength that is similar in boys and girls (Jones & Round 1990).

In adolescent girls and women, the relationship between muscle strength, height and weight is similar to that of younger children. In adolescent boys, there is an additional hypertrophy which particularly affects the upper torso and limbs and which is probably an effect of testosterone.

Peak muscle strength is reached in approximately the early 20s and in the fifth decade there is a progressive atrophy (reduction in size and strength). This affects both genders equally until the menopause, when women show a greater loss of muscle size and strength which can to some extent be prevented by hormone replacement therapy (HRT).

The progressive loss of muscle mass can be as much as 30% by 90 years. The reduction in the size of a whole muscle is said to be greater than the atrophy of individual muscle fibres (Grimby & Saltin 1983) and it may be that the loss of neurones in the brain is accompanied by a loss of anterior horn cells in the spinal cord resulting in a reduction of motor units.

There is no evidence that habitual exercise can prevent the muscular effects of ageing. However, the preservation of cardiac and respiratory function brought about by regular exercise will help the elderly to make optimal use of the remaining muscle. Muscle performance can still improve in response to strength training, although there is some indication that the improvements are brought about more by learning and less by hypertrophy than in the young (Moritani & DeVries 1979). This learning adaptation to exercise implies that the central nervous system 'forgets' how to perform with disuse and is an additional reason why the elderly should be encouraged to remain active.

Body types (somatotypes)

As well as differing in gender and height, people vary in their somatotype (Fig. 6.1) and this is another congenital determinant of musculature and, therefore, physical strength. The majority of people contain elements of more than one type, but there are some who show a clear domination of one or another.

There are correlations between somatotype, lifestyle, disease and sporting ability. Certain somatotypes dominate in particular athletic events and endomorphs are unlikely to excel in any type of athletic activity. The different ratios

between body weight and muscle mass and also the biomechanical consequences of varying the length of body segments provide a genetic advantage, or disadvantage, in different physical activities (Tanner 1964).

Alterations in body weight with diet and exercise do not overcome the basic somatotype characteristics and the basic body proportions are retained despite the most rigorous attempts to change them.

In the absence of injury, disease or training, each individual has a natural position on a spectrum of strength and physical performance (Fig. 6.2). The occurrence of pathology and also disuse may shift them temporarily towards the left (poor) end of the performance spectrum. Primary diseases of nerve and muscle may have long-lasting, permanent or progressive effects. Training can usually improve strength, although, even in the absence of pathology, each individual has a predetermined physiological ceiling which cannot be exceeded. Any increases brought about

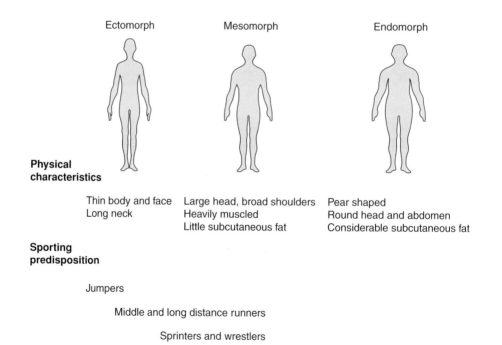

Figure 6.1 Illustration of the three basic body types and their physical characteristics. Elite athletes are usually ectomorphs (endurance events) or mesomorphs (power events). Endomorphs are unlikely to excel at any athletic activity, despite rigorous training.

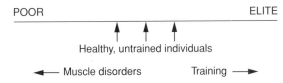

Figure 6.2 The spectrum of human performance. Healthy, untrained individuals can be pushed to the left by injury, disease and disuse or to the right by training.

by training will disappear once training ceases and the healthy individual will revert to their original place on the spectrum.

Measurements of strength

Objective

Theoretically, either size or force can be measured to indicate muscle strength. However, the only measurements of size that are useful are those of the physiological cross-sectional area (PCSA) (Fig. 6.3). As many muscles have a pennate structure and thus the fibres are not arranged parallel to the line of pull of the muscle, the anatomical cross-sectional area (ACSA) may not be the same as the PCSA. Therefore, measurements of limb circumference are of very little use as any change in the PCSA does not necessarily result in a proportional change in the ACSA (Jones & Round 1990).

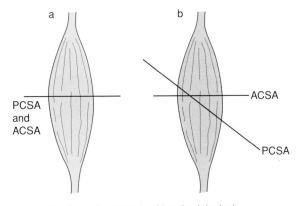

Figure 6.3 Force is determined by physiological cross-sectional area (PCSA) but measurements of limb circumference only identify the anatomical cross-sectional area (ACSA). In a muscle whose fibres lie parallel to the line of pull (a) the PCSA and ACSA are the same. Most muscles do not have this arrangement of fibres, which often lie at an angle to the line of pull and where PCSA and ACSA are very different (b). In this situation, measurements of ACSA will not detect large changes in PCSA.

A number of factors, including disease, disuse and training, can alter the thickness of subcutaneous fat as well as muscle bulk, but circumference measurements are unable to discriminate between different tissues (Stokes & Young 1986). Furthermore, there are considerable differences in measurements of limb circumference made by different people and even by the same person on different occasions (Stokes 1985). Accurate measurements of muscle CSA can only be made using ultrasound, computerised axial tomography (CAT) and magnetic resonance imaging (MRI) techniques which are normally unavailable to the therapist.

There are a number of relatively inexpensive hand-held devices that measure either force or pressure which give accurate and reliable results if the operator is trained adequately and the testing position is standardised. Their only limitation is that they rely on manual resistance by the therapist; the large muscle groups of adults cannot therefore be measured unless they are particularly weak. Some of these devices overcome this problem by having attachments that can be connected to immovable objects, such as a table leg.

An objective measurement of strength that can be made with the minimum of equipment is the 1 Repetition Maximum (RM), which may be performed under isometric or dynamic conditions using free weights. In an isometric contraction, a 1 RM is the maximum weight that the patient can hold in a particular part of the range. In a dynamic contraction, it is the maximum weight that they can move through the available range. Care must be taken to standardise the joint position during isometric testing and the velocity of movement during dynamic testing as both muscle length and angular velocity will influence the force a given muscle is able to generate. In practice, it is easier to monitor joint position more accurately than angular velocity and therefore isometric testing is probably more reliable.

Subjective

Manual muscle testing scales usually range from 0 (no contraction) to 5 (normal strength) and are based on a method devised to measure strength in infants (Martin & Lovett 1915). However, it has been well established that their accuracy and sensitivity are so poor that they are only of any use in cases of very severe weakness. Even then their use should probably be restricted to smaller muscle groups (Sapega 1990).

Manual techniques may indicate similar scores on repeated testing despite significant increases in objective strength measurements (Krebbs 1989). A strength increase of as much as 50% may not be detected (Watkins et al 1984) and a strength which is only about 10% of normal may be rated as 'good' (Agre & Rodriquez 1989).

Task 6.2

What reliable and valid techniques for measuring muscle strength are available to the therapist? Which techniques are unacceptable due to either technical reasons or lack of accuracy?

ENDURANCE

This is the ability to continue muscular activity over time and is obviously highly developed in athletic activities such as distance running. Endurance activities predominantly rely on aerobic metabolism and therefore depend on mechanisms that transport oxygen to, and metabolic waste products away from, the working muscles, as well as oxygen utilisation and the availability of energy stores within the muscles. Therefore, both the muscles themselves and the cardiovascular and respiratory systems are involved in endurance activities.

The importance of endurance capacity is that it reduces the effects of muscular fatigue. This is an inevitable consequence of activity that results in a decrease in strength or performance over time. In healthy subjects it is a temporary event, although the rate of both fatigue and recovery varies between individuals and is influenced by training. Fatigue is an inevitable consequence of activity and cannot be eliminated, but the resistance to fatigue, i.e. endurance, can be improved.

The extent of fatigue varies between a sensation of tiredness and complete exhaustion. As fatigue progresses, additional motor units and also muscle groups are recruited in an attempt to

maintain function and the energy cost of activity increases.

Fatigue can be broadly divided into two groups according to whether the underlying mechanisms are peripheral, i.e. in the muscles themselves, or central, i.e. within the central nervous system.

Peripheral fatigue

This occurs due to mechanisms in the working muscles themselves that can affect contraction, excitation or both (MacLaren et al 1989, Jones & Round 1990, Kukulka 1992). Working muscle is a highly active tissue in biochemical terms and the substances released (e.g. acetylcholine, potassium, phosphate and lactic acid) act alone or in combination to decrease force, contractile speed and power output. Active muscle often achieves internal pressures that are sufficient to occlude its own blood supply and therefore to exacerbate fatigue.

It was thought that the release of lactic acid and consequent decrease in intramuscular pH was the sole cause of metabolic fatigue, but it is now clear that this is not the case (Jones & Round 1990). Peripheral fatigue impairs the muscles' ability to generate force, even though it is maximally activated either through the nervous system or by external electrical or magnetic stimulation.

Central fatigue

This term describes mechanisms within the central nervous system which result in decreased voluntary activation, irrespective of the muscles' ability to produce force. Prolonged activity may be very boring and uncomfortable and this alone tends to increase the sense of effort and decrease motivation.

In addition, reflex mechanisms resulting in either decreased excitation, increased inhibition or an increased threshold to stimulation of the anterior horn cells can also cause central fatigue in the presence of full motivation. Both pain and joint pathology (Hurley et al 1992) also result in a reflex determined failure of voluntary activation.

The presence of central fatigue is confirmed when the superimposition of external (electrical or magnetic) stimulation upon a maximal voluntary contraction generates additional force (Rutherford et al 1986a).

Limitations and ageing

There are physiological limits to the amount of oxygen that can be taken up by the body. This is called the maximal oxygen consumption or $VO_{2\,max}$ and is influenced by a number of factors including genetics, age and gender in addition to training (Åstrand & Rodahl 1988, McArdle et al 1996).

After the mid-twenties, the $VO_{2\,max}$ steadily declines with age and by 70 years may be in the order of 50% of that at 20 years. Maximal heart rate also declines with age; a rough guide for an individual is 220 minus the age in years (Åstrand & Rodahl 1988, McArdle et al 1996). It is interesting that the decline in endurance ability with age is less than that for muscle strength.

$VO_{2\,max}$ also decreases with inactivity and particularly with bed rest (Saltin et al 1968). This is separate from any direct effects of pathology and should be remembered during treatment.

Measurement of endurance

Objective

Objective methods include the performance of maximal or submaximal activity using cycle ergometers, treadmills or step tests (Åstrand & Rodahl 1988, McArdle et al 1996). The measurements made may include the volume and composition of expired air, heart rate and blood pressure. Appropriate clinical measurements can be made using these techniques, or by measuring the number of repetitions possible with a given load or resistance, or timing a specified activity such as walking a fixed distance or climbing a flight of stairs.

All these measurements and tests involve strength as well as endurance to some degree and this is unavoidable. Without adequate muscle strength, no movement is possible and weak muscles result in slow movement. However, by using a relatively low force activity and using a high repetition number over time, a good indication of endurance capacity can be obtained and any changes observed.

An increase in endurance capacity is indicated by a reduced heart rate or sense of effort (Borg 1982) for a given amount of activity, an extension of the duration for which an activity can be carried out or an increase in the number of repetitions possible in a given time.

Subjective

Reported symptoms of fatigue are very difficult to interpret. Most patients complain of weakness, rather than fatigue, and find it difficult to distinguish between the two.

Task 6.3

What factors should be considered when a patient presents with fatigue as the main symptom? What assessments should be made?

MUSCLE TRAINING

Training may be defined as the preparation of an individual for purposeful, skilled and effective specific movements that may range from the general activities of daily living and function to specific and highly skilled activities. All activities comprise elements of:

- strength
- endurance
- flexibility
- coordination
- skill.

Training programmes need to be worked out for each individual according to their current condition and the goals and aims of training.

General principles of training

There are some principles that are common to all types of training (Fig. 6.4).

Overload

This means that a muscle, or physiological system such as the cardiovascular, is required to work harder than it is accustomed to. For strength training this applies to the force of contraction; for

GENERAL PRINCIPLES OF TRAINING

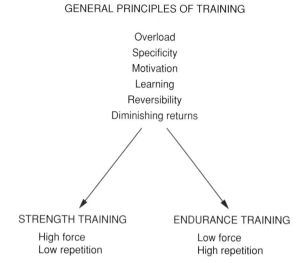

Overload
Specificity
Motivation
Learning
Reversibility
Diminishing returns

STRENGTH TRAINING   ENDURANCE TRAINING

High force   Low force
Low repetition   High repetition

Figure 6.4 The general principles are common to all forms of training, but the type of exercise required to improve strength or endurance is very different.

endurance training it means a repetition number of relatively low force contractions.

For a given stimulus to remain an overload, it must constantly be increased as muscle performance improves. The training programme needs to be kept at the same relative intensity and so must change in proportion to the changes in the muscle itself and, in the case of endurance training, the cardiovascular system.

Specificity

There is now considerable evidence that after training the greatest improvement is seen in the activity that was performed during training (Jones et al 1989, Jones & Round 1990). This is known as training specificity. It also means that an improvement in one type of activity is not automatically reflected in other activities. There is also little or no overlap between strength and endurance training: if both are to be improved, they must be individually addressed in the training programme.

Motivation

It takes considerable mental and physical effort to carry out an effective training programme and only well motivated individuals will be able to do so. One of the key roles of the therapist is to inform and motivate patients so that they can see the reason and relevance of what they are being asked to do.

Learning

There are two aspects of learning which relate to training. One is the motor learning that occurs with the practice of a motor event and is discussed later with strength training. The other is that patients must know exactly what they are required to do and what not to do. This puts the therapist in the role of educator, not only for the patients' knowledge about their own condition, but what they can do about it.

If the learning component is not addressed satisfactorily, the patient may well develop inappropriate movements and exercise programmes, but is unlikely to be sufficiently motivated to persevere with training.

Reversibility

After an acute or reversible pathological event individuals should regain their original position on the performance spectrum (see Fig. 6.2). In the absence of ongoing disease or further incidents, they should be able to maintain that position without further training.

In some cases, and particularly with athletic training, they are in a position on the spectrum that is further to the right of their natural one. Once training ceases, the tendency will be for them to revert to their original, congenitally determined position. This is why athletes need to continue training to maintain their enhanced performance.

Diminishing returns

The response to training is roughly inverse to the physical condition at the start of training. Thus it is much easier to bring about a 10% improvement in someone who is grossly weak or unfit than in an individual who is already at a high level of performance. All people have their own ceiling for physical performance and the closer one is to it, the harder it becomes to improve. This is probably one of the factors which persuades athletes to resort to illegal and often dangerous means of attempting to improve performance.

Despite these common principles, the physiological stimuli for increasing strength and endurance are very different. Strength training (Jones et al 1989) involves the generation of relatively high forces and therefore only low repetition is possible before fatigue sets in. In contrast, endurance training requires a high repetition of low force contractions.

Warm-up

Therapists and athletes commonly use a brief period of light exercise before embarking on the training or competitive event. This will certainly have the effect of increasing muscle blood flow and temperature (Åstrand & Rodahl 1988) which enhance performance. It also may allow a practice for the desired movement or activity and may possibly increase arousal and alertness.

It is also believed that a warm-up decreases the probability of strains and injury in athletes, although there is little direct evidence for this.

Warm-up regimens may take the form of a generalised, whole body activity designed to increase muscle blood flow and soft tissue flexibility (DeVries 1986). An alternative approach is to practise the specific movement to be used, but at low intensity (Shellock & Prentice 1985). There is little conclusive evidence on the relative merits of these two approaches.

STRENGTH TRAINING

The most common methods of providing resistance are by means of free weights, pulleys and springs or elasticated bands. In recent years there has been an increase in the number and type of equipment available for muscle testing (dynamometers). These tend to be isotonic or isokinetic systems which can be used to perform concentric or eccentric, isometric and dynamic contractions. Most are computerised systems that give measurements of strength and power in addition to joint angle and velocity. The display of force or power output acts as visual feedback that can aid and encourage the patient. Dynamometers are both large and expensive and will not be available to many therapists, nor are they a possibility for home use by the patient.

Table 6.1 The definition and key features of different types of exercise. A single contraction may be purely of one type or contain elements of more than one

Type of contraction	Definition	Features
Isometric	Constant muscle length	No movement May be isotonic or force may vary
Isotonic	Constant force output	May be isometric or dynamic Velocity may vary
Isokinetic	Constant velocity	Usually not isotonic

The terms *isokinetic* and *isotonic* are often used incorrectly and it is necessary that they are understood in order to avoid confusion and inaccuracy (see Table 6.1).

Types of muscle activity

Isometric exercise (Fig. 6.5a)

During these static contractions the muscle remains the same length, no external movement occurs and therefore no external work or power is performed. The contractions may be maximal or submaximal and the force generated may vary during the contraction or it may remain constant, i.e. isotonic.

If a maximal isometric contraction is maintained for more than a few seconds, the force will start to decline as fatigue sets in.

Isometric contractions are all that is available to a muscle that is immobilised. They are also useful when activity at a certain joint position or muscle length is to be avoided. They are relatively simple procedures and require a minimal amount of time to learn and perform properly. It is important that the rest of the body is well stabilised so that effort can be directed to the required activity rather than to maintaining posture.

Isometric exercises can be performed with relatively simple and inexpensive equipment and are ideal for home use when a fixed object, such as a wall or table, can be used as the resistive force.

Isometric force can be measured objectively and reliably using inexpensive equipment such as the 1 RM or hand-held dynamometers and strain gauge systems in addition to the large and expensive isotonic or isokinetic dynamometers.

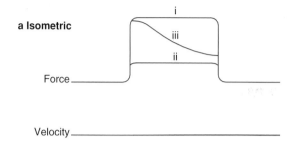

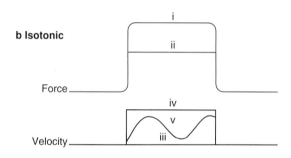

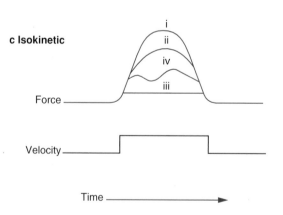

Figure 6.5 Possibilities for force and velocity in different contraction types. (a) During an isometric contraction there is no movement. The force may be isotonic at either maximal (i) or submaximal (ii) levels, but it may also vary (iii). (b) In an isotonic contraction the force remains constant at either maximal (i) or submaximal (ii) levels while the movement velocity may be zero, i.e. isometric (iii), isokinetic (iv) or variable and therefore neither isometric or isokinetic (v). (c) In an isokinetic contraction the movement velocity remains constant but the force may be maximal (i) or submaximal (ii). It may be isotonic throughout most of the contraction (iii) or may fluctuate (iv).

High force isometric contractions, particularly of the upper limbs, cause large increases in blood pressure. They should therefore be avoided with individuals in whom this might be dangerous.

Isotonic exercise (Fig. 6.5b)

It is often thought that these are always dynamic contractions, but in fact they may be either dynamic or isometric (static). The key feature is that the force generation remains constant throughout the contraction. This is what happens when lifting or holding a given weight. If movement occurs, it may be isokinetic or the velocity of movement may vary.

If isotonic contractions are dynamic, it should be remembered that they cannot be maximal throughout the entire range of movement. Due to the length:tension relationship and also the biomechanical changes occurring during movement, the greatest force is usually generated in mid-range and is less at the extremes of range. Therefore, a force which is maximal at either the shortest or longest muscle length will be submaximal at mid-range. This is illustrated by the difference between force lines i and iii in Figure 6.5c.

Isokinetic exercise (Fig. 6.5c)

This is exercise performed at a constant, predetermined velocity and controlled by the isokinetic dynamometer (a dynamometer is something that measures (metron) work (dynamics)). This then controls movement so that the preset velocity cannot be exceeded, irrespective of the strength or force generated. However, it is possible for the person being tested to move at lower velocities. The range of movement is controlled by the therapist and may be through either all or part of the available or anatomical range.

It is important to realise that there is an acceleration phase at the start of movement and a deceleration phase at the end. Therefore, the patient is only moving at the preset velocity for part of the time and the entire movement is not isokinetic. The proportion of the movement that occurs at the preset velocity decreases as velocity increases.

An important point is that the term 'velocity' refers to the angular velocity, i.e. that of the moving body parts, and not the velocity at which the muscles themselves are changing length. The relationship between angular and muscle velocity is a complex one and, in the absence of any direct measurements, no assumptions can be made about the velocity of changes in muscle length.

The maximal angular velocity available with even the most sophisticated isokinetic equipment is 300 deg/s. Whilst this feels very fast, it is relatively slow compared to the maximal physiological angular velocity which can exceed 1000 deg/s.

What is the best type of exercise to increase strength and performance?

For years this has been a subject of controversy and discussion. There are still a number of unknown issues, which are outlined below, but a reasonable degree of clarity has emerged in some areas (McDonagh & Davies 1984, Jones et al 1989, Jones & Round 1990, McArdle et al 1996). It is worth remembering that there is considerable individual variation in the response to training even in normal, healthy people and that individual variation is probably even greater in those with pathology.

It is generally true that both static and dynamic high force contractions increase strength and that there is no inherent advantage with either type. The training method used should be based on the functional requirements of a particular patient and will obviously be governed by the clinical condition and available equipment.

Manufacturers of dynamometers and advocates of particular exercise regimens claim that one form of resisted exercise, for example isokinetic, is superior to others, but there is very little evidence for this. One claim often made for both isotonic and isokinetic systems is that they are the most physiological form of exercise and therefore their effects are most likely to carry over to functional activities. These claims are rather spurious in that normal movement is composed of all types of activity; it is rarely isokinetic and is often not isotonic. Postural muscles are most likely to perform isometric contractions, but there are often small amounts of movement.

There is no evidence that one form of exercise is inherently better than another.

There has also been debate about whether eccentric exercise is best for strength training. The theoretical basis underlying this is that the greatest force is generated by a muscle under eccentric conditions and if high force generation is the stimulus for hypertrophy, then this should be the most effective type of exercise. However, the available evidence does not support this (McDonagh & Davies 1984, Jones & Round 1990), perhaps at least in part because the performance of unfamiliar high force eccentric exercise causes muscle pain, long-lasting fatigue and damage (Newham 1988). There is no reason to think that this improves the training response, in fact it seems more likely to hinder it.

Specificity

This takes the form of training and task specificity (Jones et al 1989, Jones & Round 1990).

Training specificity

There are some reports of training specificity in both muscle length and velocity. In other words, if training is carried out at a particular muscle length or velocity, the benefits are only, or mainly, seen at that particular speed or length. Theoretically, this seems unlikely as it implies an alteration in the length:tension or force:velocity relationship, which are fundamental principles of the myofilaments and it is difficult to imagine how they could be eliminated.

The solution may be that the claims for length specificity have been made after studies on whole muscle groups that comprise a number of individual muscles. The observed length:tension relationship is the product of all these muscles, which may show peak tension at different lengths. If one of these muscles hypertrophies to a greater extent, or they all show different amounts of hypertrophy, then the length:tension relationship of the whole muscle could be changed (Jones & Round 1990).

The evidence for velocity specificity is not convincing. Measurements of the force:velocity relationship are very difficult to make in large muscle groups. This is particularly so when voluntary contractions, rather than electrically stimulated ones, are used.

Task specificity

It is undoubtedly the case that being able to lift heavier weights does not necessarily mean improved performance during functional activities and that there is no simple relationship between strength and performance. People can become better at lifting weights without becoming stronger simply by practising the movements and becoming more skilled at them. Equally, people can become stronger by training with isometric contractions, but not necessarily perform better in another activity such as cycling (Rutherford et al 1986b, Rutherford 1988). Therefore, task specificity is a very important part of strength training that is brought about by a learning process in which the correct sequence of movements is laid down as a motor pattern in the central nervous system. This means that the training task must be identical, or as similar as possible, to the functional task or tasks which it is hoped to improve.

Intensity, repetition and frequency

Despite the vast number of studies that have investigated different training regimens, an optimal programme has not been identified. However, it seems that a load which exceeds 80% of maximum will produce an increase in strength if as few as 10 repetitions are carried out at least three times a week. Higher force contractions will bring about greater increases in strength. It is, therefore, essential that the resistance is increased as strength improves, otherwise it will cease to act as an adequate stimulus.

Types of strength training programmes

A number of training programmes are well established and all have their advocates. The two main categories are progressive resistance exercises (PRE) and progressive rate training (PRT) (Hellebrandt & Houtz 1958). In PRE the resist-

ance is increased proportionally with muscle strength, while in PRT the resistance remains constant and the speed at which a set number of repetitions is performed is increased. PRT is a rather complicated technique involving the use of a metronome and, theoretically, is unlikely to be effective as the resistance remains constant, irrespective of the extent of strength increases, and may cease to act as an overload stimulus.

Common examples of PRE methods are as follows:

- The Delorme programme (Delorme & Watkins 1948) is based on the 10 RM: the maximal weight which can be lifted throughout the available range 10 times. Resistance is applied by means of a weighted boot or barbell. The programme consists of 1 set of 10 lifts at 50%, 75% and 100% RM with a rest between each one. This is performed 5 times weekly and the 1 RM is used as a test of progress at weekly intervals.

- The Oxford programme (Zinovieff 1951) uses a system whereby the resistance is progressively reduced in each training session. It consists of 10 sets of 10 repetitions. The first is at 10 RM and thereafter reduced by 0.5 kg in each set. A rest is given between each set. This is recommended to be performed on 5 days each week.

- The MacQueen programmes (MacQueen 1954, 1956) consist of two programmes, one each for hypertrophy and power. The hypertrophy programme consists of three sets of the 10 RM with a rest between each set. The power programme consists of one set of 10 RM followed by a rest period and further sets in which the weight is increased and the repetition number decreased, e.g. second set of 8 lifts at 8–6 RM.

It seems that none of these programmes is inherently more effective in increasing strength than the others and perhaps the most pragmatic solution is to use the MacQueen hypertrophy programme as it is the simplest.

Changes during strength training

Strength training appears to result in a sequence of events (Jones & Round 1990). The first phase is that of motor learning when performance improves but strength remains virtually constant. It continues for 6–8 weeks. The second phase is an increase in the strength of the muscles which appears to occur without a parallel increase in muscle size. This might be because of an increased synchronisation of motor unit firing (Komi 1986), an increased ability to recruit all available motor units or changes in fibre architecture or increased packing (density) of contractile material. The final phase of true hypertrophy starts after about 10–12 weeks and thereafter there is a slow but steady increase in both muscle size and strength. The stimulus for this phase remains unclear but certainly requires the generation of high forces.

Hypertrophy or hyperplasia?

The main possibilities for increased muscle size and strength with training are either that the total number of fibres remains constant, but they all increase in size (hypertrophy), or that the fibre diameter remains constant but there is a growth of new fibres and therefore an increase in fibre number (hyperplasia). Whilst there is some evidence of fibre splitting leading to hyperplasia in animal studies, there is little human data to support this theory and it appears that hypertrophy is the main mechanism (McDougall et al 1984).

TRAINING FOR POWER

In many cases, the desired outcome of a training programme is an increase in power rather than strength *per se*. Since power is the product of force and velocity, these are the only variables that can be manipulated to improve power. The evidence is that the maximal velocity is unlikely to be affected by training and, therefore, the only practical way to improve power is by increasing strength (Jones & Round 1990).

The importance of task specificity has already been discussed. This means that the greatest increases in power output will be seen in the task used for training and not transferred equally across all activities. Similarly, strength can increase substantially during isometric exercise, but little or no improvement is seen in other,

more functional activities. Therefore, the training task should be the same as the activity that is required to improve, or should be as close as possible in terms of movement.

TRAINING FOR ENDURANCE

The common principles of training apply to endurance activities. In contrast to strength training, it is based on a high number of repetitions of relatively low force contractions and the stress (overload) is the increased metabolic demand of the working muscles. If high force contractions are used, anaerobic metabolism is utilised, a form of strength training is implemented and endurance capacity will not increase.

As a general rule, exercise should not cause heart rate values greater than those shown in Table 6.2. There may be clinical reasons to train at even lower heart rates than this, particularly for those with cardiovascular pathology.

The muscles need to contract at about 30–50% of their maximal force generation and exercise needs to be continued for about 20–30 minutes three times weekly (McArdle et al 1996) for endurance to improve.

During the sessions the individuals should be slightly breathless if they are performing activities such as treadmill walking or cycling on an ergometer, but they should not be distressed or exhausted at the end.

Individual muscle groups may be trained by the performance of either isometric or dynamic contractions, but the cardiovascular and respiratory systems are best influenced by whole body exercise.

The American College of Sports Medicine (1978) has issued the following guidelines for

Table 6.2 The maximal heart rates recommended during training at different ages. Recommendations of the World Health Organization (Anderson et al 1971)

Age (years)	Upper limit (beats/min)
20–29	170
30–39	160
40–49	150
50–59	140
60 and over	130

training to develop and maintain cardiorespiratory fitness in healthy adults. Lower levels of training may be necessary for some patients, particularly at the start of treatment:

- Frequency of 3–5 sessions each week.
- Intensity at 60–90% of maximal heart rate (measured or estimated for age) or 50–80% of $VO_{2\,max}$.
- Duration of 15–60 minutes for each session. Lower activity should be continued for a longer time. Low to moderate intensity for relatively longer duration is recommended for non-athletic training.
- Type of activity: any that uses large muscle groups, which can be maintained for the desired time, and that uses aerobic metabolism. Exercise such as walking, running, swimming and cycling are effective.

In general, endurance training which occurs less than twice weekly, at less than 50% $VO_{2\,max}$ and for less than 10 minutes per session is inadequate for training purposes.

Changes during endurance training

Endurance training affects the muscles themselves and also the cardiovascular and respiratory systems so that the delivery and utilisation of oxygen is improved (Åstrand & Rodahl 1988, Jones & Round 1990, McArdle et al 1996). Capillary density increases in the trained muscles so that the diffusion distance for oxygen decreases. The quantity and quality of mitochondria changes so that they become better able to metabolise the increased amount of oxygen delivered to the muscles.

The cardiac muscle hypertrophies so that the cardiac output increases and the resting heart rate decreases. The body switches to fat metabolism earlier, prolonging the time for which exercise can continue.

CIRCUIT TRAINING

This comprises a series of four to six activities that are performed in a single session with a rest period between each one (Åstrand & Rodahl

1988). This has the advantage that general and task specific exercises can be selected and combined for each individual. Activities planned to increase strength, endurance, flexibility, coordination and general fitness can be combined.

There is some evidence that strength training is less effective when combined with endurance training (McArdle et al 1996) but this is probably more relevant to athletic training than to clinical treatment.

As with all types of treatment, the purpose of each activity must be considered by the therapist and explained to the patient. Intensity and duration must also be increased with performance. The programme should be designed so that different types of activities and muscle groups are interspersed to avoid fatigue and boredom.

Task 6.4

What are the similarities and differences of training regimens for increasing strength and endurance?

THERAPEUTIC EXERCISE

This forms the major part of most physical therapy programmes and can be defined as the use of body movement during clinical treatment. It may include movement and use of individual joints or muscles, as well as graduated training for the activities of daily life. Exercise is often used in conjunction with other therapeutic modalities.

Assessment and measurement

Before commencing treatment, an accurate assessment must be thoroughly carried out. This should include the following:

- Diagnosis/pathology. Coexisting medical, psychological or social issues that may have an effect on management, treatment, prognosis or outcome should be determined.
- The extent of handicap, impairment and disability should be established along with the limiting factors and their underlying causes.

• Sensory, perceptual, cognitive or behavioural problems. These may affect the treatment itself or the potential for the patient to become self-managing.

• Objective measures of muscle strength, joint range, functional activity relevant to the individual, their problems and lifestyle. Examples of functional activities are measurements of the time taken to walk a fixed distance, climb a flight of stairs, move from sitting to standing or the maximal weight that can be overcome.

Objective and subjective assessments are both essential so that a complete picture of the patient as an individual is built up, allowing aims and goals for treatment to be established and progress to be monitored regularly and accurately.

It is essential that the therapist involves the patient in the assessment. Time must be taken to identify what the patient perceives to be a problem and what his expectations of therapy are. Aims and goals for treatment must be agreed between patient and therapist, otherwise it is unreasonable to expect the patient to comply and become sufficiently involved and motivated about his treatment. It is also essential that realistic goals be set to avoid disappointment and loss of motivation.

Both diagnosis and prognosis must be taken into account in addition to the patient's current state and his previous level of ability or disability. These will be revealed through a thorough examination and assessment and are the basis for treatment planning. The central questions to be asked are:

• What can the patient do?
• What can he not do and why?
• What does he want and need to do?

The assessment should include a detailed analysis of movement and any related problems. The present, absent and incorrect movements need to be identified along with the potential for improvement.

The principles of therapeutic exercise and training are the same as those used in athletic training as described previously. The difference is that both the initial starting point and the desired outcome are likely to be at a lower level of the performance spectrum. The training programme (and assessment) should take all the components of physical ability into account, i.e. strength, power, endurance, flexibility, coordination and skill.

Selecting and using an exercise programme

An exercise programme should take a holistic approach and consider the whole patient, not simply a clinical condition affecting one or more parts of the body. The exercise programme may also be part of a treatment programme by one therapy profession, or it may form part of a multidisciplinary rehabilitation plan. The latter must be carefully coordinated and effective communication with other health care professionals will avoid uneconomical use of time and unnecessary overlap in treatment.

An initial priority is to relieve pain and swelling as much as possible, since both of these will adversely affect any exercise programme.

It is important to remember that whilst the goals may be similar for different patients, the best way to achieve these will vary from one individual to another and will be influenced by present and past condition, in addition to the functional tasks involved. Therefore, each programme should be individually tailored to each patient and the therapist must be vigilant in monitoring and making changes where necessary. Change may be necessary for clinical reasons or may be used simply to avoid boredom.

Where possible, activities should be used which patients can carry on independently in their home environment. Any carers involved with a patient should also be involved in the treatment. They should be aware of the aims and goals of treatment, its expected outcome and time course. Carers can help in continued exercise programmes when a therapist is not present and they may be important in keeping up motivation and ensuring that treatment continues and progresses.

Planning a treatment programme must involve the patient directly and closely. The setting of priorities and short- and long-term goals must be agreed between patient and therapist if the patient is to be expected to become sufficiently involved. Any restrictions to functional ability must be identified and taken into account. These may include the physical condition (motor and sensory) of patients, their environment, psychological factors and also their ability to communicate, participate and learn.

A therapy programme should be developed on the basis of the individual patient's current level of performance and the desired outcome. Clear goals and aims must be set and adhered to. However, if it becomes apparent that they are no longer appropriate or realistic, they must be changed accordingly. An effective programme requires close interaction between patient and therapist so that problems are identified and a rational and mutually agreed programme is embarked upon.

The patient is required to make a considerable effort and it is unreasonable for the therapist to expect this input if the patient is not aware of, and in agreement with, the expected aims and results. The therapist must involve the patient at every stage of the treatment and take care to find out from patients what are their main problems and expectations. Any unrealistic expectations by patients must be pointed out so that they do not become disappointed and lose motivation. Care must also be taken that the programme is varied and interesting, otherwise it may become boring for all concerned.

The setting of long- and short-term goals will help both patient and therapist to plan and monitor treatment. Regular and accurate assessment and measurements are essential for this.

A problem-solving approach is the key to the optimal planning and execution of a successful treatment programme involving a number of factors and steps which are illustrated in Figure 6.6. Those involved with caring for the patient should also be involved in all stages of this process.

Preparation for treatment

If there is severe loss of movement, the circulation to the affected parts may be reduced and there may also be some pain and stiffness. Both these would impinge on treatment and may be relieved by gentle warmth, massage and passive movements.

Body positioning

The patient's kinaesthetic sense may be reduced by sensory loss or prolonged disuse and the patient may have a poor sense of his posture. Correct body and limb alignment is important in gaining accurate and efficient movement and minimising the development of secondary postural problems. The therapist should explain this clearly to the patient. Continuous monitoring and correction of posture may be necessary.

The choice of activity

This should be governed by the findings of assessment, examination and measurement. Additional factors will also play a role in determining the choice of activity for a particular individual.

Psychological factors

Patients must be motivated to make the effort necessary for exercise and training. They should have a clear idea of what is required, and why, as well as how it will affect their function or clinical condition.

There may be several possible reasons for patients not being sufficiently motivated to comply with an exercise programme, including personal or social reasons for wishing to remain in their current state. Patient behaviour patterns can be adopted (Pilowsky 1994) either consciously or unconsciously. They are not easy to break out of and may be reinforced by carers, friends and relatives (Rowat et al 1994).

Patients may be genuinely convinced that improvement will not take place, or that if it does it will be so small as to make little difference to their lives. They may be frightened of failing to improve. If legal proceedings are proposed or pending, there may also be financial reasons for poor motivation. Therapists should explore these possibilities and deal with them as best they can,

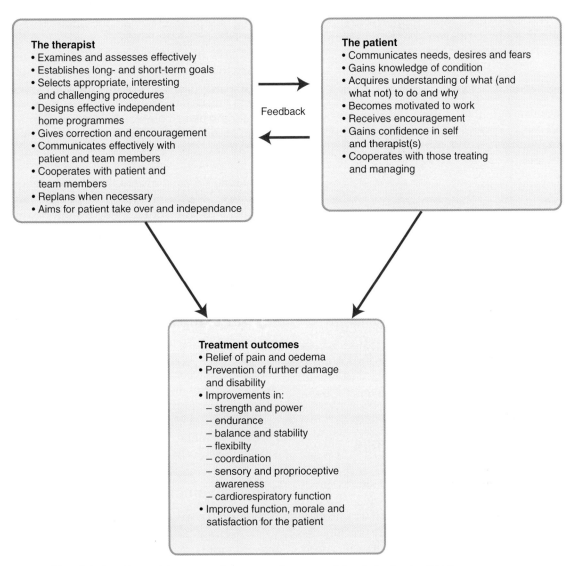

Figure 6.6 The clinical problem-solving approach necessary for successful and effective treatment.

and care should be taken not to assume that poor motivation automatically indicates a difficult or malingering patient.

Anatomical and physiological factors

The patient needs to have the following in order for the desired activity to occur:

- necessary range of movement
- adequate muscle strength to maintain posture and simultaneously perform the movement

(external stability or assistance is necessary if patients are unable to provide this themselves)

- adequate endurance and skill
- the sensory and motor components for movement control
- the cognitive and perceptual ability to understand and perform what is required.

Mechanical factors

- Gravity, friction and momentum may be utilised to assist or resist movement.

• The size of the base of support and type of supporting surface may help or hinder the desired movement.

Environmental factors

Concentration, motivation and the sense of effort can all be affected by a number of environmental influences. The most common disadvantages are:

• cramped space
• dim or over bright lighting
• excessive heat or cold
• noise and air pollution.

Patterns of movement

The technique of proprioceptive neuromuscular facilitation (PNF) utilises movement patterns relevant to normal functional activities that have diagonal and rotatory components (Knott & Voss 1968, Waddington 1976). It emphasises proprioceptive stimulation, visual, auditory, tactile and stretch, in an attempt to gain a maximal muscle response.

Irradiation, overflow and cross transfer

An attempt to make a maximal voluntary contraction of an individual muscle or muscle group will quickly demonstrate the fact that it is virtually impossible to isolate the effort to only one muscle. This may be due in part to the simultaneous need for increased stabilising forces, but it is probably also due to the fact that the central nervous system tends to activate groups of muscles, rather than individual muscles. Furthermore, the excitatory influences descending from the higher centres are unlikely to be restricted only to specific anterior horn cells forming motor units within a single muscle (Rothwell 1994). Therefore, strong voluntary efforts directed at one muscle may irradiate, or overflow, to other muscles within the same functional group or to those in a group performing a synergistic or stabilising role. For example, it is difficult to imagine being able to voluntarily activate only one muscle of the quadriceps femoris group, or to activate these muscles without including the abdominals.

Similarly, it is difficult to limit strong muscle activity to a unilateral activity. It is highly likely that a maximal effort of the right quadriceps femoris muscles takes place with the muscles of the left limb being completely inactive. A number of unilateral training studies have reported a strength increase in the apparently 'untrained' limb.

It should be remembered that such techniques are only appropriate when a patient has a problem with the voluntary activation of a particular muscle either through disease, injury or disuse. The force of contraction elicited by such means is unlikely to be sufficient to bring about hypertrophy in all but the very weakest muscles. Therefore, their role is restricted to learning or relearning to use inactive muscle. Once voluntary activation is possible, it is more effective to use direct resisted exercises of the muscle, or muscle group, in question.

In a low force contraction it is easier to restrict muscle activity to the prime movers. As force increases, synergist muscles are progressively activated and with strong activity, particularly at extremes of range, there may be co-contraction of antagonists (Rothwell 1994).

Trick movements

If the prime mover for a particular action is too weak to bring about the movement, an instinctive attempt is made to carry out the movement using other muscle groups and body movements. A common example of this is the use of the lateral abdominal muscle to lift the pelvis if the hip abductors alone are inadequate for this purpose.

Such trick movements should be identified by the therapist and pointed out to the patient. Where possible they should be avoided as they can become habitual and may lead to deformity and musculoskeletal problems. However, they can be useful in very early stage treatment by utilising the principles of irradiation and overflow. Furthermore, it is clearly unreasonable to expect a patient to restrict their activities to those that can be performed correctly. In some cases this would markedly increase the level of disability and have severe functional consequences, particularly in chronic and progressive conditions.

Muscle imbalance

The importance of the relative strength of agonist and antagonist muscle pairs is the subject of much current interest (Dirix et al 1988). This is particularly so for the knee and spine where there are claims that a disturbance of the normal balance of strength between flexors and extensors results in an increased susceptibility to musculoskeletal problems.

It remains unclear how important the balance of strength between muscles with an opposing action is, but it would not seem unreasonable to seek to correct any large discrepancies.

There is some evidence that resisted exercises of one muscle group cause greater strength increases if resisted contractions of the agonist are alternated with resisted reciprocal contractions of the antagonist, rather than with a rest period between contractions of the agonist (McArdle et al 1996). This is thought to be due to neuromuscular facilitation and the subsequent recruitment of more motor units.

Starting and finishing positions

All activity has a starting position that is the position of readiness from which activity is initiated. The finishing position may be a return to the initial starting position or might be the beginning of a new phase in a sequence of movement.

The starting position

For a movement to be accurate, it is necessary that the patient understands the need for good postural alignment, is conscious of the position of his head and body and is able to correct when necessary. This process requires constant minor adjustments unless the patient is fully stabilised by external means.

The starting position may be used:

- as a foundation for an activity

- to provide fixation for one part of the body so that localised movement can be achieved
- to train posture and balance
- as an exercise to improve the stability and safety of the required posture.

An activity can initially use a very stable starting position and then be made more difficult by performing it in progressively more unstable positions. The four basic postures, from the most (easiest) to least (hardest) stable, are lying, sitting, kneeling and standing.

The factors necessary for selecting a starting position are as follows:

- It is appropriate to the activity itself, relevant to the needs of the patient and acceptable to him.
- The supporting surface is stable, the base of support is of an adequate size and weight is distributed correctly.
- The position can be taken up, with or without help, held in good alignment and is capable of any necessary adjustment.
- The line of gravity falls within the base.
- Resistance to external forces can be withstood.

Progression may take the form of changing the starting position or modifying the current one. An activity will be made more difficult if:

- the size of the base is reduced
- the centre of gravity is raised
- the speed of movement is increased
- the supporting surface is made more soft or mobile.

A position may fail for a number of reasons:

- an inappropriate choice
- muscle weakness or fatigue
- inadequate joint range
- joint or muscle pain
- lack of coordination or balance
- disturbed proprioception
- abnormal reflex activity.

Additional support may be provided, i.e. by wall or parallel bars, straps or splints, to help ensure correct posture and movement and to aid safety and confidence.

Teaching and learning

When helping a patient to learn a movement, whether one of an isolated joint or a sequence of movement patterns, it is beneficial to use as many teaching techniques as possible.

Explanation is used to describe what is required, why it is necessary and what the benefits will be.

Demonstration by the therapist will also act as a learning aid in combination with other techniques. However, even for trained observers, a demonstration is difficult to follow in any detail (Carlsöö 1972). In unilateral conditions it may be practised on the unaffected side and should be shown, with assistance and clear guidance, on the affected side.

This procedure will clarify the proposed movement to the patient and gives him the opportunity to practise, which is important for motor learning.

Illustrations are an important aid to learning for those able to use them. They may take the form of videotapes or photographs as well as written illustrations and instructions. It is helpful to give patients some form of illustrated instruction that they may keep with them.

Review and progression

Regular reviews should assess and measure the patient's progress. Treatment should be modified according to the answers to the following questions:

- What has been achieved?
- Have the aims altered?
- What features should be added to, or removed from, the programme?

Once a contraction or movement is possible, the aim of training is to increase the intensity and complexity of the muscle contractions. Assistance should be phased out as quickly as possible and replaced by a resistance (overload) which increases with ability.

Resource management issues for therapists make it necessary for manual resistance to be replaced by other resistive forces as soon as possible in strength training. Lever length can be manipulated so that, initially, short lever arms are used and the patient progresses to longer ones. Resistance can be increased by changing the starting position so that initially gravity and then mechanical resistance is used.

Movement patterns should be increased in complexity from simple movements of individual joints to those involving multiple joints and patterns which mimic those of functional activity and aid control of movement. In this way, independent work by the patient is encouraged.

If an increase in strength is the sole aim of treatment, there is little point in increasing the number of repetitions to more than approximately three sets of ten contractions performed three times a week. An increase in the number of repetitions above this in a single session will have little effect due to the onset of fatigue, which will temporarily reduce the strength of the muscle and not induce hypertrophy.

Most training programmes will aim to increase both strength and endurance, but it is important to remember that different types of exercise will need to be performed for these two purposes.

Early re-education of movement

In the early stages of treatment a patient may be unable to perform the desired activity without assistance from the therapist, but such assistance should only be provided when absolutely necessary. Independent activity, albeit assisted by gravity or the patient himself, should be implemented as early as possible. The patients should take responsibility for their own treatment so that they may continue it when the therapist is unavailable and in their own environment. When possible, the therapist should ensure that the patient has a good understanding of the exercises that he can do without assistance and how to progress them in order for the treatment to continue without the therapist.

Active movement may be impossible because of injury, disease, disuse or immobilisation. However, weakness and atrophy need to be unusually severe for any movement at all to be impossible. Denervation of a muscle of normal strength will result in the affected motor units being unable to generate any voluntary force, although either external electrical or magnetic stimulation will generate the available force.

When active movement is not possible, it is necessary to perform passive or assisted active movement throughout the available range. This will help to prevent or reverse any shortening of the soft tissues (muscle fibres, tendons and ligaments) causing a loss of range of movement and the flexibility that is necessary for optimal function.

For hypertrophy to occur, the muscles must generate a force that is close to their maximal capacity and therefore passive movements will not increase strength. In addition to preserving or increasing joint range, passive movements in which the patient attempts to participate may act as an aid to the central nervous system in learning, remembering and practising motor patterns. It may be beneficial to perform passive and assisted active movements in patterns that involve a number of joints in patterns of activity used in daily living. Thus, movements involving whole limbs, e.g. in flexion and extension patterns, may be preferable to moving each joint individually.

The starting position

A starting position should be selected which encourages and allows the desired movement to occur freely. In the case of very weak patients, the segment to be exercised may need to be positioned so that the effects of gravity are minimised if movement is to occur. An example of this is patients with very weak hip flexors who may be unable to produce movement when lying supine. They may, however, be able to do so if they are placed on their side, lying with the affected leg uppermost and its weight supported by the therapist.

Where possible, clothing should be adjusted so that the relevant parts of the body are uncovered and both patients and therapist can use visual feedback.

Patients should be comfortable and well supported so that they are free to concentrate on the desired movement and unnecessary strains and stresses are avoided.

Body stability and support are necessary to hold the body steady and in good alignment so that nearly maximal muscle contractions can be made with the minimum of stress and strain. For example, in quadriceps strengthening exercises an ideal position is sitting with the thigh and back well supported.

Assisting and resisting forces

Manual assistance provided by the therapist is the most common form of assisting force, although it may also be provided by the patient in some cases. Assistance may also be provided by water, smooth surfaces or supporting slings.

Resistive forces may include manual resistance by the therapist. Limb weight, friction or unwanted contractions or spasm in antagonist muscle groups will also increase the resistance to movement.

The ability to develop maximum force depends on adequate proprioception. The sight of movement and correct placement of the therapist's hands, indicating the direction of movement or providing resistance, will help the patient. Clear instruction, encouragement and feedback are necessary.

Manual assistance

Ideally, the patient will gain confidence and reassurance in working closely with the therapist and it is important that manual contact is comfortable and pleasant. The therapist's hands should be warm, gentle and supportive and should help the patient understand what he is required to do. One of the therapist's hands should be used to control the proximal area and support the working part while the other is used for providing stretch, direction and assistance or resistance as appropriate.

The therapist should ensure that she moves with the patient and that her own body position is maintained in a good position which will reduce the incidence of musculoskeletal injury.

Manual resistance

The role of manual resistance is restricted to situations where other forms of resistance are not possible. This might be due to extreme weakness or cases where the force generated in different parts of the range varies more than usual. It is also useful in the very early stages of treatment when the patient needs assistance from the therapist on how to perform the movement.

In practical terms, it is very difficult, or even impossible, for a therapist to offer sufficient manual resistance to adequately challenge the large muscles of adults with anything other than extremely weak muscles. To attempt to do so is putting the therapist at unnecessary risk of physical injury.

Manual resistance has the advantage that it is quick and easy to apply. However, it is not accurately measurable and can be influenced as easily by any changes in the physical and psychological state of the therapist as by real strength changes in the patient.

Stretch and vibration

A patient may have difficulty in activating a muscle which is extremely weak or which is not normally innervated with either motor or sensory impairment. In these situations, the muscle may be facilitated by a rapid stretch or mechanical vibration. The stretch should be applied to the contracting muscle in a lengthened position, although care must be taken not to damage the weakened muscles or the joints over which they act.

Both stretch and vibration activate the extrafusal muscle fibres through the muscle spindles. They also have the additional effect of inhibiting activity in antagonist muscle groups (Rothwell 1994).

Later stage treatment

Once the patient is able to perform movement against gravity, the emphasis of training and rehabilitation should be on independent exercise. Input from the therapist will still be necessary to correct any postural errors and to ensure that the training overload is increased appropriately. The performance of exercise that does not stress the system will not act as a stimulus for a training response.

The importance of task specificity must constantly be remembered and the training task should reflect as closely as possible the function requirements of each individual. In this way the effects of increased strength can be combined with motor learning processes which will act together to optimise function.

General maintenance

During all stages of treatment the strength and function of the whole body should be borne in mind and maintained as far as possible. The prognosis may be unknown; there may be improvement for some patients whilst others will deteriorate or remain static.

The situation must be reviewed regularly using both subjective and objective assessments and treatment goals, with aims and programmes revised accordingly. In addition to the peripheral effects of exercise on the muscles themselves, the effects of exercise on the heart and circulation are important and should always be remembered.

Task 6.5

What factors should be taken into account when developing an exercise programme? Consider two individuals with an acute ankle injury: one is a competitive athlete and the other is an elderly person who has had a stroke previously.

An unsatisfactory training programme

If difficulties arise which the therapist cannot correct easily, the reason for the patient's difficulties must be analysed. Analysis should include how, why and where the movement fails. The cause may include errors such as:

- planning faults
  - an overambitious or insufficient progression
  - the movement sequence may be too complicated
  - inadequate assistance, teaching and explanation

- psychological and emotional factors
  - lack of ability of the patient to understand what is required of them
  - poor memory
  - poor awareness by the patient of their body positioning
  - boredom, lack of interest and effort
  - fear of pain and exacerbating the clinical condition
  - fear of inadequacy in the outside world
  - dislike or lack of rapport with the therapist
- teaching faults
  - poor explanation and demonstration
  - lack of suitable stimuli
  - incorrect or inadequate help and correction
- other complicating factors
  - poor vision and hearing
  - poor general health resulting in lack of energy and motivation
  - coexisting pathology
  - sensory loss
  - impending litigation
  - the patient having become used to dependency or encouraged to be dependent by others.

Task 6.6

A training programme is apparently not having the desired effect. What factors might contribute towards this? Consider this situation for a number of different individuals.

REFERENCES

Agre J C, Rodriquez A A 1989 Validity of manual muscle testing in post-polio subjects with good or normal strength. Archives of Physical Medicine and Rehabilitation 70(Suppl): A17–18

American College of Sports Medicine 1978 Position statement on the recommended quantity and quality of exercise for developing and maintaining fitness in healthy adults. Medicine and Science in Sports 10: vii–x

Anderson K L, Shephard R J, Denolin H et al 1971 Fundamentals of exercise testing. World Health Organization, Geneva

Åstrand P E, Rodahl K 1988 Textbook of work physiology. Physiological basis of exercise. McGraw-Hill, Singapore

Borg G A V 1982 Physiological base of perceived exertion. Medicine and Science in Sports and Exercise 14: 377–381

Carlsöö S 1972 How man moves. Heinemann, London

Delorme T L, Watkins A L 1948 Techniques of progressive resistance exercise. Archives of Physical Medicine 29: 263–273

DeVries H A 1986 Physiology of exercise for physical education and athletics. William C Brown, Dubuque

Dirix A, Knuttgen H G, Tittel K (eds) 1988 The Olympic book of sports medicine. Blackwell Scientific, Oxford

Grimby G, Saltin B 1983 The ageing muscle: a mini review. Clinical Physiology 3: 209–218

Hellebrandt F A, Houtz S J 1958 Methods of muscle training: the influence of pacing. Physical Therapy Review 38: 319–322

Hurley M V, Jones D W, Wilson D, Newham D J 1992 Rehabilitation of quadriceps due to isolated rupture of the anterior cruciate ligament. Journal of Orthopaedic Rheumatology 5: 145–154

Jones D A, Round J M 1990 Skeletal muscle in health and disease. Manchester University Press, Manchester

Jones D A, Rutherford O M, Parker D F 1989 Physiological changes in skeletal muscle as a result of strength training. Quarterly Journal of Experimental Physiology 74: 233–256

Knott M, Voss D E 1968 Proprioceptive neuromuscular facilitation. Harper & Row, New York

Komi P V 1986 How important is neural drive for strength and power development in human skeletal muscle? In: Saltin B (ed) Biochemistry of exercise VI. International Series on Sports Sciences Vol 16. Human Kinetics, Champaign, Illinois

Krebbs D E 1989 Isokinetics, electrophysiological and clinical functions relationships following tourniquet-aided knee arthrotomy. Physical Therapy 69: 803–815

Kukulka C G 1992 Human skeletal muscle fatigue. In: Currier D P, Nelson R M (eds) Dynamics of human biological tissues. F A Davies, Philadelphia

McArdle W D, Katch F I, Katch V L 1996 Exercise physiology: energy, nutrition and human performance, 3rd edn. Lea & Febiger, Philadelphia

McDonagh M J N, Davies C T M 1984 Adaptive response of mammalian skeletal muscle to exercise with high loads. European Journal of Applied Physiology 52: 139–155

McDougall J D, Sale D G, Alway S E, Sutton J R 1984 Muscle fibre number in biceps brachii in bodybuilders and control subjects. Journal of Applied Physiology 57: 399–403

MacLaren D P, Gibson H, Parry-Billings M, Edwards R H T 1989 A review of metabolic and physiological factors in fatigue. In: Pandolf K B (ed) Exercise and Sport Sciences Reviews 17: 29–66

MacQueen I J 1954 Recent advances in the technique of progressive resistance exercise. British Medical Journal 2: 1193–1198

MacQueen I J 1956 The application of progressive resistance exercise in physiotherapy. Physiotherapy 40: 83–93

Martin E G, Lovett R W 1915 A method of testing muscular strength in infantile paralysis. Journal of the American Medical Association 65: 512–513

Moritani T, DeVries H A 1979 Neural factors versus hypertrophy in the time course of muscle strength gain. American Journal of Physical Medicine 58: 115–130

Newham D J 1988 The consequences of eccentric contractions and their relation to delayed onset muscle pain. European Journal of Applied Physiology 57: 353–359

Pilowsky I 1994 Pain and illness behaviour: assessment and management. In: Wall P D, Melzack R (eds) Textbook of pain, 3rd edn. Churchill Livingstone, Edinburgh

Rothwell J 1994 Control of human voluntary movement, 2nd edn. Chapman and Hall, London

Rowat K M, Jeans M E, LeFort S M 1994 A collaborative model of care: patient, family and health professionals. In: Wall P D, Melzack R (eds) Textbook of pain, 3rd edn. Churchill Livingstone, Edinburgh

Rutherford O M 1988 Muscle coordination and strength training: implications for injury rehabilitation. Sports Medicine 5: 196–202

Rutherford O M, Greig C A, Sargeant A J, Jones D A 1986a Strength training and power output: transference effects in the human quadriceps muscle. Journal of Sports Science 4: 101–107

Rutherford O M, Jones D A, Newham D J 1986b Clinical and experimental application of the percutaneous twitch superimposition technique for the study of human muscle activation. Journal of Neurology, Neurosurgery and Psychiatry 49: 1288–1291

Saltin B, Blomquist J H, Mitchell R L et al 1968 Response to submaximal and maximal exercise after bedrest and training. Circulation 38 (Suppl 7): 1–78

Sapega A A 1990 Muscle performance evaluation in orthopaedic practice. Journal of Bone and Joint Surgery 72A: 1562–1574

Shellock F G, Prentice W E 1985 Warming-up and stretching for improved physical performance and prevention of sports-related injuries. Sports Medicine 2: 267–278

Stokes M 1985 Reliability and repeatability of methods for measuring muscle in physiotherapy. Physiotherapy Practice 1: 71–76

Stokes M, Young A 1986 Measurement of quadriceps cross-sectional area by ultrasonography: a description of the technique and its application in physiotherapy. Physiotherapy Practice 2: 31–36

Tanner J M 1964 The physique of the Olympic athlete. George Allen & Unwin, London

Waddington P J 1976 In: Hollis M (ed) Practical exercise therapy. Blackwell Scientific, London, Chs 21–25

Watkins M P, Harris B A, Kozlowski B A 1984 Isokinetic testing in patients with hemiparesis. A pilot study. Physical Therapy 64: 184–189

Zinovieff A N 1951 Heavy resistance exercises. British Journal of Physical Medicine. June: 129–133

CHAPTER CONTENTS

Introduction   129

Motor learning   129
Definition   129
Historical perspective   130
Types of movement   130

Motor control   131
The schema theory   131
Skill   135
Maturation approach   135
Perceptual cognitive approach   136
Memory   136
Application in the rehabilitation setting   137

Closed and open skills   137
Closed skills   137
Open skills   138
Skill acquisition   138

Conclusion   140

7

Motor learning

N. Phillips

OBJECTIVES

At the end of this chapter you should be able to:

1. **Define the term motor learning and describe the limitations to motor control**

2. **Demonstrate an understanding of the information processing model of motor control**

3. **Define the term skill**

4. **Discuss the main components involved in the skill acquisition process**

5. **Discuss how long- and short-term memory are involved in learning and performing a motor skill.**

INTRODUCTION

Earlier chapters have explained some of the biomechanical principles of movement and the musculoskeletal and neurological bases of movement production and control. This chapter aims to explain how these human movements are learned and become the skilled coordinated patterns of activity necessary for function.

MOTOR LEARNING

Definition

Motor learning has been defined as a set process associated with practice or experience leading to relatively permanent changes in skilled behaviour

(Schmidt 1988). The set process mentioned in the above definition will be explained in this chapter. The other important term to note in the definition is 'relatively permanent changes'. A change in technique of carrying out a particular task is not considered learned if it just happens once or twice, possibly by chance. Again, this concept will also be explained later in the chapter.

Historical perspective

The field of movement control has historically been studied from two entirely different areas; those of neurophysiology and psychology. More recently it has become an independent area of study in its own right. Much of the research was initially done in physical education and this work has been developed and modified to suit the medical model.

Sherrington was an important early influence in neural control and his concepts of reflex responses to stimuli causing movement of the extremities is still a foundation of many treatment approaches today. It was this formative work that highlighted some of the sensory receptors involved in proprioception and introduced the concept of reciprocal innervation of agonist and antagonist muscle. The term *final common pathway* was also introduced at this time; this is where the influences from reflexes, sensory sources and cognitive sources converge at spinal level.

Weiner first developed the information processing model and likened the brain to a computer where information is received and processed leading to an output to muscles, creating movement. This approach was termed *cybernetics*.

Since then there has been a gradual progression towards a model of cognitive information processing (Schmidt 1975).

Winstein (1991) stated that the acquisition of motor learning is fundamental to human life and consists of neural, physical and behavioural components. This statement conveniently encompasses many of the aspects which will be covered in this chapter and serves as a reminder of the different aspects that need to be considered to understand the basic concepts of motor learning.

Types of movement

As described in Schmidt's (1988) definition, motor learning is a process which leads to changes in skilled behaviour. These motor skills are demonstrated by relatively predictable patterns of movement during performance of a particular task. Before investigating motor learning any further it is therefore necessary to outline the categories of movement, as it is the coordination of these movements which produce the learned motor skills described by Schmidt.

Movement can be broadly divided into two types:

1. Reflex – these are usually inherited.
2. Learned – these do not appear to be inherited and therefore need practice.

Both these types of movement can be either simple or complex. For example a simple reflex task would be blinking in response to an object near the eye. We might not be consciously aware that this has happened until after the response, and quite possibly then only because the object, such as dust, might have caused some irritation. We certainly wouldn't remember ever having to learn how to blink at the right time.

Conversely, a simple learned task would be clapping our hands. Learning to clap requires conscious control and a number of attempts to bring the hands into contact at the right time to make a noise; the concentration on a young child's face is testament to this. Similarly, breathing is a complex motor task subject to a great deal of variation but is under reflex control. We are not consciously aware of the general rate or depth of our breathing unless it changes dramatically, such as after a fairly intense physical effort, but there is a high degree of coordination required to produce the optimum rate and depth of breathing for every circumstance. On the other hand, a gymnastic tumbling routine is a complex learned task which requires hours of practice and takes a great deal of conscious control throughout the learning process.

MOTOR CONTROL

The schema theory

The coordination of movement, whether reflex or learned, can be termed *motor control*. The different areas of the central nervous system (CNS) which deal with the reflex or learned responses have been highlighted in Chapter 4 and include spinal cord, brain stem, motor cortex and cerebellum. The study of this field is about how movements are selected in response to sensory information obtained from the environment and/or within the body, based on previous experience. The process, known as the schema theory (Schmidt 1975), is thought to be controlled by the long-term memory and then modified by other centres in the central nervous system. This process can be divided into three main parts for clearer explanation:

- **Stimulus identification** – input via interoceptors or exteroceptors is identified as stimuli at CNS level.
- **Response selection** – the appropriate movement pattern in response to the identified stimuli is chosen based on prior experience.
- **Response programming** – the motor experience is carried out with feedback to decide if it was the right choice.

Figure 7.1 is adapted from Schmidt's (1975) schema theory and shows how these stages are thought to work.

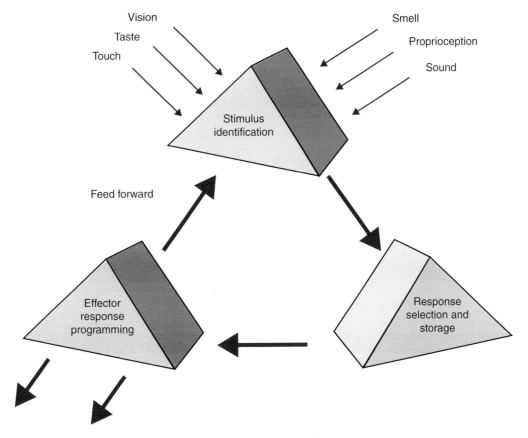

Figure 7.1 Information processing model. (Adapted, by permission, from R. A. Schmidt & T. D. Lee, 1999, Motor control and learning, 3rd edn. (Champaign, IL: Human Kinetics), 45.)

Stimulus identification

This stage can be subdivided into three separate steps.

Stimulus detection. Firstly, it should be noted that there would be a tremendous amount of information being absorbed from various sources during any simple everyday activity. For example, when walking downstairs the central nervous system is receiving information from the visual field, auditory input of the sound of each step, background noises and possibly continuing a conversation as well as proprioceptive input from joint, muscles and tendons about the depth and width of the step. This amount of information would be far too much for anyone to cope with efficiently so a filtering process takes place of what is important for that particular function and environment, based on prior experience. Any input considered irrelevant is discarded before continuing the process to conscious levels.

Consequently, there is not usually conscious awareness of this level of perception unless the brain receives input it does not recognise or is not expecting in comparison to previous similar functional tasks. For instance, during that normally familiar task of walking downstairs you don't notice the width and depth of each step, allowing you to continue your conversation, unless one step is suddenly different. You then become very aware of the steps beneath your feet. Your brain takes in the visual input and proprioceptive and tactile feedback but only alerts your conscious thought if there is a problem. How many times have you walked down a flight of steps and almost tripped because one step is slightly different to the others? You turn and look at the step and, for a while, watch each step carefully to avoid stumbling again. Normally stimuli which have been received for a while are ignored, whereas any new stimuli are passed on to the next stage of the process. This is a type of internal feedback and is termed *knowledge of performance*.

Stimulus interpretation. How you interpret information will depend on what sort of stimulation is expected and any prior experience of similar situations. This is a form of pattern recognition which is stored in the long-term memory.

The accuracy of this interpretation will depend on how efficiently the individual can retrieve previous experience from the long-term memory. For example, someone who has been on a rollercoaster many times will take in stimuli from the inner ear and the eyes but ignore input from the gut. Needless to say the first time rollercoaster rider is likely to feel quite sick if he pays more attention to the sensory information coming from his stomach.

A typical example in the sporting world would be two rugby union centres, one experienced player and one novice. The experienced player will recognise the body position and foot movements of an opponent who is about to make a dummy pass and react accordingly, successfully tackling the other player. The novice will probably miss the tell-tale visual signs allowing earlier reaction, and feel very foolish lying on the floor having missed the tackle as his opponent runs past him. In addition, the experienced player will be able to use a more parallel style of taking in external cues, which will be discussed later in the chapter. It means that instead of dealing with one stimulus at a time, which would result in quite a delay in some responses, the expert player could notice and react to a few things at once, allowing things to be taken in at a glance. This would in turn allow concentration on other skills such as tactical decision making or ball retention skills.

Task 7.1

If you can drive a car, think back to when you were learning. How many different things did the instructor tell you to pay attention to at once? How many different things did you have to do with your feet and your hands at the same time? How many lessons did it take you to be able to cope with all those tasks at the same time?

This is the difference between a learner having to deal with such challenges in a more *serial* manner whereas practice allows some challenges to be dealt with at the same time, or in *parallel*.

Stimulus selection. How much or what type of stimuli are selected to be passed on to the next stage of the decision making process will depend on how much concentration or attention is devoted to this particular function at the time. Selection of the most useful stimuli for that particular task requires the correct allocation of attention to ensure that the appropriate information is passed on. The balance of the breadth of attention needs to match the focus of attention for the correct selection of movement. For example, compare attention to a beam of light; it can be a tightly focused spotlight or a diffused beam covering a large area. The focus needs to be tight enough to increase concentration but concentrated too tightly it will create a tunnel vision, thereby missing important cues around the periphery. Someone learning to ski has to concentrate on controlling the skis and is probably not able to take in the alpine scenery and stay on her feet at the same time. Conversely, she may not take in peripheral cues, such as other skiers or trees, in time to do anything about it!

Response selection

Once the afferent stimuli have been accepted and recognised, the brain must then decide what sort of response to make. A movement plan is assembled, based on identical or similar previous performances, which is tried out in the individual's head, usually at an unconscious level, to decide if the outcome of the movement is appropriate for the task. Any necessary modifications are then made before the movement plan is passed on to the effector stage.

Imagine you are about to assess a patient in an outpatient clinic, having been given a referral with a brief diagnosis of a condition you have not treated before. First you look up the condition and different methods of treatment in a textbook (long-term memory). Then you make a rough plan of what you are going to do in the assessment (short-term memory). During your assessment you modify what you do depending on what information you receive from your patient. Once you finish your assessment you organise the subjective and objective information you have collected and formulate a treatment plan. This whole process is similar to the decision making process involved with every motor task.

From this example you will see that if the emphasis is on a thoughtful or cognitive process, as described in the schema theory, then there is likely to be a substantial delay which would be too slow for most functional tasks; this is even more the case when considering complex skills. For instance a tennis forehand takes around 200 ms to perform. An experienced tennis player does not need to consciously remember what sort of response a ball travelling towards their forehand requires but reacts to the ball immediately because the visual system is used to responding to this particular stimulus. This function is termed *perception-action coupling* and allows for the faster reaction times needed in many activities. This is a type of triggered reaction and is thought to be the way in which practice can produce the speed of reaction needed in many activities where the stimulus is similar but not always identical.

Response programming

This is the stage in the process where the selected response is coordinated by recruiting the appropriate muscles with the right amount of effort, in the right direction at the right time. At first consideration this would seem to be an insurmountable task to be performed within the time limits needed for almost all skilled movements. If every stage of all our movements had to be controlled by cognitive processes, how could we possibly be able to think of other things or be able to speak or listen at the same time?

Central programming in the motor cortex allows unconscious performance of some skills once they have been learned, allowing an individual to be able to divert cognitive processes to other areas which might be necessary at the time.

Constant monitoring of the movement through proprioceptive feedback allows knowledge of performance before knowledge of results. This means that we are able to have an awareness of how the movement is progressing by utilising sensory information from muscle spindles and joint and tendon receptors without waiting for information from visual or auditory receptors on completion of the task. Continued monitoring each time a motor task is performed means that an expert in a particular skill will know if that movement was successful before viewing the outcome. For example, experienced weightlifters will know whether they have made a successful clean and jerk attempt before the referees pass or fail the lift. They can relate the current performance to previous attempts and compare the feel of that particular movement with previous successful and unsuccessful attempts as the movement is happening, rather than waiting to view the outcome. Afferent information from joints and muscles is vital for the success of this function.

Engram

Coordination of a complex activation of different muscle groups for a specific task such as weightlifting is known as a motor programme or engram. As mentioned earlier, for a coordinated movement to be accomplished there must be an optimal combination of agonists, antagonists, synergists and fixators at the right force, in the right direction and with the right timing. These patterns of movements are thought to be stored as action memory traces in the motor cortex once they have been refined through feedback mechanisms (Vansant 1995).

Feed forward

It should be noted that some motor tasks are still too fast for this type of cognitive control, which has a refractory period of approximately 200 ms. A boxer's punch has a reaction time of 90 ms (Schmidt 1991). This is well below the reaction time necessary for a cognitive response. A *feed forward* mechanism is thought to control this type of task which relies on more of a reflex reaction, as discussed earlier in the chapter. The memory traces in the motor cortex instigate preparatory muscle stimulation in order to respond at this speed. Although this mechanism allows a faster response, the boxer does not have time to think about altering the movement once the response has been initiated. This is why a boxer has to practise each different type of punch in his repertoire until the feed forward mechanism is developed sufficiently for each response.

Realistically, the brain would never have the capacity to store individual movement programmes for each and every functional task. Schmidt's (1975) schema theory helps explain this phenomenon. He defined a motor scheme as a general motor programme that would be activated for all movements that are associated with a common task.

Limitations of motor control

Looking at how this process of motor control works, there are obviously going to be limitations within the whole mechanism. These limitations are:

- Capacity – how much information the system can process at any one time. Every individual has a limit to how much information he can cope with all at once.
- Speed – how fast it can process the information. This will depend on whether the individual has to deal with the information in series, i.e. one element at a time if it is unfamiliar, or in parallel, i.e. at the same time if it is very familiar.
- Distortion – the extent to which information is lost or distorted during the process. This limitation will often depend on concentration or attention.

Refractory period

Schmidt's original information processing model assumed that all these processes happen in series, i.e. one after the other. The process in this form would understandably involve a significant delay between stimulus and response, which is called the *refractory period* (Fig. 7.2). This delay would fit into the speed limitation of the control process described above.

In Figure 7.2 the top reaction shows the time taken for a response to be generated to a particular stimulus. If each stimulus were processed in series, when another stimulus was applied before the initial response could be generated the processing would have to wait until the first response had been dealt with, hence increasing the reaction time necessary for the second response.

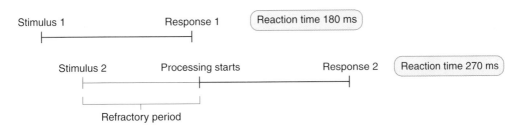

Figure 7.2 Refractory period.

More recent thinking has led to the view that some of these processes can happen in parallel, which would reduce the reaction time involved between impulse recognition and motor reaction as in the earlier example of the rugby player. This would explain the ability of an expert to perform complicated decision making processes, allowing motor skills to be performed more efficiently.

Skill

The term skill has been mentioned frequently when discussing the process of motor learning. Before explaining how skills are learned and developed it might help to define the word. Skill is the accuracy, consistency and efficiency of movement deployment (Higgins 1991).

Accuracy, consistency, efficiency

In other words, the desired outcome of the motor task has to be achieved (accuracy) in a high proportion of the attempts (consistency) and with the minimal amount of physical effort (efficiency). For example, a beginner throwing a dart at a dart board might well hit the bullseye. If she did, most people watching would put her success down to 'beginners' luck'. There would be a very slim chance of the lucky beginner reproducing her success consistently until she had learned which components of the combination of movements produced the first successful attempt.

In addition to learning the optimal coordination of movements for a task, the beginner also has to learn the optimal amount of muscle work necessary. Usually people learning a new task will hold themselves very stiffly, only moving the limb sections absolutely necessary for the task in hand. Anyone who has ever tried out a new sport will remember the feeling of aching all over despite only needing to work certain areas for that activity. Students learning a new manual technique will have to consciously relax their shoulders as they gradually get closer to their ears and their arms begin to ache. This is known as freezing degrees of freedom (Vereijken et al 1992). As the individual becomes more proficient, the limb and trunk segments are given a little more freedom of movement, making the functional task appear more fluid.

There are, once again, a variety of theories about how this learning process takes place. These fall into two main schools of thought: the maturation approach (Gessell et al 1974) and the perceptual cognitive approach (Bressan & Woollacott 1982).

Maturation approach

This approach describes alternating periods of stability and instability during maturation. The periods of instability are thought to be the times when new patterns of control are being learned and hence result in some instability or lack of control until the pattern becomes skilled. For example, toddlers learning to walk will take a number of attempts over a few months until they can control a walk without falling over. During this time the child's skill level in walking will be unpredictable; some days almost perfect and other days disastrous. Following this approach, each functional ability would develop in the same way throughout childhood, adolescence and adulthood.

Perceptual cognitive approach

The perceptual cognitive approach suggests that intellect may have a bearing on how well a motor skill is learned. Sensory input is regarded as having a significant impact on motor performance and feedback of the outcome of a particular movement. With this approach trial and error play an important part in the learning process, where the learner consciously discards the motor patterns which produced an unsuccessful outcome and retains those that produced an outcome closer to the ideal.

Memory

Whichever the approach favoured, once a motor programme has been established, it then takes repeated practice to develop that pattern into a skilled movement. For any learning to occur there must be a memory of that particular skill to allow repetition and refinement. This is thought to be controlled in the area of the cortex concerned with long-term memory.

Figure 7.3 illustrates a simplified version of how memory controls the learning process. First, sensory information is received via a variety of sources, as in the previous model of motor control. This might be a combination of sensory input such as kinaesthetic sensation, vision, sound, light, touch or pain. The relevant information is stored temporarily in the short-term memory. For something to be maintained in the short-term memory it has to be constantly repeated, rather like remembering a telephone number from the directory when you haven't got a pen to hand. Once someone speaks to you the number is often forgotten. This is when information is lost by replacement with new sensory information, which might be similar or completely different to the previous information.

To be able to recall that number you would usually remember it in chunks of numbers and associate it with a particular name which allows it to be stored in the long-term memory. The first few times you need to use that number again you still have to look it up. Eventually the number

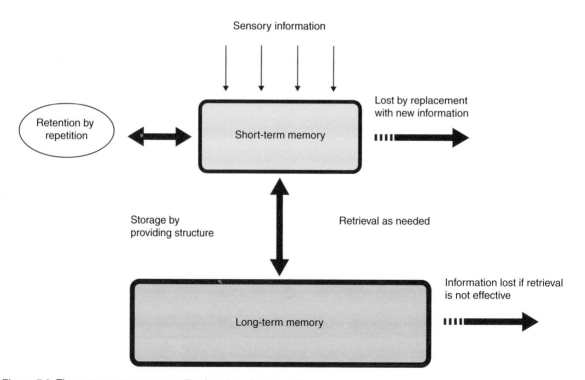

Figure 7.3 The memory process controlling learning of a new skill.

gets used frequently enough for you to remember it without looking it up. This is because you have practised retrieving the information from the long-term memory until this process becomes efficient by strengthening the memory trace of that particular skill.

Task 7.2

Working in pairs, try two slightly different tasks:

- One person reads out any line from this book, letter by letter, backwards. To give the other person a chance, only use up to 20 letters.
  - ask them to repeat the sequence of letters (without writing them down)
  - then get them to recite a nursery rhyme
  - ask them to repeat the sequence of letters.
- This time read out the same letters forwards as words.
  - repeat the same process as above.

Was the second attempt any different from the first?

Application in the rehabilitation setting

Transfer that model to a rehabilitation situation and it might explain why patients sometimes appear to retain improvement following treatment more than at other times. For example, imagine you have just spent some time trying to improve vastus medialis control in weight bearing during a gait rehabilitation session. Following repeated practice the patient can eventually contract vastus medialis in a functional weight bearing position. She is then sent home and on returning for the next treatment she appears to have forgotten everything that was taught in the previous session. This is possibly because the repetitions of the exercise were rehearsed to allow retention in the short-term memory but either not given enough structure to allow long-term memory storage or not given the practice of retrieval from long-term memory. The information then becomes lost or useless. One way to improve this process would be to:

- explain why the exercise is being given, to provide structure and assist with retention in long-term memory

- teach the particular motor skill required (vastus medialis control in standing)
- add in a new activity, possibly related to the first
- repeat the first skill/activity, requiring recall of the taught skill.

Variable practice

Changing the activity will have the effect of distracting from information stored in short-term memory. This will encourage retrieval from long-term memory to facilitate retention of the new skill which is control of knee extension in weight bearing. Repeated retention and retrieval will strengthen the memory trace. In addition to this, if the second activity performed is similar to the first it is thought that some learning is transferred between skills, thus speeding up the learning process. This type of approach is called variable practice and there is some evidence demonstrating its efficacy (Lee et al 1985, Shea & Khol 1990, Eidson and Stadulis 1991).

Task 7.3

Think about how you would teach someone an exercise as part of a rehabilitation programme and how you could improve the skill acquisition process. Think of an example for each of the following cases:

- improve understanding for more efficient storage in LTM
- provide better information on knowledge of performance
- progress to a more automatic movement.

CLOSED AND OPEN SKILLS

For the purposes of this chapter, skills are split into two broad categories:

- closed skills
- open skills.

Closed skills

A closed skill is movement which is repeated in the same way for each performance of the one task. Using the example of the weightlifter again, the technique for the clean and jerk will be identical for each attempt at the same weight. This skill requires a very high degree of spatial control with relatively little time limit in comparison to catching a ball, for instance. To demonstrate what happens when a greater temporal (time) control is applied observe what happens in a competition when a lifter has to rush out to make his attempt because time is running out. It quite often fails because he has practised the movement skill many times but at the same speed. The environment that this type of skill is performed in is said to be a *stable environment*. If any part of that environment is changed, the ability to perform that skill will be compromised. The fairly rigid sequencing that occurs in a movement such as this limits the performer to a relatively narrow choice of movements compared to an open skill, but allows very efficient performance (Browenstein 1997).

Open skills

An open skill requires a combination of both spatial and temporal control. The movement has to be practised many times as in a closed skill, but variations in speed and effort have to be applied to be able to adapt to a changing environment. This time refer back to the tackling rugby player as the example. Changes in the intended movement may well have to take place, depending on the actions of the opposing player and possibly the actions of players in the same team. This type of environment is said to be an *unstable environment*.

When re-educating a motor skill in a rehabilitation environment, both these principles need to be considered. To start progressing through a new skill, such as balancing on one leg following an ankle injury, a high degree of cognitive attention is required, using visual cues as well as input from mechanoreceptors in the limb. At this stage balancing can only be maintained as a closed skill. If any part of the environment changes, such as introducing an unstable base of support, balance reactions are challenged once more. As balance improves, secondary activities are introduced. If

balance has to be maintained whilst catching a ball or being pulled in one direction by elastic tubing, the balance strategies have to change with each different circumstance. Exercises such as this encourage skills learned as a conscious effort to become automatic and to adapt to a changing environment. This same balance activity has now become an open skill in preparation for the functional mobility required of the ankle in everyday life.

Taylor et al (1998) highlight the effects on motor performance of diverting attention in their study investigating joint position error detection during concurrent cognitive distraction. Joint position sense was reduced in subjects who received an auditory distraction whilst performing the task. They point out that this can have a positive or negative effect, depending on the timing of the distraction. For someone concentrating on mastering a very new task, distraction could reduce the safety of the activity. Conversely, appropriate distraction as a progression in later stages would supplement a rehabilitation programme.

Both types of skill need a significant amount of repetition to allow efficient retrieval from long-term memory and the development of a motor engram.

For example:

— Learning to walk (to age 6) – 3 million steps
— Parade ground marching (end of army basic training) – 0.8 million steps
— Hand knitting – 1.5 million stitches
— Violin playing to a professional level – 2.5 million notes (4500 hours of practice)
— Baseball throwing (pitcher) – 1.6 million throws
— Basketball shot from any angle – 1 million throws (Kottke et al 1978).

Skill acquisition

Bressan and Woollacott (1982) describe a model of the stages of skill acquisition (Fig. 7.4).

Skill construction

The first stage involves organisation of the skill when an approximate estimation of the move-

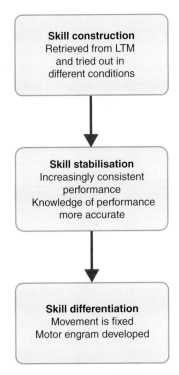

Skill construction
Retrieved from LTM
and tried out in
different conditions

Skill stabilisation
Increasingly consistent
performance
Knowledge of performance
more accurate

Skill differentiation
Movement is fixed
Motor engram developed

Figure 7.4 A model of the stages of skill acquisition. (Reproduced with permission from Bressan & Woollacott 1982.)

ment is constructed which will vary, depending on prior experience of similar activity. Similar movement patterns used in other motor tasks can be transferred to the new skill and adapted as appropriate. For example, good basketball players could transfer their ball handling skills to other sports such as rugby. This would be called *positive transfer*. In this instance hand/eye co-ordination, wide visual field and manual dexterity skills would be similar enough in both to allow modification between the two activities. However, a squash player would have problems on initially trying to play tennis as, despite the improved hand/eye coordination, the racquet action required in squash has a detrimental effect on the technique used in tennis. This is called *negative transfer*. A fair amount of trial and error will also be involved by the learner who will need to devote a relatively high level of cognitive attention to the task to appreciate an overall picture of the required movement task. This

would explain why a learner cannot always listen to a teacher or coach at the same time as attempting to perform the new skill being taught. Watching a child learning to write illustrates this point quite well.

Skill stabilisation

As learning continues and the skill begins to stabilise, successful attempts will become more frequent and movement patterns will become more consistent. Feedback providing knowledge of results is important at this stage to correct minor faults as the motor engram is becoming established; this will be difficult to change once the movement becomes automatic. In support of this, Prapavessis and McNair (1999) found that subjects who received verbal instruction and correction improved subsequent attempts at a jumping and landing task more quickly than those who used their own sensory feedback from each attempt. Hewett et al (1996) had similar findings, where subjects taken through a programme designed to improve neuromuscular control in addition to strength in the lower limb were able to reduce landing forces on the knee more efficiently than those who progressed through a strengthening programme alone.

A typical example of this would be that someone who is progressing through a gait re-education rehabilitation following a lower limb fracture will be encouraged to continue using a stick or crutches after the fracture has healed enough to bear weight. This is not just a safety aspect but it prevents an abnormal gait pattern becoming automatic, making progression to a more normal gait easier once the appropriate joint range and muscle strength have been achieved. Feedback on correct gait patterns can then be reinforced before full weight bearing is encouraged.

Skill differentiation

By the final stage the movement pattern has been established. Knowledge of performance is now being monitored and the proprioceptive feedback is routinely being filtered out from conscious awareness unless there is any significant change. This change in allocation of attention means that more can be devoted to higher processes, within the individual's capacity, during the task. Think back to the earlier example of the experienced rugby player who is able to time the tackle more appropriately and also be more aware of the tactical considerations happening around him. This ability has become possible because the actual movement skill has become automatic, freeing up more attention for anticipation or communication with team mates.

Think back to Task 7.1 about driving a car. Once you have learned to drive, you can probably listen to music, talk to a passenger, read road signs and be aware of other traffic and pedestrians whilst performing the task of driving automatically. But what if you suddenly have to drive in another country on the other side of the road? Think about what sort of things you do to be able to perform the task. Suddenly the task changes and cannot be dealt with automatically. The sorts of things you might do would be to turn the music off, stop talking and ask people to look for road signs and landmarks.

What you have done with these actions is to reduce some of the sensory input and additional cognitive tasks being performed at the same time, in order to make more capacity for a motor task that now requires cognitive attention rather than being automatic.

Any change in sensory input involved with a learned stabilised skill will have a similar effect. Injury is no exception to this. For instance, if a joint has smaller range of movement after an injury, the kinaesthetic input from joint and muscle proprioceptors will be different. The cognitive process of relearning a motor skill, whether it be walking, running or climbing stairs, will need to be repeated, albeit with some prior experience for comparison, until the task becomes automatic again.

Task 7.4

Think of ways in which the experience of some pain or discomfort following injury would affect the control process in a functional movement which had been automatic prior to injury.

CONCLUSION

Motor learning requires a combination of factors to be successful. This chapter has outlined many of the principles involved, but the reader is directed to some of the texts solely devoted to this subject for more in-depth information. These texts are listed in the reference section. The main factors to consider in the field of motor learning are short- and long-term memory, transfer of skills, knowledge of both performance and results, and practice. How we use these principles in the clinical setting will have a significant impact on the success of a rehabilitation programme, whether the ultimate goal is to walk unaided, transfer from bed to chair or return to a highly skilled activity.

You should now have an understanding about how an individual controls movement both for simpler repetitive movements and more complex skilled tasks. You should understand how these skills are learned and how the learning environment can be manipulated to facilitate this process.

REFERENCES

Bressan E S, Woollacott M H 1982 A prescriptive paradigm for sequencing instruction in physical education. Human Movement Science 1: 155–175

Browenstein B 1997 In: Browenstein B, Shaw B (eds) Functional movement in orthopaedic and sports physical therapy: evaluation, treatment and outcomes. Churchill Livingstone, Edinburgh

Eidson T A, Stadulis R E 1991 Effects of variability of practice on the transfer and performance of open and closed motor skills. Adapted Physical Activity Quarterly 8(4): 342–3556

Gessell A, Ilg F L, Ames L B 1974 Infant and child in the culture of today (revised edn). Harper and Row, New York

Hewett T E, Stroupe A L, Nance T A, Noyes F R 1996 Plyometric training in female athletes. Decreased impact forces and increased hamstring torques. American Journal of Sports Medicine 24(6): 765–773

Higgins S 1991 Motor control acquisition. Physical Therapy 71(2): 123–129

Kottke F J, Halpern D, Easton J K M, Ozel A T, Burrill C A 1978 The training of coordination. Archives of Physical Medicine and Rehabilitation 59: 567–572

Lee T D, Magill R A, Weeks D J 1985 Influence of practice schedule on testing schema theory predictions in adults. Journal of Motor Behaviour 17(3): 283–299

Prapavessis H, McNair P J 1999 Effects of instruction in jumping technique and experience jumping on ground reaction forces. Journal of Orthopaedic and Sports Physical Therapy 29: 352–356

Schmidt R A 1975 A schema theory of discrete motor skill learning. Psychological Review 82: 225–260

Schmidt R A 1988 Motor control and learning. A behavioural emphasis, 2nd edn. Human Kinetics, Champaign, Illinois

Schmidt R A 1991 Motor learning and performance. Human Kinetics, Champaign, Illinois

Shea C H, Kohl R M 1990 Specificity and variability of practice. Research Quarterly for Exercise and Sport 61 (12): 169–177

Taylor R A, Marshall P H, Dunlap R D, Gable C D, Sizer P S 1998 Knee position error detection in closed and open kinetic chain tasks during concurrent cognitive distraction. Journal of Orthopaedic and Sports Physical Therapy 28(2): 81–87

Vansant A 1995 Motor control and motor learning. In: Cech D, Martin S (eds) Functional movement development across the lifespan. W B Saunders, Philadelphia

Vereijken B, van Emmerik R E, Whiting H T A, Newell K M 1992 Free(z)ing degrees of freedom in skill acquisition. Journal of Motor Behaviour 24(1): 133–142

Winstein C J 1991 Knowledge of results in motor learning: implications for physiotherapy. Physical Therapy 71(2): 140–149

CHAPTER CONTENTS

Introduction   143

Kinematic assessment of human movement   144
Use of film for kinematic analysis of movement   144
Hand held goniometers   148
Electrogoniometers   148
Optoelectronic devices and polarised light
goniometers   150

Kinetic analysis   151
Isokinetic dynamometry   152
The isokinetic dynamometer as a measure of human
function   153

Force and pressure measurements   153
Ground reaction forces   153
Pure pressure measurements   154

Electromyography   156
The basis of EMG   156
Types of electrodes   156
Recording the EMG   156
EMG processing   157
Clinical significance of EMG for measuring human
movement   158
EMG and the phasic activity of muscles   158
EMG and force production   158
EMG and isometric tension   159
EMG and isotonic tension   159

Energy expenditure analysis   159

8

Measuring and evaluating human movement

M. Trew   T. Everett

OBJECTIVES

When you have completed this chapter you should be able to:

1. **Understand why the measurement of human movement is difficult**

2. **Discuss the range of measurement techniques available**

3. **Choose the appropriate tool for evaluating and measuring movement**

4. **Evaluate the value of the different measurement techniques.**

INTRODUCTION

At the moment there is no single, satisfactory solution to the problem of how to measure human movement and, in particular, human movement when functional activities are being undertaken. Whilst it is relatively easy to measure static parameters such as limb length or the position of a stationary joint, it is considerably more difficult to measure and analyse the performance of functional activities. The problem lies in the multifactorial, multidimensional nature of human movement which results in the need to measure not only factors such as joint movement or muscle activity but also to take into account the control and the quality of the movement. Currently, it is not possible to measure the control and quality of movement, mainly because there is no consensus about what these terms mean; they are very difficult to define. Until there is a consensus as to the exact meaning of quality, it is unlikely that satisfactory measures will be designed, and whether it will ever be possible to produce a global definition of quality of movement is open to discussion. Quality encompasses many factors such as precision, smoothness, velocity, range and appropriateness; the importance of each of these factors differs from movement to movement so that the likelihood of producing a universal measure of quality would seem remote.

Other chapters describe normal patterns of movement seen in some common functional activities and the facts that formed the bases of these chapters were obtained by collating the work of many scientists who were looking at different aspects of the same movement. The complexity of measuring human movement has made it extremely difficult to design a system whereby all the parameters involved can be measured simultaneously. Those professionals who need to analyse normal and abnormal human movement are faced with the problem that they need to consider all the factors which together contribute to normal movement, yet there is no practical way of achieving this. One solution is to undertake a subjective assessment of the activity, after which it should become clear which parameters are most important. With this knowledge a limited number of appropriate measurement tools can be chosen to specifically measure the key parameters.

KINEMATIC ASSESSMENT OF HUMAN MOVEMENT

Kinematics considers human movement in terms of position and displacement (angular and linear) of body segments, centre of gravity, and acceleration and velocities of the whole body or segments of the body such as a lower limb or the trunk.

A kinematic assessment will provide information on the relationship of parts of the body to each other. This is useful in measuring joint angles during complex movements and has provided the basis for understanding functional activities including rising from a chair or stair climbing: much of the information in Chapter 10

comes from kinematic assessments. Equally valuable is a knowledge of the acceleration and velocities of body segments; for example, in prosthetics it is important that the design of a prosthetic limb ensures that it has similar properties of acceleration and velocity as a normal limb. Knowledge of the displacement patterns of the centre of gravity during movement gives information on efficiency and this is an important factor in most rehabilitation programmes.

Kinematic assessment uses anatomical terminology and a spatial reference system where:

Y = vertical component or direction

X = anterior posterior component or direction

Z = medial lateral component or direction.

Figure 8.1 illustrates the conventions used when measuring angles in the major body planes. Angles in the XY plane are measured from 0° in the X direction with positive angles being anti-clockwise, which makes extension positive and flexion negative. In the YZ plane, angles start at 0° in the Y direction with positive angles being anti-clockwise (Winter 1990).

Use of film for kinematic analysis of movement

The simplest method of assessment and evaluation of human function is by visual observation. Whilst experienced observers can obtain a substantial amount of subjective information about human movement, they do not have the ability to observe and remember all the complex, multi-joint movement patterns that occur in even the simplest functional activities. The unassisted eye functions at the equivalent of 1/30th of a second exposure time and can only see details of slow motion; the brain, too, despite its amazing ability, has a limit on the amount of information it can absorb and remember. As a consequence, when observing complex movement only a limited amount of the detail is actually seen (Terauds 1984). The other major drawback to unaided visual observation is that only subjective information can be obtained and without baseline data, reliable measurement of change is impossible.

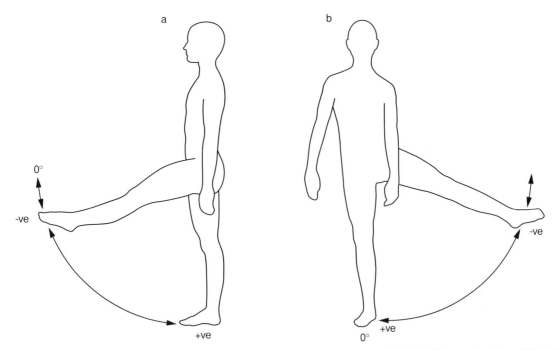

Figure 8.1 The conventions used when measuring angles in the major body planes: (a) in the XY or sagittal plane; (b) in the YZ or coronal plane.

Film has been used to enhance understanding of human movement for more than a hundred years. Cine, video or still photography are all valuable as they all enable movement to be observed in much more detail than is possible on unaided visual analysis; they also permit measurement and provide a permanent record. Whilst cine is the most accurate of these methods of movement analysis, it is expensive, difficult to use and the process of developing films is time consuming. Still photography is limited by the fact that it only captures one instant in time and the totality of movement can not be seen. Video is cheap, easy to use, very portable and the results are immediately available. These advantages outweigh the limitations of only being able to sample data 50 or 60 times a second and it is now used in preference to all other methods.

Cine film and video tape can be stored over many years and replayed repeatedly. This is particularly valuable as it allows the analysis of movement to occur after the patient or subject has left, when there is time for uninterrupted observation and analysis. Visual analysis of film is enhanced by the use of freeze-frame, slow motion facilities and computer-aided analysis software. Video and cine film of human movement enhance the acquisition of qualitative information and quantitative data, and can also be used as feedback to the patient or athlete.

The qualitative and quantitative use of film

A vast amount of qualitative information can be obtained from film. Human movement as a total pattern can be observed and re-observed. The relationship of all body parts to each other can be seen, as can the quality of the movement – whether it is fast or slow, uncoordinated or smooth. The patient can be shown the film as part of the rehabilitation process and this greatly facilitates understanding of movement difficulties. Patients who have seen their own films are frequently able to formulate their own recovery objectives and monitor their own progress. Though there is no research in this area, it is likely that this greatly improves compliance and as such is a tool that ought to be used frequently.

Case Study 8.1

Mrs Wilson, 59, had had rheumatoid arthritis for approximately 20 years when she suddenly noticed an increased clumsiness when undertaking functional activities using her hands. She had learned to cope with limited movement and pain at both shoulder and elbow joints and severe ulnar deviation of her metacarpophalangeal joints. For many years she had managed most activities of daily living despite her substantial problems, but now she found she was knocking over items as she went to pick them up and her accuracy at putting down objects like cups or a vase of flowers was seriously compromised. She reported that she had noted no change or deterioration in her physical condition so it was decided to evaluate the total upper limb joint movement patterns by use of video. When viewed in slow motion the tape revealed an inability to fully extend the joints of her index finger beyond the resting position. As she performed grip activities, the index finger became caught on the object she wished to pick up and, because of the lack of extension, she was unable to let go of objects at the end of a task. A physical examination subsequently showed total rupture of the extensor indices tendon.

Finally, the film can be kept and used for subjective comparison with films taken at a later date, enabling judgements to be made about progression or deterioration.

Quantitative data can be obtained by digitising the video image and subjecting the data to computer processing and analysis. Digitisation is the process whereby the image or parts of the image are converted to digital form so that the data can be manipulated by a computer. In order to be able to digitise film, skin markers must be placed over major landmarks prior to filming. The film is then either manually or automatically digitised. This process involves viewing each frame (or field) of the video tape and identifying and storing the coordinates for each of the skin markers, in each of the frames of the film. The data thus obtained can be called upon when calculations are required. The process of digitising can be undertaken either manually or by use of a computer programme. Experiments in the author's laboratory have shown that manual digitising is reliable, accurate and that human error is relatively small especially with experienced digitisers. Unfortunately, the process is time-consuming as only 15 to 30 points can be digitised per minute. Automatic digitisation using the computer is also accurate and reliable, though it is necessary to undertake manual checks to ensure that the computer does not confuse two different markers when they cross in space. Direct measurements of an image on video tape taken from the video screen are subject to considerable error and should not be used as a method of quantifying human movement.

Computer aided analysis of video tape can give a wide range of information and most systems now allow the analysis of movement in more than one plane.

The computer-analysis software makes it possible to plot body coordinates (centre of gravity, etc.). Knowledge of the position of the centre of gravity is important when considering the efficiency of movement. For example smooth displacements of the centre of gravity tend to indicate a more efficient movement than those where the centre of gravity is subjected to extensive vertical displacement. Figure 10.3 (see Ch. 10) illustrates the displacement of the centre of gravity and the original information that enabled this figure to be drawn was taken from computer analysis of video tape.

The computer can also generate stick diagrams and these are valuable as an initial qualitative analysis of the sequence of movement. A stick diagram of a jump is shown in Figure 8.2.

Data on joint angles in one or more planes of movement can be collected and the pattern of movement at a joint can be graphically represented and related to other joints or the whole body. Joint angle data are available for any instance in the movement sequence.

The velocity and acceleration of limb segments can be measured and the data give useful information about patterns of movement, for example when comparing the acceleration of the tibia in the swing phase of normal gait with the acceleration of the shank of an artificial limb in amputee gait.

Using video tape, it is also possible to calculate cadence, stride length and velocity in gait, but to do this it is necessary to provide some form of scaling in the filming area (Whittle 1991). In con-

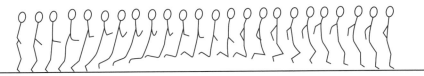

Figure 8.2 A stick diagram of a jump. This was generated from data obtained by digitising a video film and gives an overall, subjective impression of the movement.

junction with force plate data, information on joint angles can be used to calculate net joint moments as described in Chapter 3 (Winter 1990).

Filming with video is a relatively simple and cheap technique that can be undertaken almost anywhere and, because it does not require measuring equipment to be attached to the subject, it does not disrupt the movement being analysed. (Whether there is a psychological effect on movement patterns brought about by the self-consciousness of being filmed is not known, and this should not be discounted.) The value of film as a movement analysis tool has long been recognised by sport scientists, but the health care professions appear to have been less enthusiastic about its use. Film has been used to analyse human movement in a limited range of activities, for example the ability of paraplegic subjects to reach from their wheelchairs (Curtis et al 1995); the measurement of angular velocity of the leg in a patient with cerebral palsy (Winter 1982); the biomechanical analysis of swing through gait (Noreau et al 1995); and the energy transfers of children walking with crutches (McGill & Dainty 1984).

For meaningful data collection, great care must be taken in setting up the filming site and arranging the camera. For accurate spatial and temporal measurements the camera must be positioned carefully in relation to the subject, and timing and scale devices must be included in the field of view.

Frame rate. Video, unlike cine, has a fixed frame rate which in the UK and Europe is 25 frames per second (in the USA it is 30 frames per second). Each frame can be broken down into two fields which in Europe gives 50 fields per second. Some authorities (Winter 1990) feel that this rate is acceptable for all but the fastest

athletic movements and is, therefore, acceptable for work with patients. However, a low frame rate will not guarantee capture of specific moments of impact or the instant of change of direction in normal human movement, such as the instant of heel strike, etc. For detailed analysis of specific instants of the movement cycle, it may be more appropriate to use a cine camera with a variable frame rate rather than video, although the comparative difficulty and the cost of using cine has to be a counter argument.

Shutter speed. It is essential to use a camera that has a variable shutter facility. If the shutter speed cannot be controlled, fast movement will give spatial blurring and make the identification of the position of skin markers impossible. A shutter speed of a thousandth of a second will eliminate spatial blurring, but the short period when the shutter is open will result in the film being under exposed. This can be solved by using additional lighting, though that in itself may be off-putting to the patient.

Skin markers. Computer aided analysis of film requires the placement of skin markers over bony landmarks so that joints and body segments can be identified. Unfortunately, the use of skin markers introduces a number of potential errors to which there is no easy solution. Problems arise in designing markers that can be easily seen on screen and some markers will at times be obscured by the swing-through of other parts of the body or as the subject moves behind other objects in the filming area. The markers, being attached to skin, will be displaced along with the skin as joint movement occurs and will not retain a fixed position in relation to the underlying joint or bone. To complicate matters further, few joints have fixed axes and, though the skin marker might be aligned directly over the axis at one point in the joint range, as the instantaneous centre of rotation changes it will move away from the static location of the marker. All these factors are likely to introduce error into the data collected.

Filming. The camera should be placed as far from the subject as possible to reduce parallax and perspective error. There is disagreement amongst researchers as to how far the camera should be from the movement, but consensus suggests that 7 m is an acceptable distance that will not require a correction factor to be applied. The axis of the camera should be at right angles to the plane of progression and the zoom facility should be used to enlarge the image so that the markers can be easily seen. If significant movement is occurring in more than one plane, a three-dimensional filming system is needed.

Photographic methods, including cine film and video, provide valuable information, usually in one plane, but they are often time-consuming to use and the filming equipment and computer hardware is costly.

Hand held goniometers

Traditionally, joint motion has been investigated by measuring the maximum range of movement available at individual joints. This is a static measurement of the end of range position and a hand held goniometer is used for the purpose. These simple goniometers have to be aligned over the joint axis and this introduces a potential source of error if the instantaneous centre of rotation changes throughout the movement or if the goniometer becomes misaligned. Nevertheless, the reliability and validity of hand held goniometers has been shown to be fairly good (Gajdosik & Bohannon 1987). The usefulness of hand held goniometers is limited by the fact that they can only record static position and therefore have little value in the description of continuous or functional movement. Despite being used as objective measures for testing the efficacy of therapeutic intervention, they give no indication of the functional range of joint movement.

Normally, static goniometric measurements are taken, with the joint in a non-weight bearing position that allows full range of active or passive movement to be measured. However, very few functional activities of the lower limb are performed in a non-weight bearing position, and few upper limb functions are performed without the limb holding a weight, so the results obtained are not an accurate reflection of the subject's capabilities in a functional activity.

Electrogoniometers

Electrogoniometers have opened up the possibility of measuring joint movement during a functional activity. The electrogoniometer, which was introduced by Karpovitch in the 1950s, can take a number of forms (Rothstein 1985). In its most simple form it can consist of two endblocks joined by an electronic potentiometer which is encased within a protective spring. More sophisticated devices may use up to three potentiometers for each joint, thus allowing simultaneous measurement of movement in three planes. Two different types of goniometer are shown in Figure 8.3. In both cases the way in which they are designed allows measurement to take place regardless of whether the centre of rotation of the goniometer coincides with the centre of rotation of the joint. Figure 8.4 illustrates how this is possible. With these types of electrogoniometers, movement of a joint will result in movement of the potentiometer and the resultant strain on the potentiometer generates electrical signals, i.e. the resistance in the potentiometer is changed. These signals, in the form of voltage and, less commonly, current, are plotted and, after calibration, represent the angular displacement of the joint. Only angular displacements are measured. Linear movements that result in telescoping of the potentiometer do not produce strain and consequently no voltage is recorded. The joint displacement curves for the hip, knee and ankle joint which are shown in Chapter 10 were taken from data obtained from an electrogoniometer (see Fig. 10.4).

Electrogoniometers are lightweight and do not interfere to any great extent with the activity that is being tested. They are designed so that only a small force is needed to distort the potentiometer, making the instrument very sensitive. Error

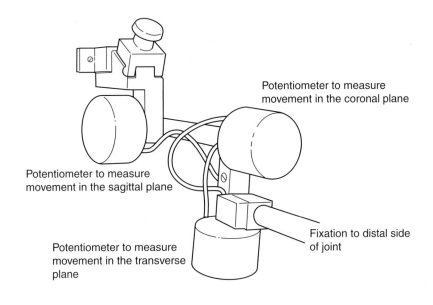

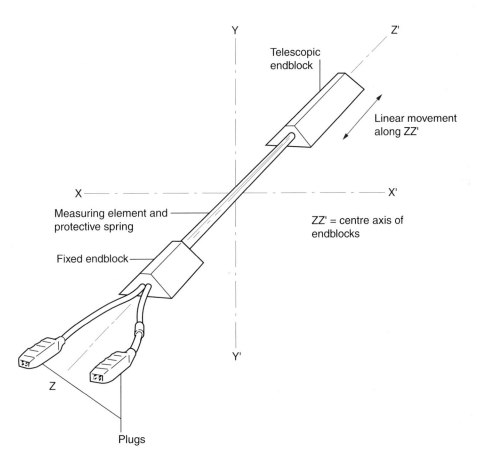

Figure 8.3 Two different types of electrogoniometers.

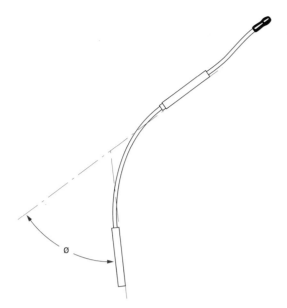

Figure 8.4 This electrogoniometer does not need to be aligned over the axis of the joint. Movement of one endblock in relation to the other enables calculation of the position of the joint.

associated with the use of electrogoniometers comes mainly from the means by which they are fixed to the subject and the method by which data are relayed to the computer for analysis. Fixation has proved to be a problem over many years as human limbs are normally conical in shape and, unless the goniometer is stuck directly to the skin, it is in danger of sliding down or round the limb during movement. When straps or bands are used to hold the goniometer onto the limb they normally need to be so tightly fastened that they are uncomfortable and restrict movement. Using adhesive tape to affix the electrogoniometer directly to the skin is a more satisfactory means, although skin movement over the joint, as discussed earlier in this chapter, may present a problem. Reliability of results using this method of fixation is reasonably good (Troke et al 1998). Some electrogoniometers relay the joint positional data to the computer via leads, and subjects can find this both off-putting and restrictive, especially on fast movements or when they are covering a substantial distance. The swinging of the leads may also introduce movement artefacts, resulting in the normal data becoming distorted

by false signals caused by the movement. Telemetry is one solution to the problem of movement artefact; in this case the electrical signal caused by the joint movement is relayed to a storage device some distance from the subject (Whittle 1991). Alternatively, some electrogoniometers have a small data logger which can be placed somewhere convenient like the subject's waistband. The data logger records data during the activity and this information can later be downloaded onto a computer and the results analysed at the researcher's convenience.

Many researchers have demonstrated the reliability of electrogoniometers (Rowe et al 1989, Troke et al 1998). Cosgrove et al (1991) found that there was a 2° discrepancy with the goniometer and no baseline drift, but more recent researchers such as Myles et al (1995) have found the hysteresis effect to be 3.6° with a residual error of 2.9° for repeated measurements of large ranges. Smaller joint ranges, however, showed discrepancy only in the order of 1° for hip and knee flexion during walking. Hazelwood et al (1995) tested the construct validity of the electrogoniometer and found the measures to be highly repeatable with little variation. All these errors can be kept to a minimum if the operational definition is implemented with care. Whilst the intra and inter tester reliability is reasonably good, the accuracy of measurement of electrogoniometers is still questionable, with different systems giving significantly different results when measuring the same subject.

Electrogoniometers have been found to be valid, reliable and easy to use. They help to measure joint ranges during activity and, therefore, represent a good picture of the functional capabilities of that joint. Although electrogoniometers are mostly used within the field of research, the costs will hopefully decrease, bringing them within the price range of clinical therapists and sport scientists.

Optoelectronic devices and polarised light goniometers

These devices use the radiation of light in the measurement of movement. Light is either reflected from or transmitted from markers placed on the subject's skin. These devices come in several forms, tend to be costly, but can produce detailed and highly accurate information relating to the movement of segments of the human body. Optoelectronic devices are based on the same principle as cine and video in that they require markers to be placed on the body, the coordinates of the markers are tracked throughout the movement and calculations can then be made. Unlike cine and video, the systems don't give a visual image of the subject, simply a frame-by-frame representation of the position and change in position of each marker. From this it is normally possible to produce computer-generated stick figures or graphs of the position of a joint showing range plotted against time. This gives good quantitative information but does not address the issue of quality of movement as there is no visual representation of the actual subject. The markers can either be active or passive.

Systems using passive markers rely on reflective markers placed on the subject's skin. Some form of light, often infra-red, is transmitted towards the subject and the rays are reflected back off the markers to a series of 'cameras' that record the marker position. Sufficient 'cameras' need to be placed around the subject so that each marker is visible to a minimum of two 'cameras'. Sampling frequency is normally 50 Hz which enables the system to track the change in position of the markers and produce a reasonable record of the gross pattern of movement. The markers have no identity, leaving the system vulnerable if cross-over of markers occurs. This is commonly seen when, for example, the marker on the wrist crosses the marker on the greater trochanter during the stance phase of gait. The accuracy of the system relies on human input to ensure that the computer accurately identifies which is the wrist marker and which is the marker on the greater trochanter, or it is dependent on a good quality computer programme that is able to correctly process the incoming data.

The more expensive systems use active skin markers. The markers each have their own small power pack that enables them to actively transmit infra-red rays to a receiving system of several 'cameras'. Because each marker has its own transmitting signal the receiver picks up not only the position and displacement of the marker but can identify which marker it has picked up. This gives the advantage of differentiating between markers and removes the potential source of error that can occur when two markers cross over each other.

For both the active and passive systems it is necessary to identify a ground reference point before measurement takes place. This enables the computer to calculate the absolute and relative positions of the markers in three dimensions.

If only one marker is placed on a segment of the body, the system can measure and record displacement of that segment in three dimensions, giving the segment's absolute and relative position. The application of two markers enables the system to calculate the distance between them relative to time and this enables calculations of velocity and acceleration. If the two markers are placed to represent the two ends of a long bone then the computer can calculate the displacement of that bone relative to the floor or another reference point. With three or more markers the angles at joints can be measured as well as the accelerations and velocities of limb segments.

KINETIC ANALYSIS

Kinetics is the description of human movement in terms of force and these forces can be internal or external (see Ch. 3). Internal forces include those resulting from muscle activity, force generated by stretch on non-contractile and elastic soft tissue and internal friction. Ground reaction forces, forces generated by other people, external loads or wind resistance would all be classed as external.

Apart from the direct information on force production obtained from kinetic analysis of human movement, it is also possible to infer information about muscle function or pain. In addition, it is possible to look at the forces generated by muscles in relationship to task performance or the way external forces impinge on an individual's ability to undertake a functional activity.

Isokinetic dynamometry

There are no direct methods of measuring the work undertaken or force generated by individual muscles during functional movements, though there are a number of mathematical approaches which can be employed to provide data on the net muscle moment at a joint (Winter 1990). Isokinetic dynamometers can record the variation in muscle torque throughout a range of joint movement and this is a major advance on manual assessment of force or hand held dynamometry.

Unfortunately isokinetic dynamometers are large machines and in order for measurements to take place the subject has to be attached to the machine; clearly this is not going to permit the measurement of muscle torque in functional activity. The isokinetic dynamometer requires the subject to be seated with the axis of the joint to be tested aligned with the axis of the machine. The limb must be strapped tightly to the dynamometer chair to ensure that misalignment of these two axes does not occur and movement can only occur through the range permitted by the fixation.

Modern isokinetic dynamometers are able to measure muscular torque, work, power, the rate of torque production (explosiveness) and endurance in movements that involve the muscle concentrically and eccentrically. The force generated in isometric muscle activity can also be measured. Information gained from the static testing position is then used to extrapolate to the moving human being.

Peak torque. This is measured in newton-metres (N.m) and represents the highest torque output achieved by a muscle as it moves its joint through range of motion. It would appear to be an accurate and reproducible measure and the most commonly collected data using the isokinetic dynamometer (Kannus 1994).

The peak torque generated by a muscle varies according to the velocity of the movement and this is known as the torque-velocity relationship. It is greatest at the lower velocities and declines as the velocity increases.

Angle to peak torque. Kannus (1994) suggests that with increasing angular velocity, the point at which peak torque is achieved occurs later in the range. In normal muscle there is an optimum part of the range when muscles are able to generate maximum force (mid-range). It is speculated that on the faster angular velocities the muscle may not have recruited all possible fibres by mid-range and the angle to peak torque may be changed. If peak torque is to be considered at different velocities then angle to peak torque should also be taken into consideration.

Angle specific torque. Torque can be measured anywhere within the range of movement and this is called angle specific torque. When angle specific torque is measured in inner or outer range, the accuracy of the measurement decreases and may fall below an acceptable level, making results inconsistent (Kannus 1994).

Figure 8.5 shows the traces taken from a normal subject who was measured during concentric contractions of the shoulder joint abductors and adductors. The traces clearly indicate that peak torque for both abduction and adduction was achieved towards the early part of the measured range. As the torque recordings do not start until the pre-set velocity has been achieved, the actual joint and muscle range is greater than that shown on the traces.

Work and power measurements. These can be obtained from the isokinetic dynamometer. In

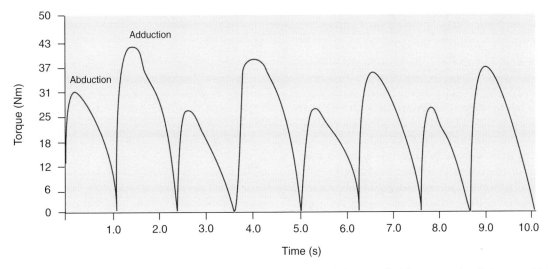

Figure 8.5 Torque curves of repeated concentric activity of the shoulder abductor and adductor muscles. Data were obtained by using an isokinetic dynamometer.

isokinetics, work is defined as the area under the torque curve where the torque curve is torque against angular displacement (work is torque × angular displacement). Work is measured in joules. Power is the rate of muscular work and increases with angular velocity. Average power is total work for a given contraction divided by the time taken and is measured in joules per second or watts.

It is also possible to measure peak torque acceleration energy, which is the greatest amount of work performed in the first 125 ms of a contraction. It is measured in joules and it is suggested that this measurement is indicative of explosive ability as it gives the rate of torque production. There is some doubt about the reliability of these data and their repeatability, especially at low speeds (Kannus 1994).

Endurance indices can be defined as the ability of muscle to perform repeated contractions against a load. An endurance index is supposed to indicate the rate of fatigue. There appears to be no agreement as to the best way to test for endurance, though most tests work on a reduction from peak torque over a specified period of time. Isokinetic dynamometers can provide this information.

The isokinetic dynamometer as a measure of human function

The isokinetic dynamometer is a popular tool because it provides information about muscle groups which may be functioning isometrically, isotonically and isokinetically. It is the only device that makes concentric and eccentric measurements possible. Unfortunately, the data obtained do not relate to human function because they have been collected from a single joint/single muscle group activity. Extrapolating from isokinetic dynamometry data to function must therefore be viewed with caution.

FORCE AND PRESSURE MEASUREMENTS

Ground reaction forces

It is possible to measure reaction forces between the human being and the supporting surface in a number of functional activities. Chapter 3 introduced the mechanics that underpin this method of measurement. This technique is most commonly seen in the evaluation of activities such as locomotion, getting out of a chair and postural sway in standing.

There are a number of different ways in which ground reaction forces can be measured; the most complex methods measure vertical forces and shear forces in the horizontal plane. In the horizontal plane they measure forces both in an anterior/posterior direction and also in a medial/lateral direction. From these three forces it is possible to calculate a single point about which these forces are said to act and also to represent these forces by a single ground reaction vector of given magnitude and angle.

Typically, force plate data are plotted against time, showing the patterns of change of force during the period of time that the foot is in contact with the supporting surface. Figure 8.6 shows the normal vertical reaction forces seen in walking plotted in two different ways.

Task 8.1

In Figure 8.7a and b, the effects of abnormal gait are illustrated. Work out how the normal gait pattern has been changed in order to produce the two force traces. What might be the possible causes of these two changes in gait pattern?

The clinical value of force plate data is debatable. Major movement abnormalities are apparent both on visual observation and on detailed examination of a force trace. The advantage that arises from using a force plate is that the data obtained enable quantification of change over time. Force plates are, however, very expensive and their use as a clinical tool is likely to remain limited.

Pure pressure measurements

These can be made by the use of pressure plates or through in-shoe devices. In both cases pressure sensors are distributed across the whole load-bearing surface of the measuring device. This enables measurements of pressure to be made over the whole of the area that is in contact with the device. Figure 8.8 shows a printout from a Musgrave footprint pressure plate. The printout is colour coded to indicate different levels of pressure and the load during any part of the stance phase can be obtained.

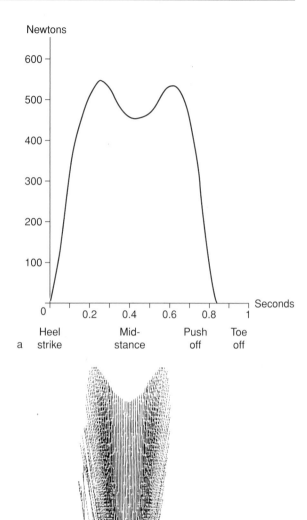

Figure 8.6 Normal force traces taken from the stance phase of walking: (a) a force curve; (b) a vector diagram.

Pressure plates take a variety of forms and different models are available to measure foot pressures and the pressures in sitting and lying. Floor mounted pressure plates provide information about standing and the different forms of locomotion but they are restrictive in that they may have to be set into the floor or into a walk-way and are normally directly linked to a computer. Pressure distribution in sitting and lying has proved useful in the design and evaluation of beds and chairs and has also provided an insight

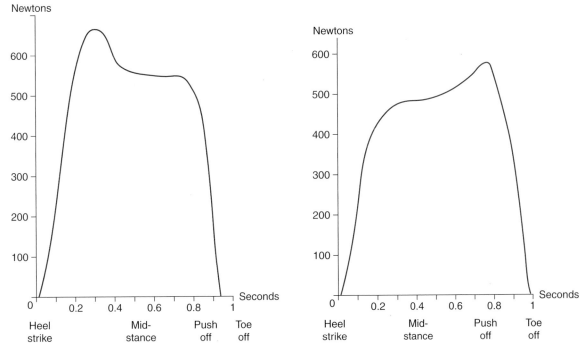

Figure 8.7 Force traces taken from patients with abnormal gait patterns.

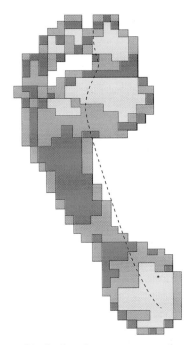

Figure 8.8 Distribution of pressure across the sole of the foot during walking. The light grey areas represent the greatest pressure.

into how pathologies can alter the distribution of pressure.

If a device is placed inside a shoe, the foot-shoe interface pressures can be measured and these provide information on pressure distribution across the foot in all functional situations (see Fig. 8.9). These in-shoe devices enable data to be collected on both pressure distribution across the

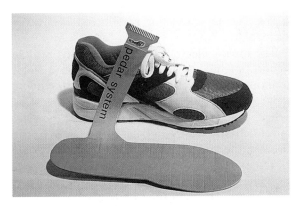

Figure 8.9 An in-shoe pressure device.

whole of the plantar surface of the foot and also across time. Most of these devices are connected by a short lead to a data logger that is normally worn on the waist belt and the data can be downloaded onto a computer for analysis at a later date.

ELECTROMYOGRAPHY (EMG)

EMG is not only the term used to describe the electrical signals produced as a result of the contraction of a muscle, but also the method of collecting these signals and the data that are produced.

When a muscle is quiescent there is little electrical activity. However, during muscular activity, electrical signals are produced and can be recorded. Electromyography will show if a muscle is active or not, the duration of that activity and, as the EMG increases in magnitude with tension, the signals will also give an indication of how much torque is being generated.

The basis of EMG

At a cellular level, the muscle fibre or cell is the unit of contraction. During muscle activity there is an electrical potential change and depolarisation and repolarisation of the surface membrane of the cell. There is transmission of impulse across the sarcolemma to the interior of the muscle cell via a complex system of tubules.

When a neural impulse reaches the motor end plate, a wave of depolarisation spreads across the cell resulting in a twitch followed by relaxation. This twitch can last from a few milliseconds to 0.25 s. The depolarisation is followed by a wave of repolarisation.

The muscle electrical potentials, called muscle action potentials (MAPs), will result in a small amount of the electrical current spreading away from the muscle in the direction of the skin, where electrodes can be used to record the electrical activity. The nearer the electrode is to the muscle, the larger the recorded signal. If muscle fibres some distance from the electrodes are conducting electrical current, the MAPs recorded will be smaller than they would have been for similar sized motor units closer to the electrodes.

Values actually obtained from muscle vary between 100 µV (microvolts) to 5 mV (millivolts). The signal can be very small and a problem may exist because electrical activity from sources other than the muscle can overwhelm the desired signal. This unwanted electrical activity is called 'noise' and a number of strategies have to be adopted to eliminate unwanted noise.

Types of electrodes

Either surface or indwelling needle electrodes can be used, though surface electrode EMG is most common in the analysis of human movement. Both types of electrodes not only pick up electrical activity which passes over their conducting surface but can also register electrical currents nearby. Surface electrodes are normally small metal discs of about 1 cm diameter, though they can be smaller if tiny muscles are being tested. The electrodes are usually made of silver/silver chloride and are sensitive to electrical signals from superficial muscles. They give a reading corresponding to the average electrical activity.

Needle electrodes are normally fine hypodermic needles containing a conductor which is insulated except for its protruding end. As two electrodes are needed, the outer part of the hypodermic forms one and the conductor inside the hypodermic forms the other. Otherwise fine wires can be used and these are less intrusive.

There is some evidence that the surface electrodes are more likely to give reliable data and, as a non-invasive technique, they are preferable (Winter 1990, Arokoski et al 1999). Subjective reports indicate that, despite the use of local anaesthetics, there is a degree of discomfort from needle electrodes and that the movement of the contracting muscle in relation to the overlying skin, when pierced by the electrode, produces some inhibition to normal movement.

Recording the EMG

In order to be able to use the data collected from muscle, the signal must be 'clean', i.e. free from noise, artefacts and distortion (Winter 1990).

Noise may come from a variety of sources. These include:

- other muscles, especially the heart
- nearby electrical machinery including the EMG recording equipment
- radio waves, e.g. ambulance/police/CB radios
- power lines, domestic electrical supply
- fluorescent lights.

Artefacts are 'false signals' which are generated or caused by the EMG machine or its cabling. Some are difficult to distinguish from the true signal coming from the muscle, but others can easily be identified. Into this latter category come movement artefacts that occur when the cables or the electrodes are moved and touched. The movement artefacts are usually at the upper and lower ends of the frequency range and can therefore be filtered out.

Distortion of EMG signals usually results as a consequence of the signals needing to be amplified before they can be of use. Distortion may occur if the signal is amplified in a way that is not linear over the whole range of the system. It is important that the larger signals are amplified to the same degree as the smaller signals.

EMG processing

After the EMG signal has been amplified it can be viewed as a raw signal or it can be processed so that it is in a form which will enable it to be compared or correlated with other physiological and biomechanical signals (Winter 1990). Computers are used for this purpose and it is important to be aware that the original signals will have been subjected to a number of manipulations before the final data are produced. This should not normally be a problem, but where the output is not what was expected then the signal processing should be checked.

Raw EMG. This is illustrated in Figure 8.10 and EMG in this form enables judgements about the onset and cessation of muscle contraction. This can provide information about the sequence of muscle activation and current thought suggests that there may be a 'normal' pattern of muscle activation which, if altered, can lead to movement problems and pain. The traces in Figure 8.10 were taken from a normal shoulder during the movement of flexion and extension and were part of a study to identify the sequence of activation of the various shoulder muscles. The trace illustrates the difficulty often experienced

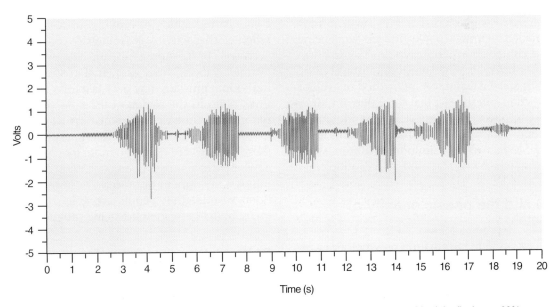

Figure 8.10 A raw EMG trace taken from supraspinatus during repeated repetitions of shoulder joint flexion at 60°/sec.

when trying to identify the instant of muscle activation.

Processed EMG. The first stage of processing the EMG signal involves rectification. Normally raw EMG has both negative and positive polarity which means that if the mean of the spikes above and below the zero line is taken it will be zero. Clearly this is of little value. Rectification converts the signal to a positive polarity so that the mean amplitude of the spikes becomes meaningful. As the mean amplitude varies with the strength of the muscle contraction, it enables judgements about whether there is more or less muscle activity in a given situation. In addition to rectification the signal can also be subjected to a low pass filter, called a linear envelope, which cuts out high frequency signals. It can also be integrated and this can take several forms. For more details a specialist EMG textbook should be consulted.

Clinical significance of EMG for measuring human movement

A question that has been puzzling researchers for at least 25 years is 'how valuable is EMG in reflecting and predicting muscle function and can findings be extrapolated to total body function?'. EMG surface electrodes are non-invasive and the method is cheap and simple to apply. Various authors have suggested that EMG will provide information on muscle power, muscle sequencing, fatigue, composition of fibre type and metabolism. The simplicity and inexpensive nature of EMG ought to make it an important method of evaluating function, but the fact that the value of EMG is still being questioned after so long indicates its limitations. There are still sufficient doubts about what EMG can reliably do to make it a measurement tool which must be used with caution.

EMG and the phasic activity of muscles

EMG can provide information on whether or not a muscle is active and for how long the period of activity or inactivity continues. There is always a small lag between the onset of electrical activity in a muscle and perceived movement of the limb;

this is in the region of 30 ms and it is probably not significant in terms of analysis of the phasic activity of muscles. The lag is partially due to the chemical changes which must take place before the muscle can contract and also due to the need of the muscle to 'take up slack' before joint movement can occur.

A similar lag occurs at the end of muscle activity. With the cessation of electrical activity, the muscle continues to contract for a short period whilst the chemical changes stabilise and the muscle is able to relax. It is likely that the period between the end of electrical activity and the cessation of contraction will vary between muscle groups and will also be dependent on the type of muscle contraction. In the normal human being the quadriceps has been studied most often and it shows a lag period of between 250 ms and 300 ms (Inman et al 1981).

It is valuable to know the duration of involvement of various muscle groups during movement, however there can be practical problems. It is not always clear from the EMG traces when a muscle starts to contract and when contraction ends. Figure 8.10 illustrates this well. All current information on the phasing or sequencing of muscles in functional activity is taken from EMG studies. These studies show when the muscles are activated and when they cease activity, but EMG is not able to provide information on whether the activity is isometric, concentric or eccentric. EMG studies of muscles involved in normal walking have shown that the input of individual muscles may only last for a very short time, often in the region of 0.2 s. As this would not give the muscle sufficient time to produce a movement at a joint, it leads to speculation that these muscles are doing no more than producing an isometric action (Inman et al 1981). With such minor involvement of muscles in normal gait, it is no wonder that people are able to walk for many hours before experiencing fatigue.

EMG and force production

There is considerable controversy about whether EMG can give reliable, quantifiable information on the magnitude of muscle activity, the recruitment of contractile elements and muscle metabolism and fatigue. Whilst it is commonly agreed that EMG can distinguish between a working muscle and a quiescent muscle, there is disagreement about whether the relationship between EMG activity and torque is consistent and linear. If the relationship is linear, EMG can be used to calculate the forces generated by muscles during functional activities. If, however, the EMG signal has an inconsistent, non-linear relationship with muscle torque, then it has little value as a measurement tool.

EMG and isometric tension

Early experiments by Lippold (1952) showed that for the gastrocnemius muscle, a linear relationship could be shown between the average amplitude of EMG and the tension developed in muscle. This appeared to indicate that EMG could be used to measure the force generated, but unfortunately in subsequent decades other workers found different results. Although the EMG increased, it was not found to do so in direct relationship to the actual amount of force generated by the muscle (Zuniga & Simons 1969, Rau & Vredenbregt 1973, Lawrence & De Luca 1983). Winter (1990) suggests that there is no more than a 'reasonable relationship' between isometric force generation and EMG activity. If this is true, the results from EMG can only be used to give a general prediction of muscle tension.

EMG and isotonic tension

Much less experimental activity has been undertaken in the field of EMG/isotonic force relationships than that of EMG/isometric relationships. On low velocity contractions there is an identifiable but inconsistent relationship between EMG and muscle torque and the faster the contraction, the more difficult it becomes to see any relationship (Komi 1973).

Mathematical calculations of muscle moment, based on force plate and joint angle data, can be made. Information gained from these calculations and from simultaneous EMG correlates very closely, suggesting that EMG is an accurate method of collecting information about whether a muscle is contracting or not during a functional activity (Olney & Winter 1985). EMG will also give some indication of the magnitude of the force being generated by that muscle, though no detail.

ENERGY EXPENDITURE ANALYSIS

There are a number of approaches which can be used to calculate energy expenditure during movement; the details are beyond the scope of this book but can be found in any advanced physiology text. Direct calorimetry produces highly accurate and repeatable results but is largely impractical as it requires the use of an airtight insulated chamber in which the activity is performed. Indirect calorimetry most commonly relies on the analysis of the oxygen and carbon dioxide content of expired air and is valuable and reasonably practical but still requires the subject to be attached to some form of device in which expired air can be collected. The need to wear a noseclip and to breathe through a fairly large mouthpiece can be rather daunting and needs quite lengthy acclimatisation. In addition, upper limb activities may be restricted by the tube leaving the mouthpiece (McArdle et al 1997, Whittle 1991).

Consideration of energy expenditure is important in patients who are frail or disabled. When individuals are already functioning at the limit of their ability, it is essential that they are encouraged to undertake activities in the most energy efficient way possible. Analysis of human movement in terms of energy expenditure provides essential information that will then inform treatment approaches.

REFERENCES

Arokoski J P A, Kankaanpaa M, Valta T et al 1999 Back and hip extensor muscle function during therapeutic exercise. Archives of Physical Medicine and Rehabilitation 80(7): 842–850

Cosgrove A P, Graham H K, Mollan R A B 1991 Gait analysis in children with cerebral palsy using electrogoniometers. Presentation, British Orthopaedic Research meeting

Curtis K A, Kindlin C M, Reich K M, White D E 1995 Functional reach in wheelchair users: the effects of trunk and lower extremity stabilisation. Archives of Physical Medicine and Rehabilitation 76: 360–367

Gajdosik R L, Bohannon R W 1987 Clinical measurement of range of motion: review of goniometry emphasising reliability and validity. Physical Therapy 67: 1867–1872

Hazelwood M E, Rowe P J, Salter P M 1995 The use of electrogoniometers as a measurement tool for passive movement and gait analysis. Physiotherapy 81(10): 639

Inman V T, Ralston H J, Todd F 1981 Human walking. Williams and Wilkins, Baltimore

Kannus P 1994 Isokinetic evaluation of muscular performance: implications for muscle testing and rehabilitation. International Journal of Sports Medicine 15: S11–S18

Komi P V 1973 Relationship between muscle tension, EMG and velocity of contraction under concentric and eccentric work. In: Desmedt J E (ed) New Developments in Electromyography and Clinical Neurophysiology 1: 596–606

Lawrence J H, De Luca C J 1983 Myoelectric signal versus force relationship in different human muscles. Journal of Applied Physiology 54(6): 1653–1659

Lippold O C J 1952 The relationship between integrated action potentials in a human muscle and its isometric tension. Journal of Physiology 117: 492–499

McArdle W D, Katch F I, Katch V L 1997 Exercise physiology, energy, nutrition and human performance, 4th edn. Lea & Febiger, Philadelphia

McGill S M, Dainty D A 1984 Computer analysis of energy transfers in children walking with crutches. Archives of Physical Medicine and Rehabilitation 65: 115–120

Myles C, Rowe P J, Salter P, Nicol A 1995 An electrogoniometry system used to investigate the ability of the elderly to ascend and descend stairs. Physiotherapy 81(10): 640

Noreau L, Richards C L, Comeau F, Tardif D 1995 Biomechanical analysis of swing-through gait in paraplegic and non-disabled individuals. Journal of Biomechanics 28: 689–700

Olney S J, Winter D A 1985 Predictions of knee and ankle moments of force in walking from EMG and kinematic data. Journal of Biomechanics 18: 9–20

Rau G, Vredenbregt J 1973 EMG force relationship during voluntary static contractions (M. biceps). Medicine & Sport Biomechanics III 8: 270–274

Rothstein J M (ed) 1985 Measurement in physical therapy. Churchill Livingstone, Edinburgh

Rowe P J, Nicol A C, Kelly I G 1989 Flexible goniometer computer system for the assessment of hip function. Clinical Biomechanics 4: 68–72

Terauds J 1984 Sports biomechanics: Proceedings of the International Symposium of Biomechanics in Sport. Academic Publishers, Del Mar, California

Troke M, Moore A P, Cheek E 1998 Reliability of the OSI CA 6000 spine motion analyzer with a new skin fixation system when used on the thoracic spine. Manual Therapy 3:(1) 27–33

Whittle M 1991 Gait analysis, an introduction. Butterworth-Heinemann, Oxford

Winter D A 1982 Camera speeds for normal and pathological gait analyses. Medical and Biological Engineering & Computing 20: 408–412

Winter D A 1990 Biomechanics and motor control of human movement, 2nd edn. Wiley Inter-science, New York

Zuniga E N, Simons D G 1969 Non-linear relationship between averaged electromyogram potential and muscle tension in normal subjects. Archives of Physical Medicine and Rehabilitation 50: 613–620

CHAPTER CONTENTS

Introduction   161

General principles of measurement scales   162
Validity and reliability   162
Methods of scoring   162
Data collection methods   163

Measurement scales for functional status   164
Defining function   164
Activities of daily living scales   164

Measurement scales for quality of life   167
Defining quality of life   167
Quality of life measures   168

Conclusion   171

9

Scales of measurement

S. Corr

OBJECTIVES

When you have completed this chapter you should be able to:

1. **Understand that loss of movement has an impact on individuals' ability to carry out everyday activities**

2. **Recognise that loss of movement can affect functional status and quality of life**

3. **Understand that measuring the effect movement loss has on function and quality of life is difficult**

4. **Identify appropriate measurement scales needed to measure the impact of movement loss.**

INTRODUCTION

Previous chapters have outlined common methods of measuring human movement. When considering human movement it is important to be aware that a loss of movement, minimal or severe, potentially has an impact on the wider aspects of an individual's life. This chapter will outline two areas that could be affected when looking at movement in a more global context. As a consequence it is necessary to consider movement as a multifactorial, multidimensional complex concept. It is important to know how the loss of movement affects an individual's ability to carry out everyday activities and the effect loss of movement has on how an individual perceives his quality of life. In essence this type of measurement is moving away from measuring impairment to measuring disability or handicap. The World Health Organization (WHO) defines a disability as 'any restriction or lack of ability to perform an activity in a manner or within a range considered normal for human beings and reflects the consequences of impairment in terms of functional performance and activity by the individual' (WHO 1981). Disability could lead to the restriction of an individual's ability to perform daily life tasks such as cooking, painting and typing. The WHO definition of handicap is 'a disadvantage, resulting from an impairment or a disability, that limits or prevents the fulfilment of a role that is normal for that individual and reflects interaction with and adaption to the individual's surroundings' (WHO 1981). Handicap could lead to the restriction in an individual's ability to fulfil social roles such as worker, student and volunteer.

There is a broad range of choices when looking at measurement scales and it is important to consider these when selecting a way of measuring the impact of loss of movement. It is critical that therapists choose one that is designed for the purpose for which it is required (Fisher 1992). A lot of measurement scales can also be used to assess the outcome of treatment and therefore are suitable to measure the impact of loss on more than one occasion. Gompertz et al (1993) suggest that in stroke rehabilitation, for example, broader issues such as mood and perceived health should be measured and not just movement loss or functional status.

GENERAL PRINCIPLES OF MEASUREMENT SCALES
Validity and reliability

No matter what measurement scale is being selected it is essential to consider the reliability and validity of that scale. Validity of a measurement scale relates to whether it measures what it is intended to measure (Bowling & Normand 1998). Scales also need to be reliable, i.e. consistent at producing the same results whether at repeated intervals (test-retest), by the same rater at different times (intra-rater) or by different raters (inter-

rater) (Gompertz et al 1993). If a measurement scale has high inter-rater reliability, different raters when measuring the same individual will produce the same results (Burton 1989). It is also important to question the sensitivity of the measurement scale. This question addresses whether the measure is able to identify changes that may occur over time (Bowling & Normand 1998). A further issue to consider is whether the scale is relevant to every person being measured (McDowell & Newell 1996). Measurement scales that have been developed for specific client groups include the Glasgow assessment schedule for head injuries (Livingstone & Livingstone 1985), Parkinson's disease disability index (McDowell et al 1970) and Robinson-Bashall functional assessment for arthritis patients (McCloy & Jongbloed 1987).

If a measurement scale is shown to be reliable and valid, then it is considered to be standardised. This standardisation process allows scales to be used to compare individuals (McDowell & Newell 1996). Once a measurement scale is standardised, the process of conducting it will be formalised, meaning that there will be procedural instructions outlining what environment the scale should be conducted in, what materials are required and the sequencing of the scale. These procedural arrangements should be clear and concise and, if followed strictly, ensure that the scale remains reliable and valid (Burton 1989, Law & Letts 1989).

The King's Fund (1988) recommends that measurement, using standard scales, should be undertaken on all patients. Although this is desirable, it is important to consider Barer's (1989) suggestion that formal measurement scales by a therapist may show what patients can do under test conditions but informal measurements made by carers are more likely to indicate what the patients do in real life. He goes on to suggest that postal surveys or interview of patients at home may reveal what they think they can do.

Methods of scoring

There are several different ways in which a measurement scale may be scored. The types of scales being described in this chapter are not interval or ratio measurements where the distance between two numbers on the scale is of a known size, like exact degrees of movement or length in centimetres (Bowling & Normand 1998). On the whole a verbal description, such as dependent or independent, will be used to identify how able an individual is to carry out an activity, or a continuum of agreement is used, based on verbal expressions such as disagree, unsure or agree. Scales using verbal definitions like this are known as ordinal scales, i.e. the options for responses are in some kind of order and have a relationship to each other (Bowling & Normand 1998). A third type of scale exists but is not commonly used in the type of measures being discussed in this chapter. These are nominal scales where numbers are used to represent labels, such as male or female, and the numbers have no value in relation to each other. It is necessary to be able to identify how a scale is measured in order to understand the appropriateness of the measurement to the question being asked. Regardless of which scoring system is used, it should be straightforward and quick. Also it needs to be easy to interpret so that the results can be used for treatment planning or measuring the outcome of treatment (Law & Letts 1989).

Task 9.1

Try to identify some examples of each of the three different types of scales. You may find some examples in everyday situations such as in supermarkets or questionnaires in magazines. For interval scales there needs to be an equal gap between two scores; for nominal scales numbers are used to label the items in the scales but there is no relationship between the numbers; and for ordinal scales there is a grading system although the intervals are not equal.

Data collection methods

Further consideration needs to be given to how information is gathered when using measurement scales. There are several options including observation, interview or self rating. Each method has strengths and limitations.

Observation

When observing it is possible to see exactly how able an individual is to carry out an activity. However, a limitation may be the effect 'being watched' has on individuals as they demonstrate their ability to perform a task. This may be positive or negative, i.e. they may make greater efforts to do something if being watched. Alternatively they may feel more anxious and lack confidence if being observed. A key to using observation as an assessment method is being clear about what is to be observed and how to match what is seen with possible scores. For example, it is important to know exactly what needs to be observed in order to rate an individual as 'able to manage most of the task'.

Interview

Interviews are another mechanism for gathering information. If this is the method used for a measuring scale often the interview is structured. This means there are particular questions to ask and even how this should be phrased may have been identified. One limitation of interviews is the reliance on the individual's perception of their ability, rather than actually observing their ability. Alternatively if it is very difficult for an individual to carry out an activity it may be easier for them to inform you of this rather than struggle to demonstrate their difficulties.

Self rating

Similarly self-rating methods of gathering information are usually very structured. The measurement scale is most likely to be in questionnaire format where the individual will answer a number of questions. It may be valid and reliable for use by post, which makes it a useful tool for research as well as clinical practice. To be used in this way it will need to be easy to complete, have clear instructions and should not take long to complete.

Some measurement scales are reliable for use by observation, interview and self rating. The Barthel activities of daily living index, which is an example of this, is outlined in the next section.

Task 9.2

Draw the following table on a sheet of paper and use it to consider the strengths and limitations of using interviews, observation and self-rating scales to measure an individual's ability to ride a bicycle.

Method	Strengths	Limitations
Interviews		
Observation		
Self-rating		

MEASUREMENT SCALES FOR FUNCTIONAL STATUS

Defining function

There are several different interpretations of functional status. According to the Collins dictionary (Harper Collins 1987) function means a natural action. This can be interpreted in humans to be the natural everyday actions that are carried out by individuals such as walking, toileting and eating. The perspective taken on function can also be influenced by the different philosophies of the professions within multidisciplinary teams. Fisher (1994) outlines them in relation to the goal of intervention (see Table 9.1). There are, of course, many overlaps among the professions but the table highlights the most unique aspects of each profession. All the disciplines share concerns related to function and functional independence; how they differ is on how they frame the patient's problems and the goal of treatment. These differences may have an influence when choosing a measurement scale. Also it is important to have an awareness of the interpretation of function that may have been adopted by those who have developed scales for measuring function.

By developing scales to measure an individual's functional status the expectation is that it will be possible to get a current picture of the individual's abilities to carry out the actions that are natural to all. According to McDowell & Newell (1996), an individual is healthy if he or she is physically and mentally able to do the things he or she wishes and needs to do.

Activities of daily living (ADL) scales

A large number of scales have been developed over the last few decades, mainly in rehabilitation medicine. This section describes two in detail, the Barthel ADL index which measures ADL and the Nottingham extended ADL scale which measures extended activities, i.e. more community based activities which also require movement in order for them to be carried out. The scales chosen are selected to illustrate the types available and are by no means the only ones available or that should be considered when identifying a measurement scale to assess function. Health care professionals need to carefully consider the options available when they are selecting a measurement scale. The choice will depend on why it is being used. It may be needed to measure ability, to evaluate the amount of help

Table 9.1 Unique perspectives of medicine, nursing, occupational therapy, physiotherapy and social work (After Fisher 1994, with permission)

Profession	Frame	Methods	Goal
Medicine	Illness	Pharmacology Surgery	Symptom elimination
Nursing	Health	Helping/Caring Interprofessional interactions	Healthy function Wellness
Occupational therapy	Occupation	Therapeutic activity Adaptation	Occupational function
Physiotherapy	Physical capacity	Therapeutic exercise and agents	Physical function Mobility
Social work	Systems	System change Helping process	Social function

patients may need on discharge, to identify treatment goals or as an outcome measure.

Barthel activity of daily living index

One of the most widely known and used measures of activities of daily living is the Barthel activity of daily living (ADL) index. It was developed in 1965 by Mahoney and Barthel, as a simple index of independence to score the ability of patients to care for themselves and, by repeating the test, to assess their improvement (Mahoney and Barthel 1965). It contains 10 items and has both a self-care and a mobility component. This scale does not measure movement in isolation but the output of movement, i.e. the ability to carry out activities. The mobility component contains items related to transfers and ambulation. The original scoring system was from 0 to 100, but this has been modified so that scores range from 0 to 20 with higher scores signifying better functioning (Collin et al 1988, Bacher et al 1990). This modified version is most commonly used in practice. Table 9.2 shows the ten items in the scales and the scoring system used. Two items, transfer and mobility, can be scored 0, 1, 2 or 3 while the remainder just 0, 1 and 2. The table indicates the interpretation of each score for all the items. A total score is then calculated.

The Barthel index is not hierarchical, meaning that it does not result in a total score that gives a clear indication of the level of disability (Gibbon 1991). This means that two people may score the same, for example 10, but it would not be possible to assume that both are independent in the same activities. The items are not in an order that reflects the complexity and difficulty of carrying out particular activities. As can be seen from Table 9.2, it also has different interpretations for the score values. For example, for bathing being independent scores only 1 whereas being independent in transfers scores 3. This does not necessarily reflect the complex movements and skills required to carry out each of these activities. Wade (1992) provides working definitions for the scores so that therapists are clear about what the individual needs to be able to do in order to be scored as independent. Using these will ensure a standardised use and understanding of the scale.

When the scores are totalled there is no single way of interpreting this total. Granger & Hamilton (1990) found that no specific total score could be regarded as adequately specific or sensitive to be used as the criteria for admission for rehabilitation services or as an indication of readiness for discharge. Rodgers et al (1993) suggest that the Barthel ADL index is most useful in assessing patients who are moderately or severely disabled. There is a ceiling and flooring effect, meaning that those scoring the maximum (20) may still be significantly handicapped but with the potential of improvement beyond the limits of the scale. As a result the Barthel ADL index lacks sensitivity to change in its upper range (Rodgers et al 1993). The same occurs at the lower end. To overcome this patients with high Barthel scores should be subsequently

Table 9.2 Barthel ADL index showing the interpretation of the scores (After Wade 1992, with permission)

Concept	0	1	2	3
Bowels	Incontinent	Occasional accident	Continent	–
Bladder	Incontinent	Occasional accident	Continent	–
Grooming	Dependent	Independent	–	–
Toilet use	Dependent	Needs some help	Independent	–
Feeding	Unable	Needs help	Independent	–
Transfer	Unable	Major help	Minor help	Independent
Mobility	Dependent	Wheelchair independent	Walks with one person	Independent
Dressing	Dependent	Needs help but can do half	Independent	–
Stairs	Unable	Needs help	Independent	–
Bathing	Dependent	Independent	–	–

assessed with another ADL scale, i.e. a scale that assesses a broader range of activities.

The Barthel index is most frequently used in clinical practice by therapists and other members of the multidisciplinary team. It has been shown to be reliable for use in this format and also for use in formal research, by post and over the telephone (Wade 1992). Law & Letts (1989) indicated that more specifically it has been shown to have adequate observer and test-retest reliability. It is a valid measurement scale for function in activities of daily living and is sensitive to measure changes in ADL after treatment in controlled research settings.

Task 9.3

Read the two case studies below. Using the information given, calculate their scores using the Barthel ADL index. Once you have completed this, consider the usefulness of the index to establish levels of function.

Mrs Smith is a 45-year-old teacher who recently had a right cerebrovascular accident (stroke). She has been discharged back to her two-storey house and is beginning to settle into some routine at home. She manages to wash and dress independently. With the aids provided by the social services occupational therapists she is independent going up and down stairs and getting in and out of the bath. Although she can manage to make a hot drink she is unable to cook a meal or cut up her food. At the moment her husband does the cooking and shopping. Mrs Smith manages to walk around the house but is unable to walk on uneven ground. She has not been outside and does not feel confident to go to the shops. She is glad that they have a downstairs toilet, which she can manage to get to and use independently.

Mr Jones is a 55-year-old car mechanic who runs his own small business. He has rheumatoid arthritis. He is currently unable to work or tend his garden due to pain and stiffness mainly in his hands. He walks to his local shop daily to get the paper. He has always been a casual dresser (T-shirts and deck shoes rather than shirt and tie or suits) and can get dressed if wearing his normal clothes. He is unable to drive at the moment but uses public transport. He has difficulty turning on the taps but can make a cup of tea if the kettle is filled for him. He is also independent showering; he has a walk-in shower rather than a bath. He is independent going up and down the stairs. Mr Jones recently bought an electric shaver and manages to shave independently with this.

Eakin (1993) suggests that the appeal of the Barthel ADL index lies in the fact that it is simple and quick to use; its results can be easily understood and communicated between different professions; and its content is perceived as relevant to both clinicians and patients. However, it needs to be remembered also that it has been thought not to have enough items to account for the impact of rehabilitation, and that the grading system is not sufficiently sensitive to reflect change, particularly in the short term.

Extended activities of daily living scale

The extended ADL scale was developed in Nottingham by Nouri and Lincoln (1987) to assess the activities which may be important to stroke patients who are living in the community. It includes activities that relate to carrying out domestic tasks and other activities that take place outside the home environment. It has been validated for administering by interview and post (Nouri & Lincoln 1987, Lincoln & Gladman 1992, Wade 1992). It consists of a questionnaire of 22 activities divided into four groups: mobility, kitchen, domestic and leisure.

The extended ADL scale is a ranked scale, meaning that all patients with the same scores are independent in the same items. Lincoln and Gladman (1992) found that an overall total score could provide an indication of overall independence in the activities if comparing groups of people. They recommend that with individual patients section scores, for example mobility or leisure scores, rather than overall totals should be used when identifying a patient's progress or change over time. They recommend this as they found discrepancies when using the total score. The scale is appropriate to use in research into the evaluation of rehabilitation.

Table 9.3 outlines the items in each of the four sections of the scale. The response options are the same for each item. The score 1 is given if activities are performed by patients on their own or on their own with difficulty. For activities which patients are unable to perform or for which they require help the score is 0.

Table 9.3 Extended activities of daily living scale (After Nouri & Lincoln 1987, with permission)

Concept	No (0)	With help (0)	On my own with difficulty (1)	On my own (1)
Mobility				
Do you:				
Walk around outside				
Climb stairs				
Get in and out of the car				
Walk over uneven ground				
Cross roads				
Travel on public transport				
In the kitchen				
Do you:				
Manage to feed yourself				
Manage to make yourself a hot drink				
Take hot drinks from one room to another				
Do the washing up				
Make yourself a hot snack				
Domestic tasks				
Do you:				
Manage your own money when you are out				
Wash small items of clothing				
Do your own housework				
Do your own shopping				
Do a full clothes wash				
Leisure activities				
Do you:				
Read newspapers or books				
Use the telephone				
Write letters				
Go out socially				
Manage your own garden				
Drive a car				

Task 9.4

Here is some additional information about Mrs Smith and Mr Jones. Use this information along with what you already know about them to calculate their scores using the Nottingham extended ADL scale.

Mrs Smith loves reading but finds she takes a long time to read the newspaper. She feels her concentration is too poor to read books. She has yet to go out anywhere mainly because she is unsteady walking and lacks confidence. She is anxious about whether she may ever return to work. She has been overwhelmed with the good wishes from her pupils and colleagues and has written several thank you notes.

Mr Jones is anxious about his business, which his son is currently running. He has been struggling of late to hold a pen to write and has done most of his communication over the telephone. His wife has traditionally done all the household tasks with the garden being his domain. He has needed help with the garden lately. At the moment his wife drives when they go out shopping or visiting friends.

MEASUREMENT SCALES FOR QUALITY OF LIFE

Defining quality of life

Like functional status, quality of life is not easy to define. There are a number of different views on the scope of what should be included in the broad consideration of quality of life. Fallowfield (1990) and De Haan et al (1993) suggest that four domains make up quality of life. These are physical, functional, psychological and social health. The physical health dimension refers to disease related and treatment related symptoms as well as pain and sleep. The functional dimension comprises self-care, mobility and physical activity level, as well as the capacity to carry out various roles in relation to family and work. The psychological dimension includes issues such as depression, anxiety and adjustment to illness, cognitive functioning, wellbeing, life satisfaction and happiness. Finally the social health dimension includes qualitative and quantitative aspects of social contacts and interactions such as relationships and participation in leisure and social activities. The inclusion of these dimensions reflects the need to ensure that when thinking of quality of life as a concept it is seen as a broad spectrum of consequences of disease, including elements of impairment, disabilities and handicaps, as well as patients' perceived health status and wellbeing. Quality of life relating to health is distinct from quality of life as a whole, which would also include adequacy of housing and income and perceptions of the local environment (Bowling & Normand 1998).

What is not clear is the balance of the four dimensions that needs to be present in order to ensure quality of life. Diener (1984) suggests that part of the influence of health on quality of life is not simply the direct effect of how people feel physically, but also what their health allows them to do. For example in two separate studies of stroke patients, Niemi et al (1988) and Wyller et al (1997) found that even when patients had a good recovery in terms of physical movement they reported a poor quality of life. This shows that the impact of a disease on health related quality of life is important but can be difficult to understand and to measure.

Task 9.5

Ask a number of friends and family of different ages to sum up what issues contribute to their definition of quality of life. If they include health as one issue, ask them to clarify what they mean by this. Also find out what level of 'ill health' they need to experience in order for their quality of life to be affected. Are there differences in views between people of different age groups?

Quality of life measures

Quality of life measures range from broad general health profiles (generic) to disease specific scales. The broad health profiles are those which have not been developed for specific target popula-

tions or patient groups. A strength of these is that comparisons of quality of life results across patient populations can be made. A limitation is that they do not always focus on the specific problems of a given patient group. Two examples of these are the SF-36 and the Nottingham health profile. Both of these will be discussed later in this section. Disease specific quality of life scales exist for a range of specific patient groups including those who have had strokes (Holbrook & Skilbeck 1983), rheumatic disorders (Liang et al 1990), cardiovascular diseases (Wenger & Furberg 1990) and cancer (Van Knippenberg & de Haes 1985). Disease specific scales do not allow cross disease comparisons but are often more sensitive to the quality of life issues particularly relevant to specific populations of patients.

Most of the available quality of life scales depend on patients to rate themselves. Quality of life is a very personal issue and therefore getting individuals to rate themselves is the preferred method of administration. It is also possible to use structured interviews or written questionnaires. It can be difficult for patients with serious cognitive, speech and language disorders to complete these (De Haan et al 1993).

Quality of life measures can be used for a number of reasons. They may be useful for patients with chronic conditions where recovery is not expected and where success of treatments may best be measured in terms of maintaining an acceptable quality of life for the patient as the disease progresses (Talamo et al 1997). They can also be used to facilitate the process of identifying which patients will likely benefit from which type of rehabilitative procedure (Mathias et al 1997). Treatment from a multidisciplinary team may include a range of interventions which individually are difficult to measure directly or to demonstrate outcome, or for which there is no sensitive measure. In these situations a quality of life measure may be the most appropriate option to demonstrate outcome from the treatment. Quality of life measures can also be used to evaluate treatment programmes. Baker & Intagliata (1982) suggest that if patients' life situations are not improved in some way and they are not happier or more satisfied after participating in treatment then ultimately it is difficult to justify the treatment.

The Short Form 36

The Short Form 36 (SF-36) health survey is an example of a measurement scale for quality of life that includes physical functioning as a component of the measurement. It has been developed from a longer medical outcomes study questionnaire, which has had the number of items reduced to 36, hence the title Short Form 36 (SF-36). The aim of reducing the items was to develop a scale that could be conducted in a short period of time and therefore lend itself to being used in a broad range of settings (Ware & Sherbourne 1992).

The SF-36 was developed to be an indicator of quality of life for population studies as well as an outcome measure in clinical practice and research (McDowell & Newell 1996). It is suitable for use with all patients as the measure addresses aspects of health that are important to all patients, rather than just those with a particular condition. It is a questionnaire that can be completed by anyone over 14 years of age in a clinical setting or at home. It can also be administered in an interview. It is easy to use and takes between 5 and 10 minutes to complete. This has made it popular (Larson 1997).

The SF-36 categorises the 36 items into eight areas relating to health concepts. These are physical functioning (10 items), role limitations due to physical problems (four items), social functioning (two items), bodily pain (two items), general mental health (five items), role limitation due to emotional problems (three items), vitality (four items) and general health perceptions (five items) (Larson 1997). The inclusion of bodily pain and vitality as concepts of health is unique to the SF-36 scale (Ware & Sherbourne 1992). The final item asks about health change over the past year. The items relating to movement (see Tables 9.4, 9.5 and 9.6) ask about levels and types of limitations when lifting and carrying groceries, climbing stairs, bending, kneeling and walking moderate distances.

Each of the eight different sections produces an individual section score ranging from 0–54. For each item there is a choice of responses on a Likert scale, ranging from 'limited a lot' to 'not limited at all' or 'all of the time' to 'none of the time' (Brazier 1995). These are not combined to form an overall score and therefore it is hard to make comparisons (Bowling & Normand 1998). It is possible to identify the scores relating to movement separately from those relating to the other concepts relating to health. As with all scales that contain sections, it is important to

Table 9.4 The ten items of SF-36 that relate to physical functioning (Reproduced with permission from Ware 2000, www.qmetric.com). The following questions are about activities you might do during a typical day. Does your health now limit you in these activities? If so, how much?

Activities	Yes, limited a lot	Yes, limited a little	No, not limited at all
Vigorous activities such as running, lifting heavy objects, participating in strenuous sports	1	2	3
Moderate activities such as moving a table, pushing a vacuum cleaner, bowling or playing golf	1	2	3
Lifting or carrying groceries	1	2	3
Climbing several flights of stairs	1	2	3
Climbing one flight of stairs	1	2	3
Bending, kneeling or stooping	1	2	3
Walking more than a mile	1	2	3
Walking half a mile	1	2	3
Walking 100 yards	1	2	3
Bathing and dressing yourself	1	2	3

Table 9.5 The four items of SF-36 that relate to role limitations due to physical problems and pain (Reproduced with permission from Ware 2000, www.qmetric.com). During the past four weeks have you had any of the following problems with your work or regular daily activities as a result of your physical health?

	Yes	No
Cut down on the amount of time you spent on work or other activities	1	2
Accomplished less than you would like	1	2
Were limited in the kind of work or other activities	1	2
Had difficulty performing the work or other activities (for example, it took extra effort)	1	2

Table 9.6 The two items of SF-36 that relate to pain (Reproduced with permission from Ware 2000, www.qmetric.com).

How much bodily pain during the past four weeks?

None	1
Very mild	2
Mild	3
Moderately severe	4
Severe	5
Very severe	6

During the past four weeks, how much did pain interfere with your normal work (including work both outside the home and housework)?

Not at all	1
A little bit	2
Moderately	3
Quite a bit	4
Extremely	5

carry out the whole scale and not just select the aspects relating to movement. These sections are not validated to be used in isolation. Higher scores indicate a perception of good quality of life (Talamo et al 1997).

There is considerable evidence for the validity and reliability of the SF-36 and its ability to measure changes in health status over time (Brazier et al 1992, Ware & Sherbourne 1992, Garratt et al 1994, Jenkinson et al 1994). This supports its use as a routine scale for monitoring and assessing quality of life both in clinical practice and research. Anderson et al (1996) found it to be valid for use in stroke rehabilitation and Talamo et al (1997) with patients with rheumatoid arthritis. However, as with other measurement scales, ceiling and flooring effects can occur.

Nottingham health profile

Hunt, McEwen and McKenna developed the Nottingham health profile in 1980 as a scale to measure health status (Hunt et al 1985). To develop it, 768 patients with a variety of health problems generated over 2000 statements. These statements were then reduced to 38. The profile consists of two parts, the first consisting of 38 statements addressing the following areas: energy, pain, emotional reactions, sleep, social isolation and physical mobility. The second part has seven statements concerning paid employment, jobs around the house, social life, personal relationships, sex life, hobbies and interests and holidays. Table 9.7 includes examples of statements that address issues relating to movement used in the profile and again, like the SF-36, these examples should not be used out of the context of the whole measure.

The Nottingham health profile is short, simple and can be self administered or carried out by interview. It takes about 5 minutes to complete. It is sensitive to change and has been tested extens-

Table 9.7 Examples of statements (Reproduced with permission from McKenna 2000, spm@galen.eng.net).

I can only walk about indoors
I find it hard to bend
I'm unable to walk at all
I have trouble getting up and down stairs or steps
I find it hard to reach for things
I find it hard to dress myself
I find it hard to stand for long (e.g. at the kitchen sink, waiting for a bus)
I need help to walk about outside (e.g. a walking aid or someone to support me)

ively for reliability and validity (Bowling 1991). Scores ranging from 0, indicating no problem, to 100 where problems in all areas have been identified, are used to score it. As a result a higher score reflects severe problems.

There are different views on whether the Nottingham health profile is actually measuring quality of life. Wade (1992) suggests that it may be recording mood rather than global quality of life, Ebrahim et al (1986) suggest it is an indicator of depressed mood while Bowling (1991) suggests that it is identifying how people feel when they are experiencing various states of ill health.

CONCLUSION

Movement cannot be considered as an isolated component of life. If there is a loss of movement for any reason, there will be implications for how everyday activities are carried out and for how quality of life is perceived. The difficulty is in quantifying or measuring these implications. Scales have been developed to try and measure these issues. Careful consideration needs to be given when selecting a measurement scale to ensure it fulfils the purpose for which it is needed.

REFERENCES

Anderson C, Laubscher S, Burns R 1996 Validation of the Short Form 36 (SF36) health survey questionnaire among stroke patients. Stroke 27: 1812–1816

Bacher Y, Korner-Bitensky N, Mayo N, Becker R, Coopersmith H 1990 A longitudinal study of depression among stroke patients participating in a rehabilitation program. Canadian Journal of Rehabilitation 4: 27–37

Baker F, Intagliata J 1982 Quality of life in the evaluation of community support systems. Evaluation and Program Planning 5: 69–79

Barer D H 1989 Use of the Nottingham ADL scale in stroke: relationships between functional recovery and length of stay in hospital. Journal of Royal College of Physicians London 23(4): 242–247

Bowling A 1991 Measuring health. A review of quality of life measurement scales. Open University Press, Milton Keynes

Bowling A, Normand C 1998 Definition and measurement of outcome. In: Swash M (ed) Outcome in neurological and neurosurgical disorders. Cambridge University Press, Cambridge, pp 14–34

Brazier J 1995 The Short-Form 36 (SF-36) health survey and its use in pharmacoeconomic evaluation. PharmacoEconomics 7: 403–415

Brazier J, Harper R, Jones N et al 1992 Validating the SF-36 health survey questionnaire: new outcome measure for primary care. British Medical Journal 305: 160–164

Burton J 1989 The model of human occupation and occupational therapy practice with elderly patients. Part 2 application. British Journal of Occupational Therapy 52: 219–221

Collin C, Wade D T, Davies S, Horne V 1988 The Barthel ADL index: a reliability study. International Disability Studies 10: 61–63

De Haan R, Aaronson N, Limburg M, Langton Hewer R, van Creval H 1993 Measuring quality of life in stroke. Stroke 24: 320–327

Diener E 1984 Subjective well-being. Psychological Bulletin 95: 542–575

Eakin P 1993 The Barthel index: confidence limits. British Journal of Occupational Therapy 56(5): 184–185

Ebrahim S, Barer D, Nouri F 1986 Use of the Nottingham health profile with patients after a stroke. Journal of Epidemiological Community Health 40: 166–169

Fallowfield L 1990 The quality of life. The missing measurement of health care. Souvenir Press, London

Fisher A G 1992 Functional measures, part 2: selecting the right test, minimising the limitations. American Journal of Occupational Therapy 46(3): 278–281

Fisher A G 1994 Functional assessment and occupation: critical issues for occupational therapy. Key note address at Annual Conference of New Zealand Association of Occupational Therapists

Garratt A, Ruta D, Abdalla M, Russell I 1994 SF-36 health survey questionnaire: II. Responsiveness to changes in health status in four common clinical conditions. Quality in Health Care 3: 186–192

Gibbon B 1991 Measuring stroke recovery. Nursing Times 87(44): 32–34

Gompertz P, Pound P, Ebrahim S 1993 The reliability of stroke outcome measures. Clinical Rehabilitation 7: 290–296

Granger C V, Hamilton B B 1990 Measurement of stroke rehabilitation outcome in 1980s. Stroke 21 (Supplement)II: 46–47

Harper Collins 1987 The new Collins dictionary and thesaurus in one volume. Harper Collins, Glasgow

Holbrook M, Skilbeck C E 1993 An activities index for use with stroke patients. Age and Ageing 12: 166–170

Hunt S M, McEwen J, McKenna S P 1985 Measuring health status: a new tool for clinicians and epidemiologists. Journal of the Royal College of General Practitioners 35: 185–188

Jenkinson C, Wright L, Coulter A 1994 Criterion validity and reliability of the SF-36 in a population sample. Quality of Life Research 3: 7–12

King's Fund Report 1988 Treatment of stroke. British Medical Journal 297: 126–128

Larson J 1997 The MOS 36-Item Short Form Health Survey. A conceptual analysis. Evaluation and the Health Professions 20: 14–27

Law M, Letts L 1989 A critical review of scales of activities of daily living. American Journal of Occupational Therapy 43(8): 522–528

Liang M H, Katz J N, Ginsburg K S 1990 Chronic rheumatic disease. In: Spiller B (ed) Quality of life assessments in clinical trials. Raven Press, New York, pp 441–458

Lincoln N, Gladman J 1992 The extended activities of daily living scale: a further validation. Disability and Rehabilitation 14: 41–43

Livingstone M G, Livingstone H M 1985 The Glasgow assessment schedule: clinical and research assessment of head injury outcome. International Rehabilitation Medicine 7: 146–149

McCloy L, Jongbloed L 1987 Robinson-Bashall functional assessment for arthritis patients; reliability and validity. Archives of Physical Medicine and Rehabilitation 68: 486–489

McDowell F, Lee J E, Swift T, Sweet R D, Ogsbury J S, Kessler J T 1970 Treatment of Parkinson's syndrome with L Dihydroxyphenylalanine (Levodopa). Annals of Internal Medicine 72: 29–35

McDowell I, Newell C 1996 Measuring health. A guide to rating scales and questionnaires, 2nd edn. Oxford University Press, Oxford

Mahoney F I, Barthel D W 1965 Functional evaluation: the Barthel index. Maryland State Medical Journal 14: 61–65

Mathias S, Bates M, Pasta D, Cistermas M, Feeny D, Patrick D 1997 Use of health utilities index with stroke patients and their caregivers. Stroke 28: 1888–1894

Niemi M, Laaksonen R, Kotila M, Waltimo O 1988 Quality of life four years after stroke. Stroke 19(9): 1101–1106

Nouri F, Lincoln N 1987 An extended activities of daily living scale for stroke patients. Clinical Rehabilitation 1: 301–305

Rodgers H, Curless R, James O F W 1993 Standardised functional assessment scales for elderly patients. Age and Ageing 22: 161–163

Talamo J, Frater A, Gallivan S, Young A 1997 Use of the Short Form-36 (SF-36) for health status measurement in rheumatoid arthritis. British Journal of Rheumatology 36: 463–469

Van Knippenberg F C E, de Haes J C J M 1985 The quality of life of cancer patients: a review of the literature. Social Science and Medicine 20: 809–817

Wade D T 1992 Measurement in neurological rehabilitation. Oxford University Press, Oxford

Ware J, Sherbourne C 1992 The MOS 36-Item Short Form Health Survey (SF36). 1. Conceptual framework and item selection. Medical Care 30: 473–481

Wenger N K, Furberg C D 1990 Cardiovascular disorders. In: Spiller B (ed) Quality of life assessments in clinical trials. Raven Press, New York, pp 335–345

World Health Organization 1981 Report 668 Disability prevention and rehabilitation. World Health Organization, Geneva

Wyller T, Sveen U, Sodring K, Pettersen A, Bautz-Holter E 1997 Subjective well-being one year after stroke. Clinical Rehabilitation 11: 139–145

CHAPTER CONTENTS

Introduction   173

Walking   174
Terminology of gait   175
Stance phase   177
Swing phase   178
Joint and muscle activity in the stance phase   179
Joint and muscle activity in the swing phase   182
Movement in the trunk, shoulder girdle and upper limbs   182
Ground reaction forces in gait   182
Energy expenditure and gait   183

Running   183

Walking backwards   184

Walking up and down stairs   184
Stance phase on ascent   184
Swing phase on ascent   185
Stance phase on descent   186
Swing phase on descent   187

Moving from sitting to standing   187
Seated phase   189
Stance phase   189

10

Function of the lower limb

M. Trew

OBJECTIVES

When you have completed this chapter you should be able to:

1. **Discuss the importance of walking**

2. **Identify the characteristics of normal gait**

3. **Describe the gait cycle**

4. **Recognise the joint movements and muscle activity that occur in normal gait**

5. **Recognise the normal patterns of movement for ascending and descending stairs**

6. **Recognise the normal patterns of movement for rising from a chair.**

INTRODUCTION

The main functions of the lower limbs are to support the body when standing and to enable locomotion. To be able to stand and move is a key part of normal, active life, and it is important for therapists to have a detailed understanding of the structure and function of the lower limbs in order to plan purposeful rehabilitation programmes. In this chapter walking, stair climbing and getting out of a chair are considered in some detail as they represent major functions of the lower limb. As you develop an understanding of the important features of these activities you should become aware of similarities in the patterns of movement and then, when you start to analyse activities not covered by this chapter, you may again notice common patterns of movement. This knowledge will be the foundation for developing an understanding of all other functions of the lower limbs.

WALKING

Human beings can perform a wide range of methods of locomotion including walking, running and, less commonly, crawling, hopping, jumping and even rolling. The diversity of locomotion is even greater when you consider that each of these movements can be performed in a variety of ways and directions. Despite this variety, all these methods of locomotion have common patterns of movement and by studying walking in detail it becomes easier to understand the rest.

Walking can be defined as a highly energy efficient method of progression involving rhythmical, reciprocal movements of the lower limbs where one foot is always in contact with the floor. People normally walk for a purpose, perhaps because they want to reach a certain place at a certain time, but they also walk for pleasure and for health. Increasingly, walking is being advocated as a safe and effective way of maintaining fitness, particularly in the later years of life (Arakawa 1993, Hardman & Hudson 1994, Pereira et al 1998), and in many countries walking for pleasure and health is a popular pastime. Providing walking speeds of more than 6 km/hr are achieved and hills are incorporated into the route, walking maintains reasonable ranges of lower limb joint motion and a functional level of cardiorespiratory fitness.

Although to most people walking is fully automatic and requires no thought, it actually comprises complex patterns of movement involving all lower limb joints. In addition, there is movement of the joints of the vertebral column, from lumbar to cervical spine and, when unrestricted, the upper limbs swing in reciprocal patterns. This involvement of all the body segments requires considerable neural control and this explains why at birth, when the nervous system is not fully developed, walking is impossible. It is not until the infant has gained control over all body parts and is able to balance that the first uncertain steps can be taken. Even then the child is unable to walk while carry-ing objects and several years will pass before the activity becomes mature and fully automatic.

In the health care professions it is quite common for the term *gait* to be used in preference to walking. Gait means the manner or way in which walking takes place and implies a detailed consideration of the kinetics and kinematics of the activity.

Basically, all people walk in the same way, with the lower limbs moving reciprocally to provide alternate support and propulsion and, if the upper limbs are unencumbered, they demonstrate a stereotyped pattern of reciprocal movement in phase with the lower limbs. The joint movements that occur in the sagittal plane (flexion and extension) are very similar in both range and direction of movement between individuals (Murray et al 1964). The differences that set one person's gait apart from another's occur mainly in movements in the coronal and transverse planes. For example the amount of hip rotation and therefore foot angle can vary dramatically between individuals, and noticeable variation also occurs in trunk lateral flexion. The range of head and trunk rotation in the transverse plane is also very variable, with some people having almost imperceptible rotation and others rotating through such a wide range that they appear to be swaggering (Murray et al 1964, Smidt 1990).

Task 10.1

It is important to develop good observational abilities. Most people are better at observing human movement than they realise. Interestingly, the general population can recognise someone they know well even when that person is too far away to make out facial details. It is likely that at a subconscious level we are aware of the small differences in the ways that people move. In the case of walking we probably store information about the transverse and coronal plane movements and use this to distinguish between different individuals when we are too far away from them to see their faces. Next time you are in a suitable place, watch the way in which people walk and see if you can work out how the gait of one individual differs from another. In particular, you should observe the degree of knee flexion and extension in the stance phase and the rotation and lateral flexion of the trunk. Are the differences in gait between individuals simply a consequence of different walking velocities?

Walking is a smooth, highly coordinated, rhythmical movement by which the body moves step by step in the required direction. The forces that cause this movement are a combination of muscle activity to accelerate or decelerate the body segments, and the effects of gravity and momentum. Walking has often been described as a fall followed by a reflex recovery of balance and, to a certain extent, this is true. To initiate the first step the anterior muscles at the ankle contract to move the centre of gravity forwards in relation to the feet and this causes a loss of balance anteriorly. Once the centre of gravity has been displaced, gravity and momentum continue the movement initiated by the muscles. In order to avoid a fall there is a reflex stepping reaction which causes one of the lower limbs to be moved forwards so that one foot can be placed in front of the other. This alters the base so that the centre of gravity is once again above the feet. If walking is to continue, the centre of gravity must again be displaced anteriorly. However, once inertia has been overcome by muscle action on the first step, all subsequent steps benefit from the momentum accrued and only a minor amount of propulsion comes from the calf muscles. For each step, balance is allowed to be perturbed so that a subsequent reflex step will occur. This continues until the purpose of walking has been achieved and, because the momentum of walking removes the need for much muscle activity, the whole process is remarkably energy efficient. Once a steady walking velocity has been reached, the actual process of walking requires low energy expenditure and it is possible to walk for long periods of time with surprisingly little fatigue (Smidt 1990, McArdle et al 1996). As would be expected, the least energy is expended when walking slowly on level ground but an increase in velocity or a change from a firm surface to a surface such as soft sand would immediately increase energy expenditure. There are two other instances in walking on level ground when energy expenditure is relatively high. Energy expenditure is higher on the initiation of movement, when inertia has to be overcome so that the body weight can be displaced forwards, than it is during a continuous sequence of steps.

Conversely, at the end of walking an increase in energy expenditure is required to stop forward movement of the limbs and trunk. The faster an individual is walking the more difficult it is to stop suddenly and the greater an expenditure of energy will occur.

Understanding the role of inertia and momentum in walking is important as the energy efficient nature of the activity is lost if the utilisation of momentum is restricted and the walker is constantly having to overcome inertia either to initiate or stop the movement. You are probably already aware of this as you must have noticed that you feel disproportionately tired after a day wandering around the shops. When people go shopping, particularly when they are not strongly focused on what they need to buy, they constantly stop to look at goods and then move on. The repeated stopping and starting involved in shopping can be surprisingly tiring. Re-education programmes should aim to develop the rhythm of gait and the smooth swinging motion of the upper and lower limbs so that the patient can benefit fully from as energy efficient a gait as possible.

Task 10.2

Analyse the effects of using a walking frame. Consider the gait of a patient using a quadruped walking frame. Is the smooth, rhythmical, reciprocal movement of normal gait preserved? Will using a walking frame conserve or increase energy expenditure? How do you think the energy expenditure needed for walking with a frame would compare with the energy needed for walking, fully weight bearing, with crutches?

Terminology of gait

Walking is a complex activity and, if it is to be fully understood, it needs to be broken down into named parts. There are a number of ways in which gait can be described and the most commonly used international terminology is given here. It is useful to consider gait in terms of both the temporal and spatial components. The temporal components are those periods of time during

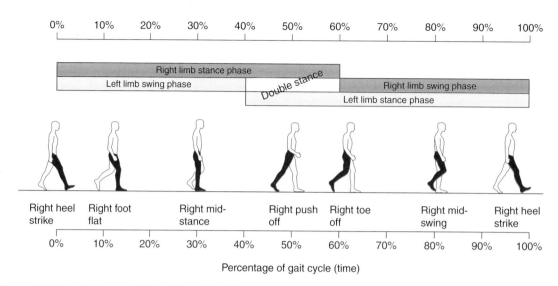

Figure 10.1 Terminology and timing of the gait cycle.

which events take place and are often measured in seconds. For example, the stance phase of walking is a temporal component and relates to the period of time that the foot is in contact with the floor. The spatial components refer to the position or distances covered by the limbs and an example of this would be step length. When analysing gait it is essential to consider both the temporal and spatial components because disease or trauma can affect either. These components are illustrated in Figures 10.1 and 10.2.

Table 10.1 illustrates two common approaches to the terminology of gait. Most of the descriptors for normal gait refer to events in the gait cycle which may be absent in pathological gait and so alternative terminology is needed. For example, a person with a painful, sprained ankle is unlikely to demonstrate heel strike, but will make initial foot floor contact with the whole foot. A person with increased tone in the lower limbs may be unable to move out of plantar flexion and so never achieves foot flat. For these reasons some authorities like to use gait terminology which is equally applicable for normal or pathological gaits.

Gait cycle

This is the period of time during which a complete sequence of events takes place. Whilst it is

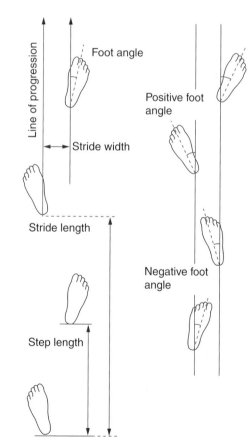

Figure 10.2 Characteristics of gait that can be measured from footprints.

Table 10.1 Alternative terminologies used to describe gait

Terminology suitable for describing the temporal components of normal gait	Terminology suitable for describing the temporal components of pathological gait
Stance phase	Stance phase
Heel strike	Initial foot-floor contact
Foot flat	Loading phase
Mid-stance	Mid-stance
Heel off	Propulsive phase
Push off	Propulsive phase
Toe off	Pre-swing
Swing phase	Swing phase
Acceleration	Acceleration
Mid-swing	Mid-swing
Deceleration	Deceleration

usual to consider the gait cycle as beginning when the heel of one foot strikes the floor and continuing until the same heel strikes the floor again, it may be measured from any moment in the gait cycle. The gait cycle is subdivided into a stance phase and a swing phase, and these terms describe the periods of time when the foot is either in contact with the floor or swinging forward in preparation for the next step. *The swing phase* is the period of time when the limb under consideration is not in contact with the floor. *The stance phase* is the period of time when the limb under consideration is in contact with the floor. In walking there is always a period of time when both feet are in contact with the floor simultaneously; this is called 'double stance' (see Fig. 10.1).

Stance phase

The stance phase is the most complex and arguably the most important phase of gait. During the stance phase the lower limb has to provide a semi-rigid support for the body weight to facilitate the maintenance of balance and allow forward propulsion. The stance limb also has a role in compensating for uneven ground and when positioned correctly, it enables an accurate swing phase on the contralateral limb to take place. The stance phase can be subdivided into the following stages.

Heel strike or initial foot-floor contact. In normal walking the leading limb initially contacts the floor by heel strike. At the moment of heel strike the fol-

lowing limb is also in contact with the floor, giving a position of double stance. This is the moment when the whole-body centre of gravity is at its lowest and the walker is most stable (Fig. 10.3).

Foot flat or loading phase. Immediately on coming into contact with the floor the stance limb takes the body weight. To achieve this in normal gait the foot has to move rapidly from the position of dorsiflexion, which allowed heel strike, to plantigrade. At foot flat the whole foot comes into contact with the floor, allowing it to accept the weight of the body as the mid-stance phase takes place. During heel strike and foot flat there is rapid loading of the limb and it is important during this phase that strategies exist to absorb the sudden imposition of ground reaction forces.

Mid-stance. In mid-stance the body is carried forward over the stance limb and the opposite limb is in the swing phase. The whole-body centre of gravity passes from behind to in front of the stance foot and it is in mid-stance that the centre of gravity rises to its highest position in relation to the supporting surface. This is the position when the walker is least stable due to the small base and the relatively high centre of gravity.

Heel off, push off and toe off, or the propulsive phase. There are now several events that happen in quick succession and all of which are designed to propel the body forwards and terminate the stance phase. Initially, the heel lifts off the ground, an event which is passive in slow gait but may require a small degree of muscle activity at faster velocities. This is usually followed by a propulsive stage when the calf muscles contract

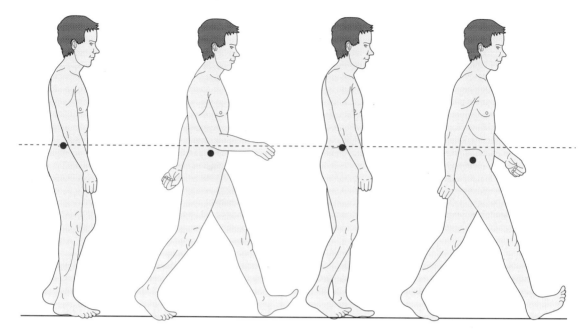

Figure 10.3 The vertical displacement of the centre of gravity during walking.

to plantar flex the fore foot against the floor, and this is called 'push off'. Finally there is the moment of 'toe off' when propulsion ends, the contact between the toes and the floor is lost and the swing phase for that limb starts.

At an average speed of walking, the stance phase takes about 60% of the gait cycle and the swing phase about 40% (Murray 1967). In slow walking the stance phase can constitute more than 70% of the gait cycle with the swing phase being less than 30%. As the velocity of walking increases, the length of time in the stance phase decreases until on very fast walking the stance phase may be reduced below 57% of the cycle (Smidt 1990). The period of double stance also decreases with increasing velocity. When walking very slowly the double stance may last as long as 46% of the total gait cycle; on very fast walking the double stance period may be reduced to 14%; and when walking develops into a run, there is no double stance period.

Swing phase

During the swing phase, the swinging limb moves in front of the stance limb so that forward progression may take place. In order to swing successfully, the limb must be shortened sufficiently to enable the foot to clear the ground and this is normally achieved by flexion of the hip and knee joints and dorsiflexion of the ankle. Clearing the ground is key to a successful swing phase but in order to conserve energy it is important that the limb is not lifted further than is necessary. In normal adult gait the average clearance of the foot from the ground in mid-swing phase is around 2 cm and with so little leeway for error it is quite remarkable that people don't catch their feet on the floor more often. The swing phase can be divided into three stages.

Acceleration. The force generated by the hip flexors, and to a lesser extent by the plantar flexors, accelerates the non-weight bearing limb forwards.

Mid-swing. This corresponds with mid-stance and at the moment the swing phase limb passes the stance limb it is at its shortest.

Deceleration. In this final stage of the swing phase, the lower limb muscles work to decelerate the swing limb in preparation for heel strike. The muscle action in this phase is usually eccentric and requires less energy than those times in the gait cycle when concentric activity is needed to accelerate a limb.

Other temporal and spatial components

Cadence. When considering pathological gait, a knowledge of the step rate is important and the term 'cadence' is used to indicate the number of steps taken per minute. The cadence mainly depends on the velocity of walking. In slow walking the cadence may be 40–50 steps per minute, whereas moderate walking will cause an increase in cadence to around 110 steps per minute and this figure will rise with increasing velocity until running occurs. If a patient has pain, joint stiffness, muscle weakness or poor balance, the cadence will be reduced. An increase in natural cadence is often taken to indicate an improvement in a patient's walking ability, but it might be more appropriate to use the patient's ability to vary cadence as an indicator of walking skill.

There are a number of spatial components that it is useful to measure as part of the analysis of gait (see Fig. 10.2).

Stride length. This is the distance between successive foot-floor contacts with the same foot. For example, this might be the distance between the first point of contact of the right heel on the floor and the second point of contact of the right heel.

Step length. This is the distance between successive foot-floor contacts with opposite feet. In this case, it could be the distance (in the line of progression) between the point of right heel strike and the point of left heel strike. There are two steps to every stride.

Step and stride length are dependent on several factors including the length of the lower limb, the age of the subject and the velocity of walking. Short lower limb length, increasing age and decreasing velocity will all reduce the step and stride length.

Foot angle. This is the degree of in-turning or out-turning of the foot: if the foot turns in there is said to be a negative foot angle; if the foot turns out, the angle is positive. The majority of the population walk with a positive foot angle of up to 30°. This angle is mainly associated with the degree of rotation at the hip joint and, to a lesser extent, the rotation between the tibia and the femur. In some cases tibial or femoral torsion will influence foot angle.

Stride or step width. This is the distance between the two feet and it is normally measured from the mid-point of the heels. This distance varies greatly between individuals but on average it is about 7 cm; however, when a person has poor balance they tend to increase their stride width to give themselves a greater base of support. It is interesting to note that on slow walking the stride width tends to be greater than on rapid walking.

Joint and muscle activity in the stance phase

As shown in Figure 10.4, the pattern of joint movement is less complicated at the hip joint than at the knee or ankle joints. Whilst the hip joint has only one phase of extension and one phase of flexion, the other two joints have two phases of each movement in each gait cycle. The range of movement at the hip and knee joints is more consistent between individuals but the movement at the ankle joint can be quite variable between one person and another.

Muscle activity, as indicated by electromyography (EMG), shows variability between subjects and also when different walking velocities are chosen. A guide to the common patterns of major muscle activity is given in Figure 10.5; the data for this were gathered from subjects walking at a moderate pace. It is interesting to note that in a substantial portion of the gait cycle there is little or no muscle activity occurring in the majority of the muscle groups. This supports the theory that gait is energy efficient.

Heel strike. At the instant of heel strike the hip joint is partially flexed and gluteus maximus and the hamstrings contract immediately to initiate hip extension. The knee joint will either be in full extension or flexed to about 5° and the quadriceps will be working eccentrically to control the knee flexion which follows immediately after heel strike. The ankle joint on heel strike is usually near the neutral position, though there

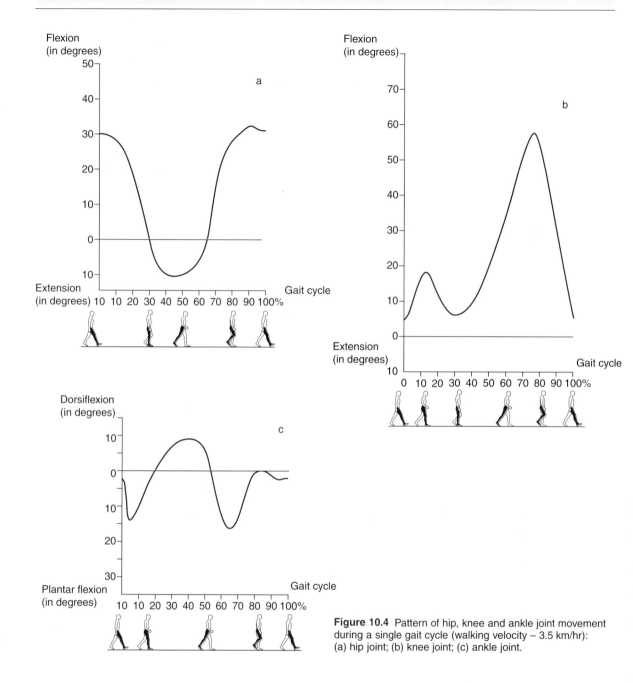

Figure 10.4 Pattern of hip, knee and ankle joint movement during a single gait cycle (walking velocity – 3.5 km/hr): (a) hip joint; (b) knee joint; (c) ankle joint.

can be a variation between individuals of up to 10° of dorsiflexion or plantar flexion. More than 10° of plantar flexion would be rare in a normal individual as it would render heel strike difficult and leave the toes vulnerable to stubbing on the floor. This position is produced prior to heel strike by concentric action of the dorsiflexor muscles and on heel strike there is an immediate change to eccentric activity to lower the fore foot to the floor. At the metatarsophalangeal joints there is a similar pattern of activity with the muscles positioning the joints in extension ready for heel strike and then lowering the toes into floor contact.

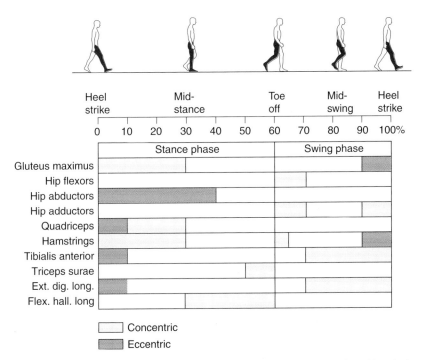

Figure 10.5 Muscle activity, as indicated by EMG, is variable between subjects. It also varies with velocity and the faster the velocity, the more muscle input will be required. This figure shows the type and duration of muscle activity which might be expected in moderate velocity walking.

Foot flat. The hip joint is beginning to move into extension by concentric action of the hip extensors, but the knee joint has flexed further in order to cushion the effect of heel strike and also to reduce the vertical displacement of the centre of gravity that would otherwise occur as the body passes over the stance limb. This knee flexion is controlled by eccentric work of the quadriceps group and measurements of knee movement taken in our laboratory show it can often be as great as 30°. At the ankle joint there is controlled plantar flexion to lower the foot to the floor, which is undertaken by eccentric work of the dorsiflexors. Without controlled plantar flexion the foot would 'slap' down uncomfortably and this can be heard in some patients. As the foot achieves good foot-floor contact there is a small amount of eversion to transfer the body weight across from the lateral border of the foot towards the great toe.

Mid-stance. Hip extension continues but by now it is being produced by momentum and the

muscles are no longer active. While the contralateral limb is in the swing phase, the pelvis is unsupported on that side and the hip abductors on the stance limb initially contract to control pelvic levels and lower the pelvis towards the swing side by eccentric muscle action. The knee joint remains in slight flexion. There is sometimes a minor burst of activity in the ankle dorsiflexors to pull the tibia forwards over the foot, but once this movement has been initiated, momentum and gravity will take over. Depending on the velocity of the movement, the calf muscles may need to exert a slowing influence on the tibia through eccentric muscle action.

Heel off, leading to push off. At the beginning of this phase, the centre of gravity is in front of the stance foot so the force of gravity will increase the range of hip extension and ankle dorsiflexion. As full range dorsiflexion is reached, the heel will rise off the floor and the plantar flexors will contract concentrically to provide the propulsive component of push off. In slow to moderate walking velocities this contraction is not usually very large as momentum is the major factor in moving the body forwards. In normal walking the hip extensors are inactive at this stage and, in fact, the hip and knee joints are usually starting to flex in preparation for the swing phase (Inman et al 1981).

Joint and muscle activity in the swing phase

Acceleration. Minor forces generated on push off by the hip flexors and the plantar flexors accelerate the limb forwards in the swing phase assisted by momentum and gravity. The hip and knee joints are both flexing and there is a rapid movement towards dorsiflexion to ensure that the toes do not catch on the floor.

Mid-swing. In mid-swing phase, flexion of the knee and hip joints continues to keep the foot sufficiently raised to avoid the toes catching on the floor. At this stage the foot may be lowered into slight plantar flexion.

Deceleration. The hip continues to flex, the movement being mainly produced by momentum, and the hamstrings act eccentrically to slow down the movement at the hip joint. The knee joint moves from flexion to extension; it is interesting to note that the quadriceps plays no part in this movement. The whole of the lower limb is being moved forwards by flexion of the hip and the resulting momentum causes knee joint extension. Towards the end of the deceleration phase, knee joint extension may have to be slowed down and this is achieved by eccentric action of the hamstrings. In preparation for heel strike, the dorsiflexors contract quite strongly to ensure that the foot is in the optimum position for heel strike.

Movement in the trunk, shoulder girdle and upper limbs

It is possible to walk with little movement of the trunk and no movement in the upper limbs, but in these circumstances gait is awkward and tiring (Murray et al 1967). Flexion and extension of the hip joints causes some rotation in the lumbar spine and, in order to keep the head facing forwards, the thoracic and cervical spine rotate in the opposite direction. Reciprocal movements of the upper and lower limbs occur, with the right upper limb flexing at the shoulder joint simultaneously with flexion at the left hip joint. Normally the shoulder joint starts to flex or extend slightly before the same movement is seen in the elbow joint. The range of movement varies greatly between individuals and in the same individual it will vary according to the velocity of walking. Whereas the patterns of movement in the lower limb are very similar between individuals, they are more varied in the upper limb (Murray et al 1967). This is not surprising as the movement of the upper limb isn't essential for the process of walking and the range of movement of upper limb joints is likely to be affected by the momentum imparted by the lower limbs and the degree of trunk rotation. There are several reasons why the upper limb moves during gait. It has been suggested that arm swing may impart momentum through the trunk to the lower limbs; subjective reports from fatigued walkers indicate that they have reduced the effort of walking by deliberately increasing their arm swing. It is also possible that arm swing acts to correct over-rotation at the lumbar spine (Murray et al 1967).

Ground reaction forces in gait

Whenever the foot is in contact with the ground there will be vertical, anterior-posterior and medio-lateral forces acting between the foot and the floor. Measurement of these forces using a force plate shows a consistent, inter-subject pattern of vertical and anterior-posterior forces. The medio-lateral forces are tiny and show much more variability between individuals (see Fig. 10.6). At the beginning and end of the stance phase the vertical ground reaction forces are normally about 25% greater than body weight, but much less than they would be in running. The anterior-posterior ground reaction forces are about 25% of body weight in each direction (Farley & Ferris 1998). The relatively small forces involved, the design of the human body that

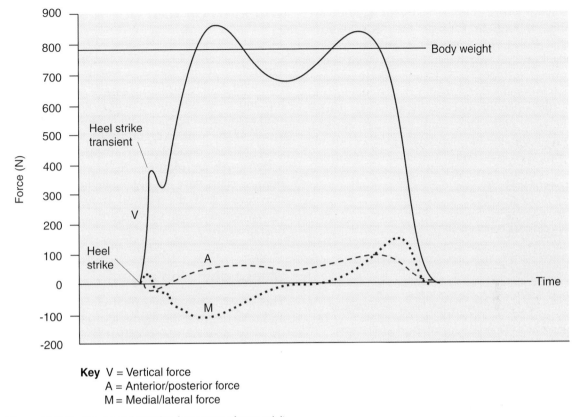

Figure 10.6 Typical ground reaction force traces for an adult.

facilitates shock absorption, and the cushioning effect of knee flexion on initial foot-floor contact mean that repetitive strain injuries caused by ground reaction forces are rare in walking.

Energy expenditure and gait

The amount of energy required to walk at a comfortable pace is very small in comparison with other activities. Normal, easy walking on a firm surface requires about 0.080 kcal.min^{-1}.kg^{-1}. A gentle run requires 0.135 kcal.min^{-1}.kg^{-1}, swimming breast stroke requires 0.162 kcal.min^{-1}.kg^{-1} and playing squash 0.212 kcal.min^{-1}.kg^{-1} (McArdle et al 1996).

Alterations in the normal structure of the human body or alterations in the normal pattern of gait are likely to increase energy expenditure significantly. In normal gait energy is conserved through the utilisation of momentum and kinetic

and potential energy. There are rhythmical, vertical fluctuations of the centre of gravity in normal gait that produce similar fluctuations in kinetic energy and gravitational potential energy. In mid-stance, when the centre of gravity is at its highest, gravitational potential energy is also at its highest and kinetic energy at its lowest. This situation is reversed during double stance and it is suggested that energy transfer mechanisms from the kinetic and potential energy contribute substantially to the overall energy requirements of gait (Farley and Ferris 1998). Figure 10.3 illustrates normal excursions of the centre of gravity.

RUNNING

Running differs from walking in the absence of a double stance phase and the addition of a period when there is no foot-floor contact at all.

In general terms, running and walking are very similar, though in running the movement is much quicker and the stride is lengthened. The vertical ground reaction forces generated are of the magnitude of 2.75–3 times body weight, which is considerably greater than walking, and heel strike may be replaced by toe strike (Farley & Ferris 1998). The trunk remains upright, although the line of gravity falls further outside the base than in walking. Movement of the upper limbs becomes essential and the elbows are more flexed than in walking.

Clinical considerations 10.1

Failure of one or more muscle groups to work can result in quite dramatic gait abnormalities. Weakness of the hip abductor muscles is quite common and will make it difficult for the patient to keep his pelvis level during the stance phase. Under these circumstances the pelvis may drop to the unsupported side producing a 'Trendelenburg gait'. Such a gait is often quite uncomfortable for patients; to avoid discomfort, they may laterally flex their trunk towards the stance side. This shifts their centre of gravity over the stance limb and the pelvis no longer drops painfully to the unsupported side. A very obvious lateral movement of the upper trunk is apparent when observing this sort of gait.

Paralysis of the dorsiflexors will lead to a high stepping gait. Dorsiflexion is normally needed to ensure that the toes will clear the floor in the swing phase and dorsiflexion is also needed to facilitate heel strike. When patients cannot dorsiflex, they have to increase the range of hip and knee flexion in the swing phase in order to avoid dragging their toes on the ground. Under these circumstances, heel strike is not possible and the patient's toes hit the ground first with the heel slapping down immediately afterwards. If you look at the shoes of a patient who has paralysis of the dorsiflexors, you will find that the toe area on the affected side is excessively scuffed and worn.

WALKING BACKWARDS

Although it is uncommon for anyone to walk backwards for any great distance, it is necessary in everyday life to be able to take one or two steps in that direction. The pattern of joint movement is very similar to normal gait but the step length is reduced and heel strike is replaced by toe strike (Vilensky et al 1987).

WALKING UP AND DOWN STAIRS

This is a modified walking activity using similar patterns of joint movement and muscle action. There is a stance phase, a swing phase and a period of double support (Fig. 10.7). The range of hip and knee joint movement is greater than in walking and there is considerable vertical translation of the centre of gravity (Andriacchi et al 1980, McFadyen & Winter 1988) making it an activity which requires high energy levels. Because stairs vary greatly in height, the range of movement and the vertical translation of the centre of gravity will vary according to the height of stair tread.

Stance phase on ascent

This phase is sometimes referred to as 'pull up' and it starts from the moment of foot contact on the step above. It normally requires a longer stance period than flat walking. Weight is initially taken on the anterior and middle third of the foot and then transferred to the remainder of the foot in readiness for full weight bearing.

On weight acceptance there is strong concentric contraction of the hip and knee extensors to extend the lead limb and raise the body up to and over the step. Gastrocnemius and soleus also work during 'pull up', moving the tibia posteriorly on the talus. As the single support phase is entered, the hip abductors on the stance limb work strongly to prevent the pelvis dropping to the unsupported side and to pull the trunk laterally over the supporting limb.

In the latter part of the stance phase, when body weight is fully on the stance limb and the knee extended, the quadriceps works isometrically to maintain joint position as the centre of mass passes in front of the stance foot. In some subjects the dorsiflexors undergo a low magnitude contraction at this stage to facilitate the movement of the centre of gravity forwards.

In the final stages of the stance phase there is plantar flexion produced by strong contraction of gastrocnemius and soleus to push the body forwards and upwards onto the new weight bearing limb. At this stage there is minimal activity in the

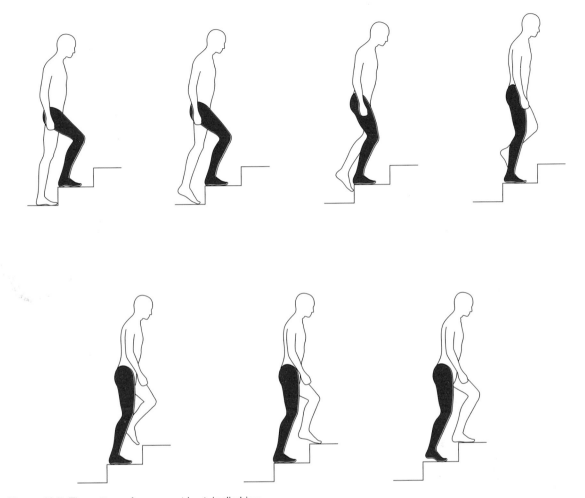

Figure 10.7 The pattern of movement in stair climbing.

knee and hip extensors (Andriacchi et al 1980, McFadyen & Winter 1988).

Swing phase on ascent

The swing limb must swing past the intermediate step and over the top step on which its stance will occur before the foot can be placed on that step. For this to occur there has to be a flexion of the whole lower limb involving concentric work of the hip and knee flexors and the dorsiflexors. In early swing the hip joint flexes and the hamstrings flex the knee joint to pull the leg and foot posteriorly to achieve intermediate step clearance.

By mid-swing the knee flexors are no longer contracting because the hip joint is sufficiently flexed to ensure intermediate step clearance. At this stage there may be some eccentric work of the quadriceps to control unwanted knee flexion.

In the later swing phase the hamstrings contract again to increase knee flexion so that the foot clears the top step, where it will eventually be placed. In order to avoid the foot catching on the top step, the amount of hip and knee flexion is quite extensive and this results in the foot being well above the step immediately before foot-step contact. To gain step contact the foot has to be lowered onto the step and this is achieved by slight hip extension controlled by eccentric activity of the hip flexors.

Through most of the swing phase, tibialis anterior works isometrically to hold the ankle joint in dorsiflexion so that the toe will not stub on the steps. Immediately before foot contact the dorsiflexors work eccentrically to lower the fore foot onto the step ready for weight acceptance on the fore foot (Andriacchi et al 1980, McFadyen & Winter 1988).

Stance phase on descent

The patterns of movement which occur when going downstairs are illustrated in Figure 10.8 and for convenience they are subdivided into the weight acceptance phase and the lowering

phase. On weight acceptance, the initial foot contact is made with the anterior and lateral border of the foot. The ankle joint moves from the initial step-contact position of plantar flexion into a neutral or dorsiflexed position controlled by eccentric work of the calf muscles. The hip joints are in very slight flexion and the knee joint may flex up to 50° to cushion the instant of foot-step contact. This is controlled by eccentric work of the hip and knee extensors. The quadriceps then contracts concentrically to extend the knee about 10° whilst the trunk moves horizontally to carry the centre of gravity over the stance limb. Tibialis anterior co-contracts with the calf muscles to control ankle position and to maintain weight bearing on the lateral border of the foot.

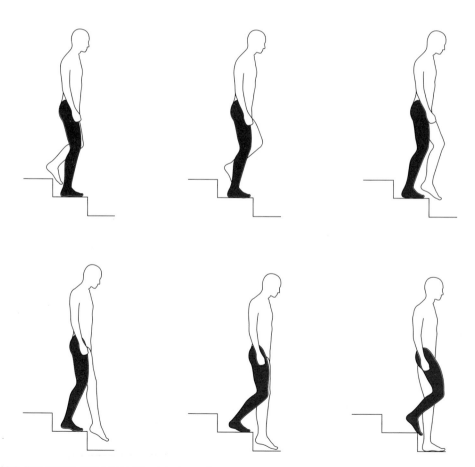

Figure 10.8 The pattern of movement in stair descent.

To lower the body weight (mid-stance) to the next step entails controlled hip and knee joint flexion and ankle joint dorsiflexion. This mainly involves eccentric action of the quadriceps and, to a lesser degree, the calf muscles and hip extensors. The stance ankle is in maximum dorsiflexion with the body weight tending to force the movement further. To prevent over dorsiflexion at the joint, the plantar flexors may need to contract. Throughout this phase the hip abductors on the stance side maintain the level of the pelvis and pull the trunk over the stance limb.

Swing phase on descent

In the swing phase, the limb has to be raised off the higher step and swung forwards and downwards, clearing the intermediate step, until it is in position to take weight at the start of the next cycle. The hip and knee flexors work concentrically to raise the foot off the top step and pull the limb forwards. Then the limb starts to extend ready for foot placement with eccentric work of the hip flexors controlling hip extension and the hamstrings working eccentrically to decelerate the extension of the knee joint. The ankle joint drops into plantar flexion, controlled by eccentric work of the anterior tibial muscles which also maintain the foot in inversion in preparation for weight to be taken on the lateral border of the foot. The hip abductors contract just before the end of the swing phase in preparation for maintaining pelvic levels on weight acceptance (McFadyen & Winter 1988).

The amount of joint range needed for ascent and descent of stairs depends on the depth of tread, but for standard sized tread (16.5 cm) the hip joint must be able to move between full extension and about 60° of flexion, the range required at the knee joint is 0°–100° of flexion and the ankle joint needs full dorsiflexion (Tata et al 1983, McFadyen & Winter 1988).

In addition to muscle strength, good balance ability is also needed for ascent and descent of stairs. When going up stairs the period of peak muscle torque and greatest instability occur simultaneously at the start of the swing phase. The hip and knee joints of the stance limb are in considerable flexion and substantial effort is needed from

---

Clinical considerations 10.2

You will be aware from your own personal experience that stair climbing requires much more energy than walking on the flat. The vertical component of stair climbing causes the main problem, but if you are to get to the top of the stairs you have no option but to go up. In contrast, walking on the flat involves components specifically designed to avoid or reduce any vertical movement. The energy expenditure required of stair descent is less because the movement is in the direction of gravity and mainly requires control through eccentric muscle activity.

---

the extensor muscles to raise the body; at the same time effort must also be directed to the maintenance of balance (Tata et al 1983).

When these facts are taken into consideration, it is no wonder that elderly and frail people find stair climbing difficult. To be able to use stairs safely it is necessary to have a wide range of movement at hip, knee and ankle joints, muscles capable of generating considerable force through a wide range, and a good sense of balance. Rehabilitation programmes for patients who have difficulties with stairs should always include activities which will increase joint range and the torque generating capacity of muscle, and will improve balance.

MOVING FROM SITTING TO STANDING

The ability to rise from sitting to standing is essential for the achievement of many everyday activities, but the movement has not been studied in the same depth as walking and contradictory evidence has been produced.

For the majority of the population, getting out of a chair is an automatic activity requiring no thought unless the chair is particularly low or the individual is feeling tired or weak. As with gait, the main patterns of joint movement are usually stereotyped with the differences being mainly caused by the initial position of the feet and the height of the chair. It is self-evident that the lower the seat height, the greater the necessary range of lower limb joint movement and the higher the level of energy.

Whether the upper limbs are involved in the process of getting out of a chair depends on the strength of the individual, the height of the chair and the presence of armrests. Under normal circumstances the situation is similar to walking in that the upper limbs are not essential to the activity and can be used for carrying or manipulating objects during the activity of standing up or sitting down. However, if weakness, balance problems or pain are factors then the upper limbs will be utilised to assist in raising the body out of the chair, thus reducing the load on the hip and knee extensor muscles.

The movement of sitting to standing can be divided into two phases, a seated phase and a stance phase, both of which occur whether or not the chair arms are used. In the seated phase, the subject prepares for standing by adjusting the position of the limbs and trunk so that the centre of gravity moves forward until it is almost over the feet.

In the stance phase, weight is taken through the lower limbs and the centre of gravity is transferred forwards and upwards. There are two main features to the stance phase: firstly the centre of gravity needs to be transferred forwards until it is slightly anterior to the lateral malleoli; and then the lower limbs must extend until the erect posture is achieved (Fig. 10.9).

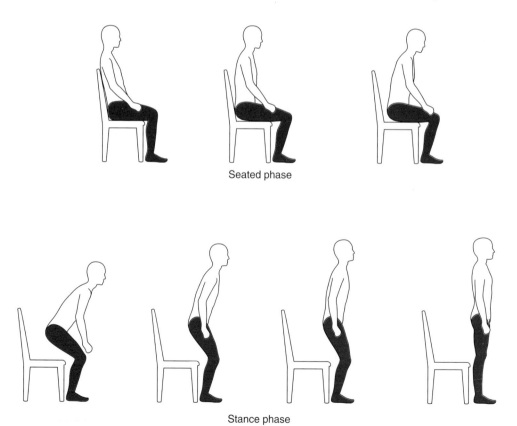

Seated phase

Stance phase

Figure 10.9 The pattern of movement when rising from a chair.

The period of time needed to complete both phases is very variable but takes, on average, 1–3 seconds (Kerr et al 1991, Baer and Ashburn 1995). The sitting phase consists of about 30% of the total movement time and in the stance phase the transfer and extension components take 20% and 50% respectively.

Seated phase

Usually people sitting in a relaxed manner lean against the back of the chair with their centre of gravity well behind their feet. It is not possible to rise with the centre of gravity in this position, and so it must be moved horizontally towards the feet before standing up can occur. The ideal preparatory position for standing up is either with the knees flexed to at least 90° so that the feet lie directly under the knee joints, or with the knees flexed up to 115° thus placing the feet approximately 10 cm posterior to a perpendicular line dropped from the knee (Ikeda et al 1991, Shepherd and Koh 1996). By positioning the feet well back, the horizontal distance that the centre of gravity has to travel is minimised and energy is conserved. Conversely, if the feet are placed too far back the knee extensors will be in a lengthened position and may not be at their optimum length to generate force. If the feet are not correctly positioned, knee flexion has to occur before a successful attempt at standing up can begin.

By the start of the stance phase the centre of gravity needs to be about 2 cm anterior to the ankle joints. To achieve this up to 55° of hip flexion from the upright sitting position is needed to cause the head and trunk to move anteriorly (Shepherd and Koh 1996). It is suggested that in normal subjects there is an initial minor burst of activity in the hip flexors in order to initiate the movement. Once that has been achieved, the flexors stop acting and the force of gravity takes over the movement. Towards the end of the hip flexion phase there may be slight eccentric work of the hip extensors to control the forward movement (Kelly et al 1976, Ikeda et al 1991). It is probable that in obese subjects or those who have 'stiffness' of the hip joint, the activity of the hip flexors will continue longer into the movement.

Knee flexion may increase slightly at this time and there is some dorsiflexion.

Very little motion is seen in the joints of the vertebral column. Schenkman et al (1990) reported between 0° and 16° of flexion in this phase and Baer & Ashburn (1995) found negligible trunk lateral flexion and rotation. Visual analysis suggests greater ranges in the cervical spine, which appears to extend to keep the vertex of the skull uppermost. If the upper limbs are not being used to push up from the chair arms, they usually flex between 11° and 53° at the shoulder joint. This combination of trunk and shoulder movement serves to move the centre of gravity forwards and also provides horizontal momentum which will contribute to the transfer of body weight onto the feet and be translated into a vertical movement as the lower limbs extend (Riley et al 1991).

The seated phase ends with the lift off from the chair. There is considerable variation in the degree of flexion at the hip and shoulder joints during this phase and also in the exact position of the head. The velocity of the movement also varies between individuals and under different circumstances. Possible explanations for such variety include the height of the chair relative to the lower limb length of the subject, the age of the subject and the degree of joint mobility and muscle strength (Kerr et al 1991).

Stance phase

The stance phase can be subdivided into transfer and extension.

Transfer

This begins on lift off from the seat and continues until the centre of gravity is about 7 cm anterior to the ankle joints, where it will remain until the erect posture is achieved (Kelly et al 1976, Ikeda et al 1991). The transfer is short and is completed in advance of hip and knee joint extension. There is peak quadriceps activity at the instant of lift off when the knees extend slightly to raise the body off the seat and this is sometimes accompanied by hip extension. Dorsiflexion of the ankle joints reaches its maximum during this phase.

Clinical considerations 10.3

Elderly and disabled people who have a limited range of joint movement and a significant degree of muscle atrophy frequently find getting up out of a chair a problem. This is partially because of the large range of lower limb movement required but also because a large muscle force is needed to overcome inertia and move the body in a direction opposed by the force of gravity. In addition, the extensor muscles of the lower limb have to generate peak torque when the hip and knee joints are in more than 90° of flexion; in this joint position the muscles are working in outer to middle range and are not at their strongest. A standard seat has a height of between 43 cm and 46 cm. To rise from such a chair the subject needs to have a range of knee flexion which is greater than 90°.

Raising the chair height, providing armrests to push on, and keeping the feet under the knees if not posterior to them all facilitate the process of rising from sitting to standing (Kelly et al 1976, Kerr et al 1991). As the height of the seat increases, the maximum angle at the hip, knee and ankle joint decreases.

The force the lower limb muscles need to generate decreases as the height of the seat increases and the chair arms are used. The largest decrease in force would appear to be in the knee extensor muscles, though some decrease around the hip has been noted. Interestingly, no decrease in ankle moment is seen. Rising from a chair which has a motorised lift on the seat or is spring assisted requires significantly less muscle force until the subject's body loses contact with the seat. At this moment there is a sudden increase in force which has been found to be greater than any force generated by rising smoothly from a normal chair (Kerr et al 1991). Frail patients find the sudden requirements to generate high levels of muscle force very difficult and it is for this reason that spring or motor assisted chair seats are not as successful as might have been expected.

The trunk and upper limbs continue the horizontal movement begun in the seated phase and the momentum developed in the seated phase carries the centre of gravity forwards until it is anterior to the ankle joints.

The transfer of weight forwards is relatively short, taking approximately 20% of the total stand up time, but it is vital to the whole process as standing is not possible without transference of the centre of gravity over the feet. It is a time of peak muscle activity in the quadriceps and the hip extensors (gluteus maximus and the hamstrings) and also a time of instability because the body is no longer supported by the seat and the centre of gravity is moving forwards. Failure to complete the transfer phase is one of the main reasons why patients are unable to stand up from a chair.

Extension

Once the centre of gravity is over the feet, horizontal movement is replaced by vertical movement. Extension of the hips and knees begins in earnest and there is also slight plantar flexion of the ankle joints. As the joints become progressively extended, the trunk also starts to extend and the cervical spine flexes slightly to keep the vertex of the skull uppermost. The upper limbs return, by eccentric muscle work, to their normal resting position.

Rising from a chair is an important functional activity which requires greater joint range and muscle torque than walking and most stair climbing (Kelly et al 1976). To be successful, it is necessary to have more than 90° of flexion at the hip and knee joints and virtually full range dorsiflexion. It is also necessary to have good balance because the centre of gravity is moving in relation to the base of support. If the relationship of the centre of gravity to the feet is not correct, the individual is likely to lose balance and fall. Flexibility of the cervical spine is particularly important because balance requires correct head positioning and, if the vertebral column is stiff, then the appropriate positions may not be achieved.

The individual must also have the strength and the balance ability to complete the transfer phase, which is arguably the most crucial part of the whole process.

REFERENCES

Andriacchi T, Andersson G, Fermier R, Stern D, Galante J 1980 A study of lower limb mechanics during stair climbing. Journal of Bone and Joint Surgery 62A: 749–757

Arakawa K 1993 Hypertension and exercise. Clinical & Experimental Hypertension 15: 1171–1179

Baer G D, Ashburn A M 1995 Trunk movements in older subjects during sit to stand. Archives of Physical Medicine and Rehabilitation 76: 844–849

Farley C T, Ferris D P 1998 Biomechanics of walking and running: centre of mass movements to muscle action. Exercise and Sport Sciences Reviews 26: 253–285

Hardman A E, Hudson A 1994 Brisk walking and serum lipid and lipoprotein variables in previously sedentary women; effect of 12 weeks of regular brisk walking followed by 12 weeks of detraining. British Journal of Sports Medicine 28: 261–266

Ikeda E, Schenkman M, Riley P, Hodge W 1991 Influence of age on dynamics of rising from a chair. Physical Therapy 71: 473–481

Inman V, Ralston H, Todd F 1981 Human walking. Williams and Wilkins, Baltimore

Kelly D, Dainis A, Wood G 1976 Mechanics and muscular dynamics of rising from a seated position. In: Komi P (ed) Biomechanics. V B International Series on Biomechanics, University Park Press, Baltimore

Kerr K, White J, Mollan R, Baird H 1991 Rising from a chair: a review of the literature. Physiotherapy 77: 15–19

McArdle W D, Katch F I, Katch V L 1996 Exercise physiology, energy, nutrition and human performance, 3rd edn. Lea & Febiger, Philadelphia

McFadyen B, Winter D 1988 An integrated biomechanical analysis of normal stair ascent and descent. Journal of Biomechanics 21: 733–744

Murray M P 1967 Gait as a total pattern of movement. American Journal of Physical Medicine 46: 290–333

Murray M P, Drought A B, Kory R C 1964 Walking patterns of normal men. Journal of Bone and Joint Surgery 46A: 335–359

Murray M P, Sepic S B, Barnard E J 1967 Patterns of sagittal rotation of the upper limbs in walking. Journal of the American Physical Therapy Association 47: 272–284

Pereira M A, Kriska A M, Day R D, Cauley J A, LaPorte R E, Kuller L H 1998 A randomized walking trial in postmenopausal women; effects on physical activity and health 10 years later. Archives of International Medicine 158: 1695–1710

Riley P O, Schenkman M, Mann R W 1991 Mechanics of a constrained chair rise. Journal of Biomechanics 24: 77–85

Schenkman M, Berger R S, Riley P O, Mann R W, Hodge W A 1990 Whole body movements during rising to standing from sitting. Physical Therapy 70(10): 638–652

Shepherd R B, Koh H P 1996 Some biomechanical consequences of varying foot placement in sit-to-stand in young women. Scandinavian Journal of Rehabilitation Medicine 28: 79–88

Smidt G L 1990 Gait in rehabilitation. Churchill Livingstone, New York

Tata J, Peat M, Grahame R, Quanbury A 1983 The normal peak of electromyographic activity of the quadriceps femoris muscle in the stair cycle. Anatomischer Anzeiger (Jena) 153: 175–188

Vilensky J A, Ganiewicz E, Gehlsen G 1987 A kinematic comparison of backward and forward walking in humans. Journal of Human Movement Studies 13: 29–50

CHAPTER CONTENTS

Development of the upper limb   193

Development of the use of the upper limb   194

Function   195
Structures permitting function   195
Hand function   196
Sensory functions   198
Forearm/arm function   199
Pectoral girdle function   200
An example analysis   201

Acknowledgement   202

11

Function of the upper limb

A. Hinde

OBJECTIVES

At the end of this chapter you should be able to:

1. **Outline the development of the upper limb**

2. **Describe how the upper limb contributes to the development of the whole person**

3. **Explain the classification of functional activities of the upper limb**

4. **Describe the structure of the upper limb**

5. **Discuss how this structure and the function of the upper limb are interrelated**

6. **Discuss the functional aspects of the individual segments of the upper limb.**

DEVELOPMENT OF THE UPPER LIMB

The upper limb is usually considered to be the clavicle and the scapula, the bones distal to the glenohumeral joint, with the muscle groups controlling those bones, the periarticular structures and the neurovascular structures. The only joint between the limb and the axial skeleton, as Moffat (1994) points out, is the sternoclavicular joint, the scapula being sandwiched between layers of muscle against the upper part of the posterior surface of the thorax.

At approximately 4 weeks, limb buds appear on the fetus and growth occurs until the eighth week when the limb shape is fully formed (Williams et al 1995). From then until birth the tissues differentiate to form the bone, the periarticular and the musculotendinous structures of the limb. There is some migration of the musculotendinous structures of the axial skeleton to become attached to the limb, e.g. latissimus dorsi. Radiographs of the upper limb at birth show ossification in the long bones but not in the short bones, these still being cartilaginous. Comparison of the proportions of the segments, either from radiographs or photographs at birth, shows the hands to be much larger in comparison with other segments (upper arm, forearm) than during childhood, adolescence or adulthood. Ossification is usually complete between the ages of 20 and 25 years.

Task 11.1

Look at a series of 'family' photographs of a developing child (yourself or a relative) and by estimation plot a histogram of the proportions of the upper limb segments over time. Then compare the results with the results of colleagues.

DEVELOPMENT OF THE USE OF THE UPPER LIMB

The work done by Illingworth (1987) to identify the sequences of behaviour and the change in ability over time has produced the concept of 'milestones of development' as a method of identifying progress in an individual's development by comparing actual with expected performance. From this work it is clear that there are two avenues of development to be followed:

- the development of activities of the upper limb as a discrete unit
- the development of the whole individual as a result of the use of the upper limb.

To illustrate the first point: the grasp reflex is present until approximately the eighth week and it is only when the reflex is disappearing that intentional activity can start, including exploration of 'things' (teething rings, cubes, paper) or environment (splashing water in the bath). These unrefined activities lead on to play and the gradual refining of movement. To illustrate the second: once the upper limb is useful, the rest of

the body benefits, e.g. by supporting the body on the forearms when placed prone (at approximately 12 weeks) or by taking weight on the hands when crawling or pulling the body into standing (at approximately 40 weeks). During this period and succeeding weeks the upper limb is also used in play and to communicate needs by gesture, and the child begins to develop self-help abilities during dressing. Van der Meer et al (1995) describe how the purposeful arm movements, under visual control in neonates, commence soon after birth, and speculate on the consequences of lack or inhibition of these movements for the individual.

An interesting point about the developmental sequence and the upper limb is that the upper limb often contributes heavily to the acquisition of abilities by other body segments and then reduces its contribution to those segments; it has an enabling function. For example, before the ability to sit unsupported has developed, the upper limbs act as props until the reflex control of the head and trunk is sufficiently matured to hold the body upright unaided. The limb then moves on to another task. Its contribution is not only in these concrete actions but also in its contribution to the cognitive ability, socialisation and habituation of the individual. The importance of these contributions is highlighted when a specific function does not itself develop, either leaving a void to be filled by compensatory techniques (equipment or trick movements) or halting progress in some specific aspect of the individual's development. McClenaghan (1989) describes a situation where poor development of sitting ability has been compensated for by the use of the upper limb as a support (i.e. as a direct replacement for an undeveloped postural ability) and the consequences of that adaptive behaviour for the accurate performance of tasks requiring both upper limbs later in life.

Task 11.2

Try to identify, then list, the uses to which you put your upper limb. This might seem initially to be infinite but if you look for 'common denominators' you should be able to produce a smaller list of 'generalities'.

FUNCTION

...function
Is smother'd in surmise, and nothing is
But what is not.
                (William Shakespeare, Macbeth I. iii. 141)

Structure and function are inextricably linked, each determining the other: although the structure allows the function, the function in its own right demands the structure. However, this chapter will work from structure to function.

In order for accurate movements to take place there must normally be a stable base about which the limb segments may move. At the other end of the limb will be the 'active' segment, i.e. that which is 'doing something'. While undertaking Task 11.2 you should have become aware that some of the uses involved the hand being moved freely in space and that others involved the hand becoming the fixed point for the movement of the rest of the body. If you did not appreciate this point look back through the list or think back to the uses again.

The appropriate way to describe these movements is to use the term *open chain* for free movements of the hand and *closed chain* for those movements where the hand is the fixed base. The open chain movements enable some manipulative activity: the hand is the focus of the activity being moved or positioned by the other segments of the upper limb, for example when using tools or cutlery, or washing hands. The closed chain movements enable the body to be moved by allowing the segments of the upper limb to act to compensate for underactivity of some other body segment. Examples of closed chain activity include pushing on chair armrests to assist rising from a chair and holding stair handrails to help maintain balance. Maki & McIlroy (1997) and Woollacott & Tang (1997) note the use of the upper limb in 'change-in-support' strategies in reaction to perturbations in balance when walking or standing. In these strategies the upper limb begins open chain movements within 90–140 ms of a loss of balance (Maki & McIlroy 1997) which apply restorative effects to the movement of the centre of gravity. If the hand is holding on to something for support, a closed chain is created and the effect is to enlarge the base of support, helping to ensure the centre of gravity remains positioned over the base of support. Crutch walking while the crutches are weight bearing and wheelchair–toilet/bed transfers are examples of closed chain compensatory use in dysfunction.

Task 11.3

Repeat Task 11.2 (or revisit your list from Task 11.2) but this time note the type of activity (open or closed chain) and the base of support and moving segments. Divide the upper limb into three components: hand, forearm/arm and pectoral girdle. Tabulate the results, e.g.

Activity	Type	Hand	Forearm/ arm	Pectoral girdle
Biscuit to mouth	Open chain	Grip on biscuit	Freely moving	Fixed base

---

You should by now be more aware that upper limb function goes beyond being the support and mover of the hand in the way that the springs, joints and arms of an 'Anglepoise' desk lamp serve only to position the light. Consider the example of a bicyclist: when pedalling seated there is open chain upper limb movement to guide the direction of travel but when a steep upward incline is reached the cyclist will often rise from the saddle to add body mass to the down-thrust of the lower limbs. At this time the hands on the handlebar grips become the fixed base and the upper limb is now engaged in closed chain movement, controlling the movement of the thorax, abdomen and pelvis.

Structures permitting function

There are three types of structure in the upper limb which permit function to occur:

- levers, i.e. bones
- joints about which levers move (including ligaments which restrict range or direction, or control movement)

- muscles causing or controlling movements of the levers (with their associated neural controls).

Each type of structure has its own specific properties and limitations and the reader is directed to other chapters in this book and to the References section of this chapter for more detail about these. It is the combination of these structures that permits the whole limb to be more than the sum of the parts, i.e. that gives the limb its ability to undertake functional use.

Hand function

The carpals are short irregular bones which lock together to form a stable block. During most actions involving the hand and needing long flexor and long extensor muscle activity, the carpals are in compression proximal to distal. Transverse section through the carpals shows the arching form of the group of bones which protects structures anteriorly from damage by items pressed into the palm and helps to maintain arterial supply and nerve conduction when gripping strongly. During movement the carpals work as a disc so that movements at the wrist joint have their axes through the carpals, with the scaphoid and lunate sliding laterally during ulnar deviation and medially during radial deviation. During flexion the articular surfaces of the scaphoid and lunate glide posteriorly and during extension, anteriorly. Cailliet (1984) explains and Tubiana et al (1998) illustrate how the many facets on the distal surfaces of the trapezoid and capitate lock the second and third metacarpals into a fixed unit, with the first metacarpal, and the fourth and fifth mobile to either side.

A transverse section through the metacarpals also shows an arched formation, concave anteriorly. This arch is more mobile than the carpal arches and will allow flattening or cupping of the hand with the medial metacarpal bones moving about the more rigidly anchored second and third metacarpals. The metacarpal heads have condylar shapes with an articular area on the distal and anterior aspects, giving a sweep area or surface arc for the proximal phalanx of approximately 180°. The surface arc of the base of the proximal phalanx is approximately 20° and this bone glides across the surface of the metacarpal head to give a range of movement between 90° of flexion and 20° hyperextension. The joint is very stable at 90° of flexion because the tension in the collateral ligaments is at its maximum (i.e. in the close pack position). When in extension the collateral ligament laxity allows abduction and adduction to occur. Each of the phalanges is similarly structured with proximal bases and small surface arcs articulating with condylar heads and large surface arcs. In these joints, however, the collateral ligaments are in tension in extension at the joint, making this the close pack position. Salter (1987) emphasises the importance of these details when splinting the hand and fingers. Flexion and extension are the only movements produced by direct muscle action but rotation does occur as an accessory movement when the metacarpophalangeal (MCP) and interphalangeal (IP) joints are not in their close pack position.

The static function of the hand is usually called 'grip' and the grips are classified by different authors in different ways; for examples see Backhouse & Hutchings (1989), Salter (1987) and Tubiana et al (1998). All grips have three features:

- a stable foundation to locate the levers
- the ability to arrange the levers appropriately
- the ability to apply forces through the levers.

Task 11.4

Observe a colleague for approximately one hour and identify the functions undertaken by that person's dominant hand. Once again classify them into the 'common denominator' type of lists.

The stable foundation will normally be provided by the carpals providing a closely packed foundation upon which the metacarpal bases will be anchored. When arranging the levers, the arch of the metacarpals is actively or passively adjusted. Intrinsic muscles of the hand actively pull the bones into a transverse arch. This positions the phalanges so that their tips converge towards a central point for gripping between thumb and finger pads, or gripping larger, roughly spherical objects between the palm and phalanges. The arch might be passively flattened during gripping so that the phalanges can move along parallel pathways to grip cylindrical or cuboidal shapes. Bray et al (1989), Wirhed (1988) and Tubiana et al (1998) indicate that the force of contraction of a muscle depends directly on its physiological cross-sectional area. The forces that can be generated during gripping can be very high but there is no space in the palm of the hand to hold an object and have large muscle bellies. The upper limb reconciles these requirements by placing the source of the forces (long flexor muscles) outside the hand and using tendons (with very much smaller volumes) and pulley-like arrangements to transmit the forces to the levers (phalanges). Cailliet (1984) and Tubiana et al (1998) have some very clear illustrations of normal and dysfunctional arrangements. Backhouse & Hutchings (1989) illustrate and describe the actions.

The long (extrinsic) muscles controlling the movements of the thumb and fingers are each named anatomically by their actions. The intrinsic muscles are named by their location (interossei), action (opponens pollicis) or appearance (lumbricals). Each group has its own function: to provide force (extrinsics), or to position the bones for the efficient application of that force (intrinsics). However, the true functions of the muscles of the hand do not become apparent until the combinations of actions are studied, i.e. it is the interplay of intrinsic and extrinsic actions that give functional ability to the hand rather than merely anatomical movement. The work of Cailliet (1984), Salter (1987) and Tubiana et al (1998) provides details of these interplays and their results. Winspur & Wynn Parry (1998) considered the role of the hand in playing a musical instrument and they provide a wide range of examples within musicianship of the complexity of the intrinsic/extrinsic relationship.

It is worth examining the combination of the concepts of types of grip and the arches of the hand. The *power grip*, for example, places the tool handle across the supports of the indicis-digiti minimi arch and then clamps between these

points with the third support (from the pollicis). The *lateral pinch grip* and the *tip grip* use only the indicis-pollicis arch supports, while the *span grip* uses all three arch supports in a centripetal motion. The *dynamic tripod grip* uses the indicis-pollicis arch to hold the tool (e.g. a pen); some of these are illustrated in Figure 11.1. Salter (1987) emphasises the role of the digiti minimi as a support for the 'working' arch. Tubiana et al (1998) show the metacarpal to distal phalanx rays for the fingers. It is possible to transpose these rays into arches between the distal phalanx of the thumb and each of the fingers, as shown in Figure 11.2.

Task 11.5

Place a ruler on a piece of paper and draw a line; look at the arches formed by the 'supporting' hand on the ruler and compare them with the arches formed by the 'drawing' hand. An understanding of these arches, the bones which comprise them and the muscle actions which cause and maintain them is essential when splinting or otherwise treating a dysfunctional hand, whatever the cause of the dysfunction.

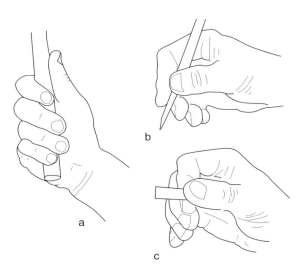

Figure 11.1 Illustrations of grips: (a) power grip; (b) dynamic tripod grip; (c) pinch grip.

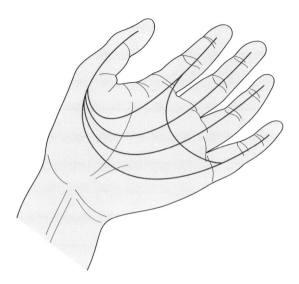

Figure 11.2 An illustration of the three 'tripod' arches and four 'ray' arches.

As a means of communication the hand and fingers may parody the spoken word, replace the spoken word or express (as body language) otherwise concealed communication. These communication gestures may take the form of pointing out features, e.g. on a poster, chalkboard or in a landscape. They might involve the hands being used to indicate the shape of, or relationship between, objects. A formalised sign language has been developed by the Association of Sign Language Interpreters and is in use to compensate for dysfunction of speech or hearing. Tubiana et al (1998) offer an example of a tetraplegic patient preferring a mobile hand to one that has undergone arthrodesis in order to retain a function in his sexual relationship.

Activities that are intentional movements have their origins in the cerebral cortex. There are many unconscious movement patterns that express an individual's values and subconscious judgement. Moods may be indicated by hand activity, but mood may also modify hand activity by the influences on the anterior horn cells through the medial pathways and limbic system. Pain (local and distant) and anger may inhibit movement by increasing muscle tone, lassitude or relaxation having the opposite effect.

Sensory functions

Review of the sensory homunculus (see Ch. 4) will show the relatively large area of sensory cortex (approximately one-third) 'allocated' to the hand. This offers a clue about the importance of the hand as a source of exteroception and proprioception information for the central nervous system.

The types and function of sensory end organs are described more formally elsewhere (Williams et al 1995), but their functional uses are worth consideration in more detail. Whether surfaces are hotter or colder than skin temperature can be identified by exteroceptors; surface texture can be similarly identified.

Task 11.6

Carry out two-point discrimination tests of a colleague's hand, palmar and dorsal aspects and forearm, anterior and lateral aspects. Prepare an outline of the hand and forearm and shade in the results in 'contours' of perhaps 2 mm. What conclusions can be drawn from these diagrams for sensory function or re-education?

The proprioceptive function of the lumbrical muscles is essential for accurate functional activity from the hand and fingers. Beyond this, the sensory data are generated by the combination of extero- and proprioception; movement, shape, dimensions and weight all require information from proprioceptive nerve endings in joint capsule, muscle and tendon as well as receptors in the skin. Most importantly, experience and practice are necessary for the data to be correctly interpreted: this differentiates the skilled craftsman or Braille reader from the beginner, for example (see Ch. 15). It is worth reflecting at this point about Illingworth's (1987) indication of the importance of maximal sensory experience during development and the consequences for children with congenital dysfunctions compared to those with acquired dysfunctions. Van der Meer et al (1995) make a similar point from a therapeutic perspective.

Combinations of motor and sensory activity applied within specific contexts can now be seen within a wider definition of function. Maslow (1954) classified the needs of individuals into a hierarchy of five levels:

- physiological (to satisfy the needs of homeostasis)
- safety or security (shelter, protection)
- belonging (social grouping or position)
- self-esteem (having a sense of 'value')
- self-actualisation (achieving full potential).

Task 11.7

Using each subgroup of Maslow's (1954) hierarchy of needs, identify two hand functions that may be undertaken to satisfy a need at that level.

The same functional activity may apply to any number of these needs at different times or in different contexts, e.g. shaking hands with someone, painting a wall or preparing a meal.

Forearm/arm function

This part of the upper limb is made up from the three long bones and their intermediate joints; further to this there is a synovial joint with the adjacent segment at each extremity, the wrist joint distally and the glenohumeral joint proximally. The forearm/arm has three main functions:

- lever systems for movement or positioning
- the location of muscle attachments
- the ability to become rigid and play a part in support functions.

The wrist joint separates the hand from the forearm and, because only two degrees of freedom are available at the joint, the extensors and flexors carpi assist in the alignment of the hand in readiness for use, or stabilise the carpals for activities using the fingers. Where problems of muscle insufficiency (active or passive) occur, the mobility of the wrist increases the range of the movements possible at the fingers. The third degree of freedom (rotation about the long axis of the forearm), sacrificed by the wrist joint, is transferred to the radioulnar joints. This arrange-

ment increases the stability of the carpal/forearm joint without the loss of potential positions for the hand. The major tension forces applied to outside loads at the hand are applied through the long flexor or extensor muscles and the phalanges. The loads on the carpals and metacarpals are relatively low and are close to the joint axis. The mechanical arrangement is further assisted by the pisiform bone acting as a sesamoid bone to alter the alignment of the flexor carpi ulnaris tendon for mechanical advantage.

The elbow joint is a complex of three articulations where two have given up freedom of movement for stability and the third is a compromise between movement and stability. The humerus/ulna articulation has a single degree of freedom (flexion and extension) as does the superior radioulnar joint (rotation). These are both very stable joints. The humerus/radius articulation offers both rotation, and flexion and extension. The complex serves to assist the wrist and inferior radioulnar joints to place the hand in a required position and to move the hand and any load to a new position.

The muscles acting on the elbow joint have an attachment close to the axis, cross the joint and attach the length of the forearm or arm away. This makes the lever system very disadvantageous in terms of effort applied, but this is compensated for by the advantageous velocity ratio giving large distance and rapid movement for the extremities of the segments in return for small length changes in the muscle during contraction. Tubiana et al (1998) use the term 'excursion' for this change in muscle length. The need to produce high forces in contraction is satisfied by having the muscles work in two groups; those in the arm attached close to the elbow on the radius and ulna, and those in the forearm attached close to the elbow on the humerus. Each group will cross the joint and attach to the further extremity of the opposite long bone. The combined action can be represented by drawing triangles of force to estimate their cumulative effect.

When the hand is used in open chain functional movements, elbow extension will usually be caused by gravity under the control of the flexor muscles in eccentric contraction. For closed chain actions, elbow extension is usually produced against resistance and so the elbow extensor muscle comes into action. The effect of the division of the triceps muscle into three heads can be estimated by drawing polygons of force, but more importantly the division allows an increase in the physiological cross-sectional area and therefore the capacity to generate high forces increases. When the hand is fixed and the triceps muscle is moving the body (as when pushing on chair arms to assist rising to standing), the lever system is of the second order and triceps has a slight mechanical advantage. From a practical point of view, the distance between the olecranon process and the trochlear notch is small when expressed as a proportion of the length of the forearm, so mechanical advantage is minimal. The advantageous velocity ratio still remains and for a physically small excursion by triceps the body is raised considerably.

Task 11.8

Return once again to your notes for Task 11.2 (or carry it out again). This time identify the axis and plane of the movements of the upper limb.

The glenohumeral joint has three degrees of freedom (about the vertical, sagittal and transverse axes) permitting the hand to describe almost the whole surface of a sphere (the axial skeleton occupying the missing part). In order to achieve this range of movement the joint sacrifices some stability and relies on muscle action to maintain congruity of the surfaces when under load.

For many of the activities involving the upper limb there are two components at the glenohumeral joint:

- the primary purpose of the movement, e.g. writing, stirring a cup of coffee
- a synergistic positioning of the segments to allow more efficient performance of the primary purpose.

The muscles acting for the synergistic purpose are the deltoid and the rotator cuff muscles, which typically need only to work against gravity's action on the mass of the upper limb. The large muscles attached to humerus and thorax or humerus and scapula usually generate primary activity. This arrangement allows large forces to be generated in either flexion/adduction or extension/adduction at this joint. The importance of these relationships is well illustrated in the case histories chosen for publication by Bullock (1990).

For many activities of the upper limb, the axis and plane of movement between the glenoid fossa and humeral head remain the same even when the direction moved by the limb changes. This apparent contradiction is explained by the adjustment in the plane of the glenoid fossa when the scapula is moved in relation to the thorax. Although the limb may be swinging in flexion/extension movements at the glenohumeral joint, the movement seen in relation to the axial skeleton may be across the front, parallel to the sagittal plane, or forwards and outwards depending on the degree of protraction/retraction of the pectoral girdle.

Pectoral girdle function

Finally the role of the pectoral girdle in permitting function in the upper limb must be considered. It has only one synovial joint with the thorax, at the sternoclavicular joint; the acromioclavicular joint is fibrous with limited available movement and the scapula lies sandwiched between layers of muscle. The girdle acts like the jib of a crane (especially when viewed from above) to position the glenohumeral joint in preparation for activity in the arm, forearm and hand. The glenohumeral joint cannot slide around on the thorax in a horizontal plane because the clavicle acts like the spoke of a wheel (unless fractured) and props the acromion outwards. When the scapula does move laterally the glenoid is moved forwards in the movement called protraction, retraction pulls the scapula towards the vertebral column and the glenoid moves backwards, always a clavicle-length from the sternum. The muscles joining the scapula to the thorax may act together to produce rotation of the scapula about a sagittal axis, raising or lowering the glenoid in elevation or depression, respectively. These four movements have the advantage of increasing the volume of space falling within the reach of the hand in the way a telescopic arrangement would in a machine.

The number, size and alignment of these muscle groups would seem at first to be excessive for open chain movements of the upper limb. It is in closed chain movements when the axial skeleton is being moved in relation to the upper limb that their purpose becomes apparent. Anthropologically, a major function of the upper limb was to transport the body, as it still is in primates. When hanging from an overhead support the animal needs to move 93.5% of its body mass. The upper limb makes up 6.5% of body mass and therefore to fulfil its locomotor functions the limb needs muscles of large physiological cross-sectional area and mechanically advantageous arrangements in terms of force production and lever systems (Wirhed 1988). Latissimus dorsi and pectoralis major are examples of such muscles. Although humans no longer rely on this form of transport, the potential retains therapeutic usefulness. This can be seen when the upper limb needs to compensate for lower limb dysfunction. For example, when using walking aids to relieve lower limb weight bearing, the axial skeleton is slung between the bilateral props of the upper limbs and the crutches. A second example is seen when people with spinal cord lesions use their upper limbs to propel wheelchairs or undertake transfers.

An example analysis

The example is intended to be an outline of an analysis of a violinist playing her instrument. It has been undertaken at a relatively superficial level without the anatomical detail, for example, of the specific working muscles. Instead it is intended as a framework onto which the reader can transpose these details.

Left arm

The pectoral girdle has elevated to enable the violinist to fix the instrument between the girdle and left mandible. Once the violin is held the pectoral girdle remains relatively stationary. The degree of elevation will be modified by the depth of the shoulder rest fitted to the body of the instrument, this being the choice of the instrumentalist.

The arm, forearm and hand serve to position the fingers to enable them to make appropriate contact with the strings. In this function they are working in open chain movements. The joint angles and the ranges of movement will depend on the size relationship between the violinist and violin, the string to be touched and the position of the touch.

The fingers are working with the 'ray' arches; the finger tips making or releasing contact with the string(s) and the thenar eminence providing counter pressure on the neck of the violin. The metacarpophalangeal joints are most active in this activity, being moved in the directions of flexion, extension, abduction and adduction. Once again open chain movements are being undertaken.

Right arm

The pectoral girdle moves to adjust the position of the glenoid fossa to maximise the efficiency with which the limb performs its role in open chain movement to enable the effective use of the right hand in bowing. Protraction and retraction are the main movements but there will be some elevation and depression as the musician varies the string in contact with the bow.

The arm and forearm move about the glenohumeral joint, principally in adduction and abduction but also at varying degrees of flexion, to enable the musician to choose the specific string across which the bow is drawn. The elbow moves in flexion and extension: there is very little movement at the radioulnar joints.

The wrist is moving in radial and ulnar deviation as the hair of the bow is drawn across the string, in order to maintain the hand moving in a straight path rather than circumferentially about the glenohumeral joint. In this action the bow, forearm and arm are moving as though they were three sides of a parallelogram.

The fingers and thumb are working with the 'tripod' arches almost in a 'fine' power grip to hold, with the digital pads, the handle of the bow as it is drawn across the strings; there is little change in position except a rolling action to adjust the contact point between the hair of the bow and the string. In this there is open chain movement.

ACKNOWLEDGEMENT

Acknowledgement is made to Mary Hinde, undergraduate at the Royal College of Music, Kensington, London for permitting photographs of her hands from which the drawings were made and for permitting an analysis of her movements during a period of practice on her violin.

REFERENCES

Backhouse K M, Hutchings R T 1989 A colour atlas of surface anatomy: clinical and applied. Wolfe Medical Publications, London

Bray J J, Cragg P A, Macknight A D C, Mills R G, Taylor D W 1989 Lecture notes on human physiology, 2nd edn. Blackwell Scientific, London

Bullock M I (ed) 1990 Ergonomics: the physiotherapist in the workplace. Churchill Livingstone, New York

Cailliet R 1984 Hand pain and impairment, 3rd edn. F A Davies, Philadelphia

Illingworth R S 1987 The development of the infant and young child, 9th edn. Churchill Livingstone, New York

McClenaghan B A 1989 Sitting stability of selected subjects with cerebral palsy. Clinical Biomechanics 4: 213–216

Maki B E, McIlroy W E 1997 The role of limb movements in maintaining upright stance: the 'change-in-support' strategy. Physical Therapy 77: 488–507

Maslow A H 1954 Motivation and personality. Harper and Row, New York

Moffat D B 1994 Lecture notes on anatomy, 2nd edn. Blackwell Scientific, London

Salter M I 1987 Hand injuries: a therapeutic approach. Churchill Livingstone, New York

Tubiana R, Thomine J-M, Machin E (eds) 1998 Examination of the hand and wrist, 2nd edn. Martin Dunitz, London

Van der Meer A L H, Van der Weel F R, Lee D N 1995 The functional significance of arm movements in neonates. Science 267: 693–695

Williams P L, Bannister L H, Berry M M et al 1995 Gray's anatomy: the anatomical basis of medicine and surgery, 38th edn. Churchill Livingstone, Edinburgh

Winspur I, Wynn Parry C B (eds) 1998 The musician's hand: a clinical guide. Martin Dunitz, London

Wirhed R 1988 Athletic ability and the anatomy of motion. Wolfe Medical Publishing, London

Woollacott M H, Tang P-F 1997 Balance control during walking in the older adult: research and its implications. Physical Therapy 77: 646–660

CHAPTER CONTENTS

Introduction   203

Support for the head, upper limbs and thoracic
cage during movement and weight bearing
activities   204
Vertebral body support   205
Intervertebral disc support   206
Vertebral arch support   210
The thoracic cage support   210
The pelvic girdle support   211

Protection for soft tissues and vital organs during
physiological movements and weight bearing
activities   211
Vertebral canal structures   211
The intervertebral foramen as a protective
structure   212

Provision of attachments for the muscles of the
abdomen and thorax and for some muscles of the
upper and lower limbs   213
Segmental stabilisation of the spine during movement
and normal posture   213
Production of gross movement over a large number of
segments   215
Stabilisation and physiological movement of the limbs
relative to the trunk   215

Spinal movement   215
Atlanto-occipital joint (C0/1)   218
Atlantoaxial joint (C1/2)   218
Lower cervical region (C2–C6)   218
Cervicothoracic junction (C6–T2)   218
Thoracic region (T3–T10)   219
Lumbar region   219
Sacroiliac joints   220

Enhancement of movement of the upper and
lower extremities and enhancement of visual and
hearing fields   221

The spine as a shock absorber   221

Giving shape to the human body in static and
dynamic postures   222

The spine facilitating changes from static to
dynamic postures   222

12

Function of the spine

A. P. Moore   N. J. Petty

OBJECTIVES

**When you have completed this chapter you
should be able to:**

1. **Describe how the spine functions to give
   support to the body during movement
   and weight bearing activities**

2. **Discuss how the spine is able to give
   protection to soft tissues and vital organs
   during weight bearing and physiological
   movements**

3. **Describe how the spine gives attachment
   for the muscles of the abdomen, thorax
   and upper and lower limbs**

4. **Explain how the spine allows movement
   of the human body**

5. **Explain how the spine contributes to the
   enhancement of movement of the upper
   and lower extremities**

6. **Describe how the spine is able to act as a
   shock absorber**

7. **Describe how the vertebral column gives
   shape to the human body in static and
   dynamic postures**

8. **Describe how the spine contributes to
   changes from static to dynamic postures.**

INTRODUCTION

The spine is a complex, multisegmented structure which has many functions. It will be seen

from this chapter that the spine is essential for weight bearing, protection and movement of the human body. A knowledge of the relationship of structure and function of the spine is of great importance to the clinician. The reader of this chapter is assumed to have a knowledge of the basic structure of the spine.

The spine as a whole functions in a variety of ways. It gives support to the head, upper limbs and thoracic cage during movement and weight bearing activities. It gives protection to the vital organs such as the heart and lungs and to soft tissues such as the spinal cord during physiological movements and weight bearing activities. It provides attachment for the muscles of the abdomen and thorax and for some muscles of the upper and lower limbs. It allows movement to occur throughout its length and enhances movement of the upper and lower extremities. It enhances the visual and hearing fields. In addition, the spine gives shape to the human body in static and dynamic postures and facilitates changes from static to dynamic postures. Finally, it acts as a shock absorber. Each of these functions will now be considered in turn.

SUPPORT FOR THE HEAD, UPPER LIMBS AND THORACIC CAGE DURING MOVEMENT AND WEIGHT BEARING ACTIVITIES

Normal movement can only take place if adequate support is available for the head, upper limbs and thoracic cage (Fig. 12.1). Such support is offered by the vertebral column and is discussed in this section.

The spine is composed of 33 vertebrae (Fig. 12.2), most of which comprise a vertebral body and a vertebral arch (Fig. 12.3). The vertebral bodies are, in the main, separated from each other in life by an intervertebral disc. The exceptions to this are found at the atlanto-occipital joint and the atlantoaxial joint, where no such disc exists, and in the sacrum, where the five sacral vertebrae are fused and do not contribute to spinal movement. At the atlantoaxial joint there is a large range of rotation available, and the inclusion of an intervertebral disc at this level would severely limit

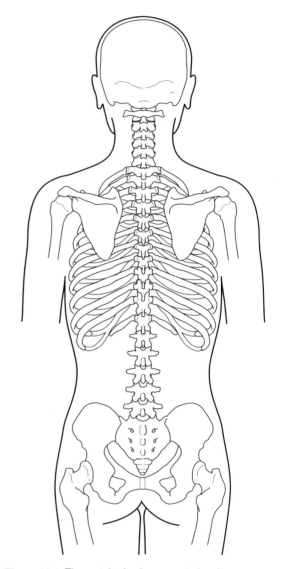

Figure 12.1 The vertebral column, posterior view. (Reproduced with permission from Kapandji 1974.)

range. It is also important that, in an area where the emerging brain stem is potentially vulnerable, this junction is well supported by ligamentous tissue. The union is, therefore, completed by the upward projecting dens fitting into the osseofibrous ring rather than through a discal union. Similarly, at the atlanto-occipital joint a large range of flexion extension movement is permitted since there is no intervertebral disc restricting range of movement. The sacral vertebrae are fused in order to contribute to a solid and stable osseous pelvic ring which has to support the forces generated in weight bearing and locomotion. The vertebral column is completed by the coccygeal region, which is composed of four vertebrae linked together by fibrous tissue: there is variable osteophytic union between either the first and second, second and third or third and fourth bones. The coccyx plays no supporting role in terms of spinal function but its movements are important in order to allow defaecation to occur.

Vertebral body support

The vertebral body consists of a cylinder of cancellous bone with trabeculae surrounded by a thin layer of cortical bone. The trabeculae act like struts strengthening the vertebral body: the vertical trabeculae resist compressive forces and horizontal trabeculae resist bowing of the struts and thus increase its strength (Bogduk 1997). This arrangement of the trabeculae can be seen in Figure 12.4. The vertebrae are thus able to resist the compressive and torsional stresses during movements of the spine and the tension caused by contraction of muscles which attach to it. The structure resembles a cardboard box full of packing material that prevents its collapse under compression during everyday movement. The compact bone represents the cardboard box and the trabeculae the packaging inside.

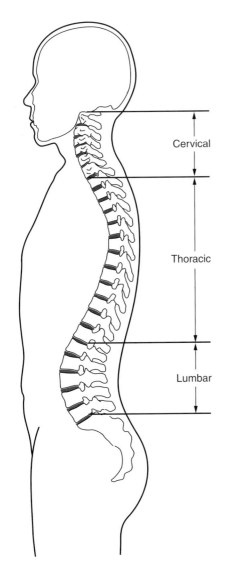

Figure 12.2 The vertebral column, lateral view indicating the spinal regions. (Reproduced with permission from Oliver & Middleditch 1991.)

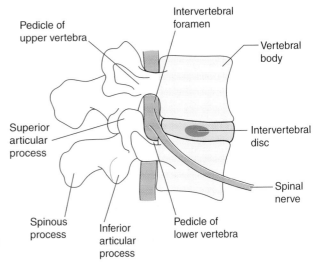

Figure 12.3 A lateral view of a spinal motion segment. The anterior weight bearing part is shaded.

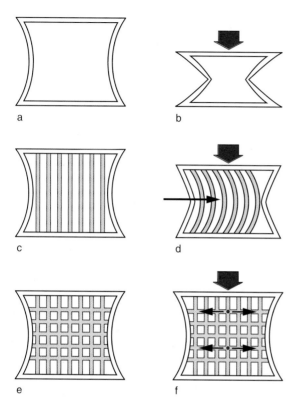

Figure 12.4 Reconstruction of the internal architecture of the vertebral body. (a) With just a shell of cortical bone, a vertebral body is like a box. (b) It collapses when a load is applied. (c), (d) Internal vertical struts brace the box. (e) Transverse connections prevent the vertical struts from bowing, and increase the load-bearing capacity of the box. (f) Loads are resisted by tension in the transverse connections. (Reproduced with permission from Bogduk 1997.)

Task 12.1

Have a look at sagittal and coronal sections of a vertebral body and the distribution of the cancellous bone. Your university may have ready prepared sections or alternatively you can obtain animal vertebrae from a butcher who will cut it into sections as needed. At first sight it might appear that the cancellous bone is randomly dispersed; in fact, it is distributed along the lines of weight bearing to enhance its strength. Look carefully at your sections and see if you can identify the way in which the trabeculae are organised.

Vertebral bodies throughout the vertebral column vary in size and shape depending on their position in the column. The lumbar vertebrae are larger and more heavily constructed

than the thoracic vertebrae which, in turn, are more substantially built than the finer and more intricate cervical vertebral bodies (see Fig. 12.2). The size of the vertebrae appears to be directly related to the amount of body weight that they must support. The cervical spine supports the head which accounts for approximately 10% of normal body weight; the thoracic spine supports the head and the weight of the upper limbs and thoracic organs; the lumbar spine supports the weight of the head, neck, thoracic cage and abdominal contents and functions to transmit all this body weight through the sacroiliac joints via the sacrum to the pelvis and hence to the lower limbs in static and dynamic postures.

Task 12.2

Look at a vertebral column and identify differences in the size and shape of the vertebral bodies in the five regions. See if you can suggest reasons for the features that you can see, noticing in particular the upward projections at the lateral aspects of the upper surfaces of the cervical bodies and the reciprocal bevelled surfaces of the lateral aspects of the lower surfaces of the cervical vertebrae. The upward projections are called uncinate processes and articulate with the vertebrae below at what is known as the uncovertebral joint (joints of von Luschka). These joints influence the degree and direction of movement and are thought to have a protective function for the lateral aspects of the intervertebral joints.

Intervertebral disc support

The intervertebral discs are interspersed between the vertebrae from the second cervical vertebra to the sacrum and constitute approximately one-fifth of the total length of the vertebral column. The shape of each disc corresponds to the shape of its adjacent vertebral body. The discs both allow and restrict movement between the vertebral bodies and transmit loads from one vertebral body to the next. The discs vary in shape and size in the different regions of the spine. They are wedge shaped, thicker anteriorly than posteriorly in the cervical and lumbar spine, which contributes to lordosis in these regions. They are thinnest in the upper thoracic region and thickest in the lumbar region in order to bear a greater proportion of body weight. In proportion to the height of the vertebral body, the discs are thickest in the cervical region and this, in part, enables the cervical spine to have a greater range of physiological movement than the other regions of the spine. The discs form the main connection between adjacent vertebral bodies and are held in place around the periphery by Sharpey's fibres (Jackson 1966). The discs serve to keep the vertebral bodies apart during the maintenance of static and dynamic postures and therefore are well placed to contribute to the support mechanisms provided by the vertebral column.

The disc is composed of three parts:

- end plate
- annulus fibrosus
- nucleus pulposus.

The end plate is permeable and lies between the disc and vertebral body (Fig. 12.5). It is composed of hyaline cartilage (Ghosh 1990a). Water and nutrients pass between the nucleus and the cancellous bone of the vertebral body through the end plate.

The annulus fibrosus is a ring-shaped structure composed of concentric layers (or lamellae) of collagen fibres bound together and prevented from buckling by a matrix of proteoglycan gel. Approximately 70% of the annulus is composed of water, although this amount varies according to the load on the disc and its age. The inner annulus is attached above and below to the vertebral end plate and the outer part of the annulus is attached to the periosteum and epiphyseal ring of the vertebral body and is strengthened by the anterior and posterior longitudinal ligaments.

The annular collagen fibres run parallel to each other and obliquely at 40–70° to the horizontal, lying in opposite directions in adjacent layers giving the annulus a lattice-like appearance (Fig. 12.6). The annulus contains both Type I and Type II collagen fibres (Ghosh 1988). Type I is found in tissues that are designed to resist tensile and compressive forces, and Type II is found in tissues designed to resist compressive forces (Bogduk 1997). The presence of Type I and II reflects the tensile and compressive loads applied to the annulus during static and dynamic postures. The lattice-like arrangement of the lamellae helps to limit movement between adjacent vertebrae. For example, during rotation half the fibres of the lamellae are stretched and the other half are relaxed (Fig. 12.7). On flexion, all the fibres posterior to the axis of movement are stretched and all the fibres anterior are relaxed. On extension, the anterior fibres are stretched and the posterior fibres are relaxed. On lateral flexion, the fibres ipsilateral to the direction of the motion are relaxed but on the contralateral side they are stretched.

The nucleus pulposus is a semifluid gel making up 40–60% of the disc and lies adjacent to the vertebral end plates of the vertebrae above

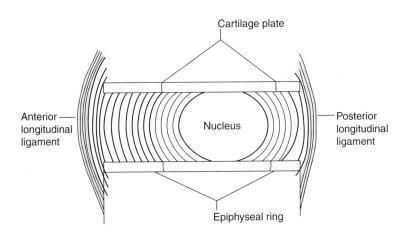

Figure 12.5 The cartilage end plate lies between the intervertebral disc and the vertebral body. The nucleus lies adjacent to the end plate. The anterior and posterior fibres of the annulus are attached to the anterior and posterior longitudinal ligaments respectively. (Reproduced with permission from Macnab I 1977 Backache. © Williams and Wilkins.)

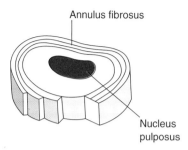

Figure 12.6 Horizontal section through a disc showing lattice-like arrangement of the annulus fibrosus. (Reproduced with permission from Oliver & Middleditch 1991.)

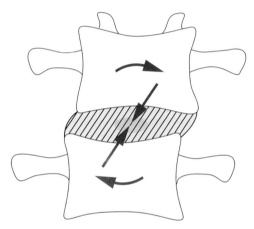

Figure 12.7 Anterior view of a spinal motion segment in the lumbar spine showing half the annular fibres stretched during rotation. (Reproduced with permission from Kapandji 1974.)

and below. At its periphery the nucleus blends with the annulus in such a way that there is no distinct separation between the two components. The nucleus is made up of a loose network (not in layers like the annulus) of mainly Type II collagen fibres (to resist compression) and a proteoglycan/water gel with some elastic fibres. Approximately 70–90% of the nucleus is composed of water.

The main property of proteoglycan gel is its water-imbibing capacity: by giving the disc a high osmotic pressure, water content is maintained even under high compressive loads generated in normal weight bearing postures and movement. The disc imbibes water and nutrients

through the end plate from the vertebral body; the imbibition of water creates a hydrostatic pressure within the disc which keeps the annulus under tension and helps to keep the vertebral bodies separated. The hydrostatic pressure varies according to the level of the disc, the posture adopted, and any weights which are lifted. Nachemson (1976) measured intervertebral disc pressure in the lumbar spine during the maintenance of various postures and during various activities; the results can be seen in Figure 12.8.

A knowledge of how posture and load bearing can influence hydrostatic pressure within the disc is important to the clinician as it explains why, in some pathological states, some postures may be more painful and unachievable by the patient than others. For example, in a patient with an acute disc lesion, sitting is often very difficult to maintain for more than a minute; such a patient would prefer to lie in a weight relieving posture in order to minimise pain. Pain in this situation may be caused by a rise in hydrostatic pressure within the affected disc. Raised hydrostatic pressure may create or increase the symptoms arising from a disc lesion, the extruded disc material being brought into closer proximity with pain-sensitive structures and giving rise to local and referred pain.

The water content of the nucleus varies with age: at birth the water content is over 85% but drops to around 70% in the mature disc. The water content does not vary very much in the annulus and is about 70% throughout life. In humans, total body height reduces by approximately 19 mm (1% of stature) from the morning to the evening (Tyrell et al 1985) due to the loss of fluid from the discs on weight bearing and the imbibition of fluid in non-weight bearing positions, particularly when recumbent.

Nutrition of the disc

The disc is avascular after the first decade of life so it then receives its nutrition mainly via tissue fluid exchange through the vertebral end plates and also from small blood vessels at the periphery of the annulus. The anterior annulus receives a better supply of nutrients than the posterior annulus.

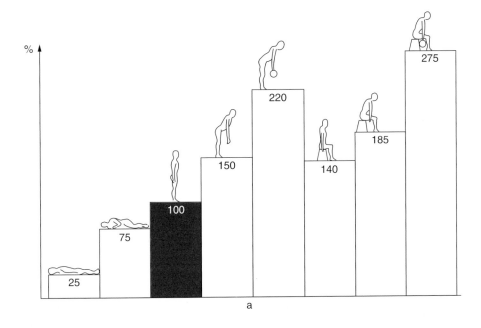

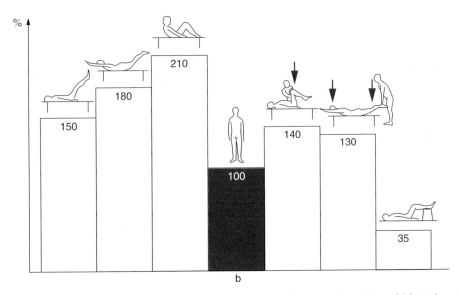

Figure 12.8 Relative change in pressure (or load) in the 3rd lumbar disc: (a) in various positions; (b) in various muscle strengthening exercises. (Reproduced with permission from Nachemson A L 1976 The lumbar spine: an orthopaedic challenge. Spine 1: 59–71.)

Fluid exchange is enhanced by movements of the spine, particularly movements in the sagittal plane (Adams & Hutton 1986), and reduced by static postures, particularly loading at end range flexion or extension (Adams & Hutton 1985). If the nutrition of the disc is inadequate, disc degeneration may then occur (Ghosh 1990b). It is therefore vital to the health of the disc that the spine changes posture throughout the day, and that prolonged static postures are avoided.

The intervertebral discs, together with the vertebral bodies and the supporting ligaments, particularly the anterior and posterior longitudinal ligaments, are well designed to support the body weight of the head and the upper limbs. The reader should note that this description is based on anatomical studies of the lumbar intervertebral disc. While a detailed description of the cervical disc is beyond the scope of this chapter, the reader should note that in the cervical spine the nucleus pulposus consists of fibrocartilage and the nucleus is not fully surrounded by the annulus fibrosus (Bland & Bushey 1990, Mercer 1995).

Vertebral arch support

The vertebral arch, lying behind the vertebral body, is made up of two pedicles and two laminae from which the spinous processes, two transverse processes, two inferior and two superior articular processes project (see Fig. 12.3). The nature, shape and direction of these processes vary in different regions of the spine. The spinous processes and transverse processes function as points of attachment for supporting ligaments and muscles to increase their leverage. The articular processes bear an articular surface called an articular facet. The superior facet of one vertebra articulates with the inferior facet of the vertebra above, forming a zygapophyseal (apophyseal or facet) joint. These zygapophyseal joints are synovial joints and therefore have a synovial membrane lying deep to the fibrous capsule. The capsules which surround the joints are fairly lax to allow movement to occur. Zygapophyseal joints are plane joints. When they are viewed in the dissected state, however, the articular surfaces are not completely flat – they undulate slightly and in life these undulations are evened out by the presence of small meniscoid inclusions. These inclusions are particularly well defined in the cervical and lumbar spines and are found in the superior and inferior recesses of each zygapophyseal joint. The role of the meniscoid inclusions is to increase surface area for distribution of loads acting through the joints and they may have a protective function for articular

surfaces. They are composed of fatty cartilaginous and synovial tissue and are firmly attached to the fibrous capsule which surrounds the zygapophyseal joint. The ligamentum flava lies in close proximity to the joint, connecting the laminae of adjacent vertebrae and attaching to the anterior margin of the fibrous capsule. This highly elastic ligament is thought to assist the back extensor muscles initiate restoration of the fully flexed spine to a more upright position. During this movement the elasticity of the ligament causes it to return to its normal length so that there is no buckling which could compromise the lumen of the vertebral canal. In addition, in the lumbar spine it protects the intervertebral disc by not allowing full flexion to be achieved too abruptly (Oliver & Middleditch 1991). Other supporting ligaments lie remote from these joints; they are the supraspinous, interspinous and intertransverse ligaments and can be seen in Figure 12.9.

The thoracic cage support

The thoracic cage forms a semi-rigid structure composed of 12 pairs of ribs which, apart from the two lower pairs of floating ribs, are united anteriorly by their costal cartilages to the sternum (see Fig. 12.1). The cage is completed posteriorly at the junction of the ribs with vertebrae, the upper 10 ribs articulating with the vertebral bodies and the transverse processes of each of the upper 10 thoracic vertebrae. The thoracic cage forms the basis of attachment for muscles which link and give support to the upper limbs, via the shoulder girdle.

Due to its position relative to the spine and its relative inflexibility, the thoracic cage serves to restrict the physiological movements of flexion, extension and lateral flexion of the spine.

Movement of the thoracic cage occurs during respiration. Small movements of the ribs at the costovertebral joints produce large movements anteriorly of the sternum and laterally of the rib shafts. Because of the long leverage of the rib shafts and the direction and shape of the costotransverse joint surfaces, these changes in anteroposterior and transverse diameters of the

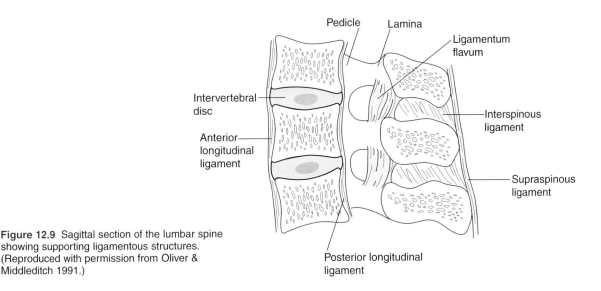

Figure 12.9 Sagittal section of the lumbar spine showing supporting ligamentous structures. (Reproduced with permission from Oliver & Middleditch 1991.)

thoracic cage increase its volume, reduce intrathoracic pressure and enable inspiration to occur.

The pelvic girdle support

The pelvic girdle comprises the two pelvic bones, the sacrum and the articulations between them (see Fig. 12.1). Posteriorly, the sacrum is wedged between the massive ilia of the pelvis and articulates with it via the two sacroiliac joints. The pelvic rim is completed anteriorly by the union of the two pubic bones at the symphysis pubis. The sacroiliac joints, which are synovial, are supported by some of the strongest ligaments in the body in order to maintain stability of the pelvic girdle. The symphysis pubis is a fibrous junction which is equally stable. Together, these articulations allow minimal movement during weight bearing and locomotion and maintain a solid base of support for the spine, head and upper extremities. The pelvic girdle is intimately linked with the lower extremities via the hip joints. Body weight is transmitted via the pelvis to the lower extremities, likewise impact from ground reaction forces during weight bearing and locomotion are transmitted via the lower extremities through the pelvis and on to the spine.

PROTECTION FOR SOFT TISSUE AND VITAL ORGANS DURING PHYSIOLOGICAL MOVEMENTS AND WEIGHT BEARING ACTIVITIES

Task 12.3

List for yourself all the possible soft tissue structures which may be protected by the spine, including the structures which lie anterior to it. As you read the rest of this chapter you will be able to check the accuracy of your list.

Also have a look at a vertebral column and work out how it is adapted to fulfil a protective role in relation to soft tissue structures which pass through or lie near to it.

Vertebral canal structures

The vertebral canal serves to support and protect the spinal cord and cauda equina with its accompanying spinal meninges, blood vessels and lymphatic drainage vessels. During movement of the spine, the spinal cord, together with its meninges, undergoes changes in length, tension and position. From spinal extension to spinal flexion there is 5–9 cm elongation, with most of the movement occurring in the cervical and lumbar regions

(Breig 1978, Louis 1981), and increase in tension (Butler 1991). On flexion, the spinal cord and meninges elongate, become thinner and move anteriorly in the spinal canal. On extension they become shorter and fatter and move posteriorly (Breig 1978). With right lateral flexion, the right hand side of the spinal cord shortens on the right and elongates on the left hand side (Breig 1978). Thus, with normal physiological movements the space taken up by the spinal cord and nerve roots in the spinal canal will vary. If pathology causes any encroachment into the spinal canal, the spinal cord or nerve roots may be compromised and this may be accentuated by certain physiological movements. It must be remembered that any blood vessels accompanying the spinal cord and its meninges or the nerve roots and their dural sleeves may also be compromised by pathology. Limb movements can also affect the neural tissue in the spinal canal, for example the straight leg raise (SLR) increases tension in the lumbar and sacral nerve roots and their meningeal covering.

The boundaries of the vertebral canal formed by the vertebral body anteriorly and the vertebral arch posteriorly are well adapted to protect the spinal cord and its meninges as they are made of compact bone which is very resistant to compressive forces.

The lumen of the vertebral canal varies in its shape in different parts of the spine depending upon the size of the neuromeningeal tissue passing through it. It is triangular and large in the cervical spine to allow for the enlarged spinal cord close to the brain stem; in the thoracic spine it is smaller and circular; and in the lumbar region the lumen widens and becomes more triangular in shape to accommodate the cauda equina (Fig. 12.10). Within the vertebral canal are small clusters of fat pads which fill in the recesses of the canal and act as cushions to the soft tissue structures during movements of the spine. This is a very important function during rapid spinal movement when the spinal cord moves forwards in the canal during flexion and backwards during extension and also when physiological movements are accompanied with compression, for example when jumping. The fat pads protect the sensitive neuromeningeal tissues from sudden impact.

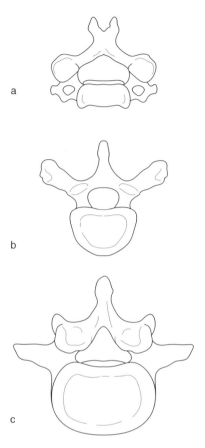

Figure 12.10 Segmental variations in the shape of the spinal canal: (a) cervical; (b) thoracic; (c) lumbar. (Reproduced with permission from Butler 1991.)

The intervertebral foramen as a protective structure

The intervertebral foramina are gaps between the vertebrae and lie laterally (see Fig. 12.3). The posterior wall of an intervertebral foramen is formed by the zygapophyseal joint, the anterior wall by the vertebral bodies and intervening disc, and the superior and inferior walls by the pedicles of the vertebrae above and below, respectively.

Within each intervertebral foramen lie the spinal nerve, sinuvertebral nerve, adipose tissue, blood and lymphatic vessels. The adipose (fatty) tissue, together with the osseous fibrous ring, serves to protect the structures in the intervertebral foramen during physiological movements when the diameter of the intervertebral foramen is altered. The cross-sectional area alters significantly during flexion and extension; in the lumbar spine flexion increases the area by 30% and extension decreases the area by 20%, whereas rotation and lateral flexion reduce the area (on the side to which the movement is directed) by 2–4% (Panjabi et al 1983).

Normally the spinal and sinuvertebral nerves occupy one-third to one-half of the cross-sectional area of the foramen, and in normal circumstances the alteration of the intervertebral foramen with movement does not adversely affect the enclosed tissues. However, certain individuals have transforaminal ligaments in the lumbar spine which are vestigial ligaments and have been described in detail by Golub and Silverman (1969). They span the intervertebral foramen and so reduce its vertical height and cross-sectional area. They occur quite naturally to a variable extent in some individuals but are absent in others. If they exist in association with minor pathology, during physiological movements the foraminal space may be significantly reduced and compression of the soft tissue structures may occur, leading to clinical signs and symptoms of a large space-occupying lesion. In other words, the presence of these ligaments may give a false impression to the diagnostician in terms of the true nature and size of the lesion. Transforaminal ligaments may also be present in the thoracic and cervical spines, but the evidence for this is far from extensive at the present time.

In the thoracic cage the vertebral column, which lies posteriorly, is perfectly positioned to offer protection to the vital organs and their protective membranes, i.e. lungs, pleura, heart and pericardium. In addition, the descending thoracic aorta is well protected from external trauma as it lies deep within the thorax on the anterior surface of the vertebral column.

In the cervical spine the transverse processes are punctuated by the foramen transversaria for the passage of the vertebral arteries. The vertebral arteries on the left and right join anterior to the brain stem to form the basilar artery and this feeds into the circle of Willis which supplies a large area of the brain (Fig. 12.11).

The foramen transversaria offer the two vertebral arteries protection from compression during physiological movements and external trauma. This protective device can, however, create some difficulty during physiological movements in the pathological state, when osteophytic growth from zygapophyseal joints can impinge on the vertebral artery, impeding blood flow and producing vertebrobasilar insufficiency. The most common symptom is dizziness; other symptoms which depend on the area of the brain stem affected can include: 'drop attacks', visual disturbance, diplopia, nausea, disorientation, dysarthria, dysphagia, ataxia, impairment of trigeminal sensation, sympathoplegia, hemianaesthesia and hemiplegia (Bogduk 1994).

PROVISION OF ATTACHMENTS FOR THE MUSCLES OF THE ABDOMEN AND THORAX AND FOR SOME MUSCLES OF THE UPPER AND LOWER LIMBS

The spine via its many bony processes offers direct or indirect attachment to muscle structures that have one or more of the following functions:

- segmental stabilisation of the spine during movement and normal posture
- production of gross movement over a large number of segments
- stabilisation and physiological movement of the limbs relative to the trunk.

Segmental stabilisation of the spine during movement and normal posture

Muscles whose function relates to segmental stabilisation and posture lie much closer to the vertebral column than muscles which produce gross movement. By virtue of the length of the vertebral processes, muscles increase their mechanical advantage because of the greater leverage that is available.

A spinal motion segment consists of two adjacent vertebrae with their intervening disc as shown previously (see Fig. 12.3). Each individual

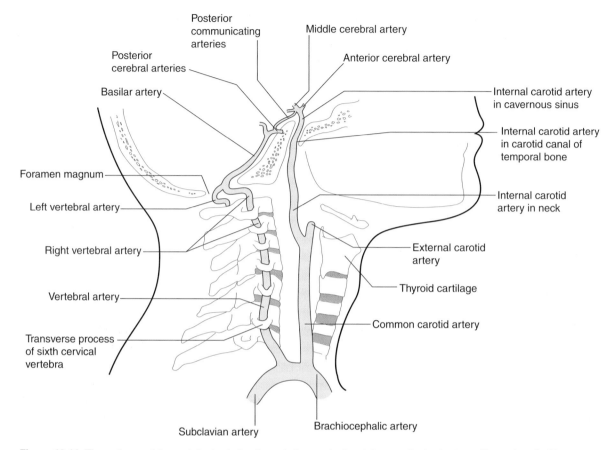

Figure 12.11 The pathway of the vertebral arteries through the cervical vertebrae to the brain stem. (Reproduced with permission from Palastanga et al 1994.)

motion segment is potentially unstable without its supporting ligaments and muscles. The muscles which span the motion segment are very important in stabilising adjacent vertebrae during gross movements of the spine which are produced by larger muscle groups. The deep stabilising muscles include multifidus, rotatores, interspinales and intertransversarii. Multifidus spans from one to three or four vertebrae and the latter two muscles link adjacent vertebrae. The main actions of multifidus are to produce posterior sagittal rotation of the vertebrae which occurs during extension, and to control this movement during flexion (Macintosh & Bogduk 1994). During rotation of the trunk the contraction of the prime movers, the oblique abdominal muscles, would tend to produce trunk flexion. Multifidus

in the lumbar spine acts with erector spinae to oppose the flexion pull of the obliques ensuring pure axial rotation (Macintosh & Bogduk 1986).

The rotatores, interspinales and intertransversarii muscles are thought to act as stabilisers. One suggestion is that they act as large proprioceptive transducers since they have been found to contain two to six times the density of muscle spindles found in the longer muscles (Peck et al 1984, Nitz & Peck 1986, Bastide et al 1984). They would thus provide feedback on spinal position and movement.

In standing, the spine is well stabilised by its joints and ligaments so that there is little back muscle activity; individuals vary, however, and there may be slight continuous activity, intermittent activity or no activity (Valencia & Munro

1985). Back muscle activity in sitting is similar to that in standing (Andersson et al 1975) but with the arms supported or with the backrest reclined there is reduced back muscle activity (Andersson et al 1974).

The degree of lumbar lordosis and the position of the pelvis are interdependent and are to some degree controlled by the surrounding muscles. Contraction of the back extensors and hip flexors will tend to increase lumbar lordosis and cause an anterior pelvic tilt; contraction of the abdominal muscles and hip extensors, on the other hand, will produce a flattening of the lumbar lordosis and posterior pelvic tilt. The balance of contraction of these muscle groups can be influenced by pathological processes of the spine (Jull & Janda 1987, Aspinall 1993, Cooper et al 1993, Hides et al 1994) and, therefore, assessment of the muscle function is important in the examination of a patient with spinal pain (Richardson et al 1999).

Production of gross movement over a large number of segments

Muscles which produce this type of gross movement tend to be more remote from the vertebrae, for example it is the more superficial members of the erector spinae group which are concerned with the gross movement of the trunk. This is because these superficial members of the erector spinae group span up to five or six vertebral segments and are thus able to produce more gross segmental movements. In the upright position the trunk muscles, notably the abdominals and back extensors, initiate movements into flexion, extension and lateral flexion. Once the centre of gravity is displaced, the antagonistic group will contract eccentrically to control the movement against gravity. For example, on spinal flexion the trunk flexors will initially contract to displace the centre of gravity forwards, then the movement will be controlled by eccentric work of the back extensors, which increases with increasing angles of flexion (Shultz et al 1982). It should be noted that because of the direction of the back extensor muscle fibres (being parallel to the spine), activity in these muscles causes a proportional increase in intradiscal pressure.

The abdominal muscles, which lie some distance from the spine, achieve the movements of physiological flexion, side flexion and rotation of the trunk in combination with other muscles of the trunk and in association with the deeper muscles of the back. None of the abdominal muscles is attached directly to the spine: however, transversus abdominis and the internal abdominal oblique muscles have attachments to the lower thoracic and lumbar spines via the thoracolumbar fascia. Together these three abdominal muscles and their fascial attachments provide a complex bracing mechanism to protect the lumbar spine during flexion movements and lifting activities. The exact mechanism of lifting still remains unclear, despite much research in this area. A detailed discussion of the various mechanisms put forward is beyond the scope of this chapter.

Stabilisation and physiological movement of the limbs relative to the trunk

The spine gives attachment for levator scapulae, serratus anterior, latissimus dorsi, trapezius and rhomboids minor and major which are all important muscles for the production of shoulder girdle movement and for stabilisation of the scapula in order to facilitate movements of the upper limb. In addition, the spine affords attachment for psoas major and piriformis, muscles which have direct influence on the lower extremity during gait.

SPINAL MOVEMENT

Functionally, the spine is considered to consist of a large number of spinal motion segments which contribute to overall spinal movement (see Fig. 12.3). The motion segment consists of the interbody joint, which allows movement to occur under compression, and the two zygapophyseal joints, which are concerned with guiding the direction of the movement that takes place. We have considered these two joints earlier in the chapter. The motion segment is well developed to allow movement to occur between adjacent segments since the collagenous fibres of the annulus are compressible to a small extent, are capable of being torsioned and are also capable of being stretched longitudinally.

In addition, the nucleus pulposus acts rather like a water cushion stabilised by the surrounding annulus and adjacent vertebral segments and is capable of deforming in response to changes of both static and dynamic postures (Fig. 12.12). The size of the intervertebral disc varies according to vertebral level. The discs are thickest in the most mobile segments of the vertebral column, i.e. in the lumbar and cervical spine, and thinnest in the thoracic spine.

The two synovial zygapophyseal joints together complete the triad motion segment. Their structure has been described earlier in this chapter.

Task 12.4

Look at the vertebral column and notice the changes in the direction of the articular surfaces in each region of the spine.

It is to be noted that in the cervical region (apart from C0/1 and C1/2) the inferior articular facets face downwards and forwards at an angle of approximately 45° (Fig. 12.13). The superior articular facets of the vertebra below lie in a complementary position, facing upwards and backwards. In the thoracic spine the zygapophyseal joints are orientated so that the inferior facets of the vertebra above face forwards and slightly medially, lying

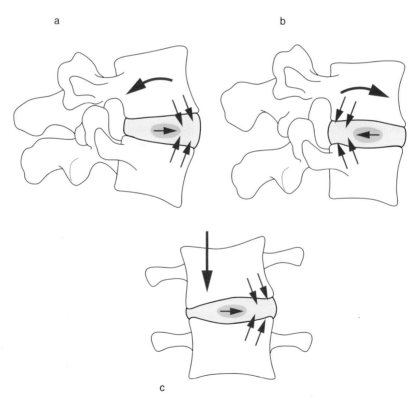

a   b

c

Figure 12.12 Effect of movement on deformation of the intervertebral disc. (a) Extension: the upper vertebra moves posteriorly and the nucleus increases the tension in the anterior part of the annulus. (b) Flexion: the upper vertebra moves anteriorly and the nucleus increases tension in the posterior part of the annulus. (c) Lateral flexion: the upper vertebra tilts towards the side of flexion and the nucleus moves in the opposite direction, increasing tension in that part of the annulus. (Reproduced with permission from Kapandji 1974.)

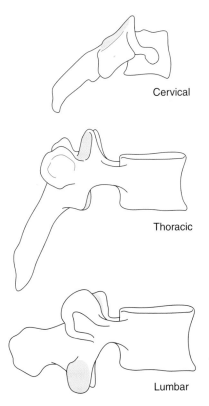

Figure 12.13 Orientation of the articular facets (shaded) in the cervical, thoracic and lumbar regions. (Reproduced with permission from Palastanga et al 1994.)

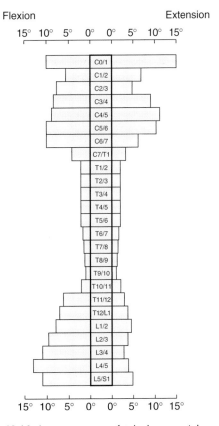

Figure 12.14 Average ranges of spinal segmental movement (flexion and extension). (Reproduced with permission from Oliver & Middleditch 1991.)

almost in a coronal plane, and therefore the superior facets of the vertebra below face backwards and laterally. By contrast, the facets of the lumbar spine are curved so that the inferior articular facets face both laterally and forwards; the superior facets face medially and backwards.

As segments are viewed progressively from C2 to the sacrum it will be noted that the change in the direction of the articular facets is a gradual process. The inclination of zygapophyseal joints will affect the range and direction of the motion available at each segmental level, as can be seen below (Figs 12.14 and 12.15).

The upper cervical joints, the atlanto-occipital (C0/1) and atlantoaxial (C1/2), are atypical motion segments since there is no intervertebral disc present between these two junctions and the direction of the facets is quite different to the rest of the cervical spine. The C0/1 articulation is the

only joint within the vertebral column which does not have a triad joint, there being only two articulations at this level which are synovial condylar joints. The superior facets of C1 are significantly expanded to enable the condyles of the occiput to be supported. They are elongated and cup-shaped, facing slightly medially, and in the anteroposterior direction lie at 45° to the sagittal plane. The configuration and direction of the joint surfaces facilitate anteroposterior sagittal rotation and translation of the occipital condyles on the superior articular facets of C1, allowing a large range of flexion and extension at this level. The C1/2 joint is formed by a pivot joint between the odontoid peg of the axis and the anterior arch of the atlas. This junction creates a very mobile joint in terms of physiological ranges of rotation, as can be seen from Figure 12.15.

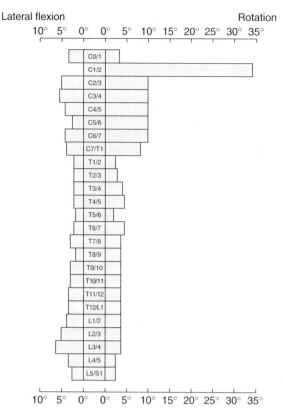

Figure 12.15 Average ranges of spinal segmental movement (values given to one side) for lateral flexion and rotation. (Reproduced with permission from Oliver & Middleditch 1991.)

There are 6 degrees of freedom at each spine motion segment: sagittal rotation and translation, coronal rotation and translation, horizontal rotation and translation (Fig. 12.16). Flexion consists of anterior sagittal rotation and anterior translation; extension consists of posterior sagittal rotation and posterior translation.

Atlanto-occipital joint (C0/1)

Flexion and extension are the largest ranges available at this segment, with slight lateral flexion also being available. During flexion of the head on the neck, the occipital condyles roll on the lateral masses of C1 and also translate forwards. The atlas translates backwards and tilts upwards and posteriorly. In extension the reverse movements occur.

Atlantoaxial joint (C1/2)

Rotation is the largest range available. During rotation to the left, the right inferior facet of C1 moves forwards and slightly upwards on the superior facet of C2 and the left inferior facet of C1 moves backwards and slightly downwards. The forward and backward movements constitute rotation and the upward and downward movements constitute lateral flexion, therefore rotation is accompanied by some lateral flexion movement. Some flexion, extension and lateral flexion movements are also available at this level (see Figs 12.14 and 12.15).

Lower cervical region (C2–C6)

Flexion and extension, lateral flexion and rotation are all possible at these levels. During flexion the vertebrae undergo anterior sagittal rotation and anterior translation. The intervertebral foramina increase in size during this movement.

During extension the vertebrae undergo posterior sagittal rotation and posterior translation. The intervertebral foramina decrease in size during this movement.

Rotation is coupled with lateral flexion to the same side. For example, with rotation to the right the left inferior articular facet of the upper vertebra glides superiorly, anteriorly and laterally on the superior articular facet of the vertebra below; the right inferior articular facet of the upper vertebra glides inferiorly, posteriorly and medially on the superior articular facet of the vertebra below. The anterior, posterior, medial and lateral movements constitute rotation movements and the inferior and superior movements constitute lateral flexion.

In the same way lateral flexion is accompanied by rotation. With lateral flexion to the right, the left and right inferior articular facets of the upper vertebrae glide in a similar way to right rotation. The inferior and superior glides produce the lateral flexion; the anterior, posterior, medial and lateral movements produce the rotation.

Cervicothoracic junction (C6–T2)

Similar movements occur in this region as above.

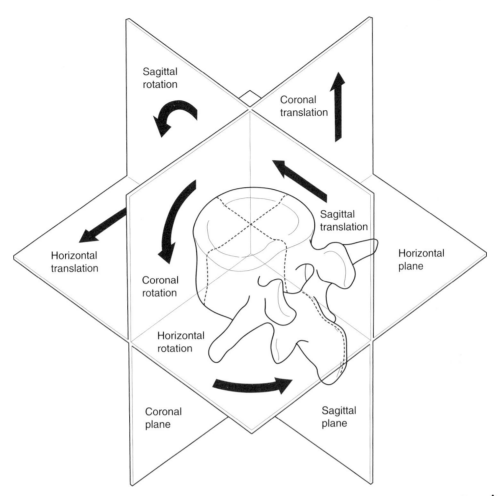

Figure 12.16 Planes and directions of motion showing the 6 degrees of freedom at a spinal motion segment. (Reproduced with permission from Bogduk 1997.)

Thoracic region (T3–T10)

This is the least mobile area of the spine. During flexion the inferior articular facets of the superior vertebra slide superiorly with a small amount of forward translation. In extension the reverse movements occur.

Rotation is always coupled with lateral flexion; the zygapophyseal joints slide relative to each other. In lateral flexion to the left, the inferior facets of the superior vertebra on the right glide superiorly and translate slightly forwards and, on the left side, slide interiorly and translate slightly backwards.

Lumbar region

Flexion is the freest movement. In the lumbar spine there are around 10° of anterior sagittal rotation and 2 mm of anterior translation during flexion and around 3° of posterior sagittal rotation and 1 mm of posterior translation on extension (Pearcy et al 1984). Movements during lateral flexion and rotation are less clear.

Lateral flexion is always accompanied by a degree of rotation. Lateral flexion to the left, for example, is accompanied by axial rotation to the opposite side at the upper lumbar levels. At the two lower levels, lateral flexion to the left is accompanied by rotation to the left (Pearcy & Trebewal 1984). Figure 12.17 depicts the overall pattern of movement of the lumbar spine during the active physiological movement of lateral flexion in standing of a young asymptomatic male subject. It can be seen that lateral flexion to the left is accompanied by rotation to the left and with lateral flexion to the right, there is rotation to the right. The lateral flexion movement in this case is accompanied by flexion; however, in other subjects lateral flexion may be found to be accompanied by extension.

It should be noted that range of movement is not static; there is a reduction in range with increasing age. The lumbar spine, for example,

has a reduced range of movement, in both males and females, with increasing age (Leighton 1966). This is due to an increase in stiffness of the intervertebral disc (Twomey & Taylor 1983). Range of spinal movement also varies between males and females, although there is conflicting evidence from the literature. One study found that up to the age of 65 men had a greater sagittal mobility than females, but the reverse was true after 65 (Sturrock et al 1973).

Sacroiliac joints

Movement of the sacroiliac joints occurs during flexion and extension movements of the trunk.

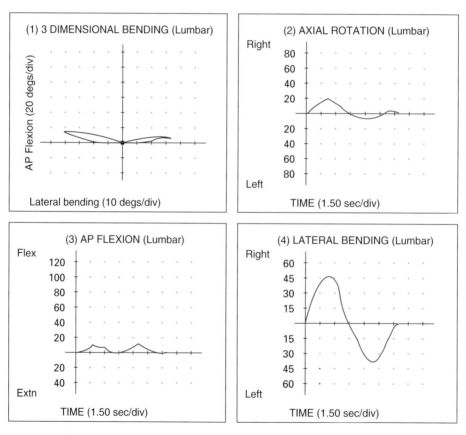

Figure 12.17 These graphs demonstrate the accompanying flexion, extension and rotation movements that occur during lateral flexion movement of an asymptomatic subject. The bottom right graph shows lateral flexion (the primary movement). The top left graph shows the overall movement as if looking from above; the bottom left graph shows accompanying flexion and extension movement; the top right shows accompanying rotation to the left and right. The CA 6000 spine motion analyser is able to measure three-dimensional spinal movement in real time. (Reproduced with permission from Orthopaedic Systems Incorporated, Hayward, California, 1993.)

Anterior rotation of the base of the sacrum with posterior rotation of the apex is termed *nutation*. The reverse movement is known as *counternutation*. There is approximately 1° of nutation during flexion and 1° of counternutation during extension of the lumbar spine in standing (Jacob & Kissling 1995). The direction of the movement varies between individuals: in some flexion is accompanied by nutation and in others by counternutation.

This movement does not occur as a result of muscle activity but as a result of mechanical forces placed upon the base of the sacrum during load bearing through the lumbar spine. The movement is restricted by the sacrotuberous and sacrospinous ligaments and also by the interosseous ligaments which bind the sacrum together with the ilia. These nutation and counternutation movements occur readily during gait and weight bearing activities.

During stance phase, the upward pressure from the supporting limb causes a reaction force from the ground to be transmitted via the femur through the hip to the ipsilateral pelvic bone. This causes a tendency for shear (sliding) to take place at the symphysis pubis and the SI joint (Fig. 12.18). This shearing force is enhanced by the weight of the dependent leg on the contralateral side. Also during gait, anterior and posterior rotation of the pelvis relative to the sacrum occurs. It should be noted, however, that due to the very strong ligaments supporting the sacroiliac joints the range of movement is extremely small.

ENHANCEMENT OF MOVEMENT OF THE UPPER AND LOWER EXTREMITIES AND ENHANCEMENT OF VISUAL AND HEARING FIELDS

The spine serves to enhance movement of both the upper and lower extremities; for example, in reaching activities the range of motion of the upper limb can be significantly enhanced by rotation and side flexion of the trunk, and an example relating to the lower limb can be seen in hurdling activities where the trunk side flexes above the flexed hip and knee in order to gain clearance of the hurdle.

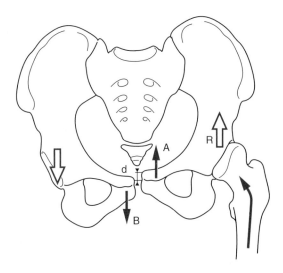

Figure 12.18 The forces around the pelvis when standing on the left leg (stance phase) and taking the right leg forward in walking. The ground reaction force (arrow R) elevates the left hip while the right hip is pulled down by the weight of the free leg. This causes a shearing force at the pubic symphysis (d is distance moved due to shear) tending to raise on the left (A) and lower on the right (B). The forces will be in the opposite direction at the sacroiliac joints, the left ilia will tend to lower and the right ilia will tend to be raised. (Reproduced with permission from Kapandji 1974.)

The trunk also serves to increase the field of vision. This is accomplished by rotatory movements of the head on the neck or of the trunk as a whole, allowing the eyes to be brought into a more optimal position for viewing the targeted object. Trunk movements can also enhance hearing fields in the same way.

Movements of the spine generally aid maintenance of balance by allowing the subject's centre of gravity to be brought over the base of support; for example, in one leg standing the trunk will side flex, rotate, flex and extend in whatever sequence is necessary to maintain the upright posture.

THE SPINE AS A SHOCK ABSORBER

Impact forces, e.g. during running and jumping, are transmitted upwards to the spine through the lower limbs and pelvis. Downward forces due to body weight are transmitted through the spine to the pelvis; these are reduced significantly by the presence of the spinal curvatures which help to stagger the transmission of these forces. These forces are absorbed to a degree by the trabeculae of the cancellous bone and the cartilaginous components of the intervertebral discs.

GIVING SHAPE TO THE HUMAN BODY IN STATIC AND DYNAMIC POSTURES

The spine in normal subjects takes on a characteristic appearance in both dynamic and static postures. If spinal contours are enhanced or lost, it can be a manifestation of poor postural control, muscle weakness or imbalance, bony deformity or bony and/or ligamentous pathology. It can also relate to habitual postural stances which can be related to work or leisure pursuits, or these habitual postures can be a manifestation of a psychological disturbance. For example, in depression the upper cervical spine is often extended so that the chin is poked forward, the lower cervical and thoracic spine is flexed, the lumbar spine is flexed producing a flattened lordosis, there is some flexion of the hips and knees and the patient walks with a shuffling gait. A change in the contours of one region will often be accompanied by compensatory changes in other regions.

The spine also moves in a characteristic way. Analysis of spinal movement is important for the clinician in order to assess the presence of pathology or spinal dysfunction. It is important that contributions by all segments of the spine are monitored in terms of a total regional/spinal movement. If one spinal motion segment is blocked (hypomobile), movement of the whole spinal region may be affected causing limited or abnormal movement, and this is sometimes compensated for by the development of an area of hypermobility in adjacent segments.

THE SPINE FACILITATING CHANGES FROM STATIC TO DYNAMIC POSTURES

The spine serves a useful function when the body requires movement from a static to a dynamic posture or from one static posture to another static posture. The mobility in the spine allows the subject's centre of gravity to be brought over the base of support; for example, when getting up from a chair the thorax and trunk move forwards over the pelvis, towards the knees, so that the lower limbs can raise the trunk from the chair, whilst the trunk remains in a stable posture.

It is likely that the trunk can be used to produce deceleration of a moving body in conjunction with the lower limbs; for example, in running the trunk flexes slightly over the lower limbs. When the runner decelerates, the trunk is brought into a more upright, slightly extended position which increases air resistance by increasing turbulence and also moves the centre of gravity posteriorly. This in itself retards motion.

In most circumstances the trunk, head and neck can initiate gross movements of the body, e.g. in rolling where either the head and neck or the pelvis can initiate the movement followed by the upper or lower extremity.

Until recently, equipment for accurate and reliable measurement of dynamic spinal motion and static posture has not been readily available. The last decade has seen an upsurge in production of three-dimensional real time instrumentation (for example CA 6000 spine motion analyser, Isotrak, Coda, Vicon and Spinatrak) which will in the future revolutionise our understanding of spinal motion. More recently researchers (Dopf et al 1994, Dvorak et al 1995, McGregor et al 1995, Troke et al 2001, Van Herp et al 2000) have been involved in testing the reliability and validity of this instrumentation, analysing spinal motion and in some cases producing normative databases (mainly in the lumbar spine).

REFERENCES

Adams M A, Hutton W C 1985 Gradual disc prolapse. Spine 10: 524–531

Adams M A, Hutton W C 1986 The effects of posture on diffusion into the lumbar intervertebral discs. Journal of Anatomy 147: 121–134

Andersson B J G, Jonsson B, Ortengren R 1974 Myoelectric activity in individual lumbar erector spinae muscles in sitting: a study with surface and wire electrodes. Scandinavian Journal of Rehabilitation Medicine (suppl) 3: 91–108

Andersson B J G, Ortengren R, Nachemson A L et al 1975 The sitting posture: an electromyographic and discometric study. Orthopaedic Clinics of North America 6: 105–120

Aspinall W 1993 Clinical implications of iliopsoas dysfunction. Journal of Manual and Manipulative Therapy 1: 41–46

Bastide G, Zadeh J, Lefebvre D 1989 Are the 'little muscles' what we think they are? Surgical and Radiological Anatomy 11: 255–256

Bland J, Bushey D R 1990 Anatomy and physiology of the cervical spine. Seminars in Arthritis and Rheumatism 20: 1–20

Bogduk N 1994 Cervical causes of headaches and dizziness. In: Boyling J D, Palastanga N (eds) Grieve's modern manual therapy, 2nd edn. Churchill Livingstone, Edinburgh

Bogduk N 1997 Clinical anatomy of the lumbar spine, 3rd edn. Churchill Livingstone, Edinburgh

Breig A 1978 Adverse mechanical tension in the central nervous system. Almqvist & Wiksell, Stockholm

Butler D S 1991 Mobilisation of the nervous system. Churchill Livingstone, Edinburgh

Cooper R G, Stokes M J, Sweet C, Taylor R J, Jayson M I V 1993 Increased central drive during fatiguing contractions of the paraspinal muscles in patients with chronic low back pain. Spine 18: 610–616

Dopf C A, Schlomo S M, Geiger D F, Mayer P J 1994 Analysis of spine motion variability using a computerised goniometer compared to physical examination. Spine 19: 586–595

Dvorak J, Vajda E G, Grob D, Panjabi M M 1995 Normal motion of the lumbar spine as related to age and gender. European Spine Journal 4: 18–23

Ghosh P 1988 The biology of the intervertebral disc, Vol 1. CRC Press, Boca Raton, Florida

Ghosh P 1990a Basic biochemistry of the intervertebral disc and its variation with ageing and degeneration. Journal of Manual Medicine 5: 48–51

Ghosh P 1990b The role of mechanical and genetic factors in degeneration of the disc. Journal of Manual Medicine 5: 62–65

Golub B S, Silverman B 1969 Transforaminal ligaments of the lumbar spine. Journal of Bone and Joint Surgery 51A: 947–956

Hides J A, Stokes M J, Saide M, Jull G A, Cooper D H 1994 Evidence of lumbar multifidus muscle wasting ipsilateral to symptoms in patients with acute/subacute low back pain. Spine 19: 165–172

Jackson R 1966 The cervical syndrome. Thomas, Springfield, USA

Jacob H A C, Kissling R O 1995 The mobility of the sacroiliac joints in healthy volunteers between 20 and 50 years of age. Clinical Biomechanics 10: 352–361

Jull G A, Janda V 1987 Muscles and motor control in low back pain: assessment and management. In: Twomey L T, Taylor J R (eds) Physical therapy of the low back. Churchill Livingstone, Edinburgh, pp 253–278

Kapandji I A 1974 The physiology of the joints. Vol 3: The trunk and the vertebral column. Churchill Livingstone, Edinburgh

Leighton J R 1966 The Leighton flexometer and flexibility test. Journal of the Association for Physical and Mental Rehabilitation 20: 86–93

Louis R 1981 Vertebroradicular and vertebromedullar dynamics. Anatomica Clinica 3: 1–11

McGregor A H, McCarthy I D, Hughes S P P 1995 Motion characteristics of the lumbar spine in the normal population. Spine 20: 2421–2428

Macintosh J E, Bogduk N 1986 The biomechanics of the lumbar multifidus. Clinical Biomechanics 1: 205–213

Macintosh J E, Bogduk N 1994 In: Boyling J D, Palastanga N (eds) Grieve's modern manual therapy, 2nd edn. Churchill Livingstone, Edinburgh

Macnab I 1977 Backache. Williams and Wilkins, London

Mercer S R 1995 Clinical anatomy of cervical disc instability. Proceedings of the Manipulative Physiotherapists Association of Australia 9th Biennial Conference, November. Gold Coast, Australia, pp 101–103

Nachemson A L 1976 The lumbar spine: an orthopaedic challenge. Spine 1: 59–71

Nitz A J, Peck D 1986 Comparison of muscle spindle concentrations in large and small human epaxial muscles acting in parallel combinations. American Surgeon 52: 273–277

Oliver J, Middleditch A 1991 Functional anatomy of the spine. Butterworth-Heinemann, Oxford

Palastanga N, Field D, Soames R 1994 Anatomy and human movement, structure and function, 2nd edn. Butterworth-Heinemann, Oxford

Panjabi M M, Takata K, Goel V K 1983 Kinematics of lumbar intervertebral foramen. Spine 8: 348–357

Pearcy M, Portek I, Shepherd J 1984 Three dimensional X-ray analysis of normal movement in the lumbar spine. Spine 9: 294–297

Pearcy M J, Trebewal S B 1984 Axial rotation and lateral bending in the normal lumbar spine measured by three-dimensional radiography. Spine 9: 582–587

Peck D, Buxton D F, Nitz A 1984 A comparison of spindle concentrations in large and small muscles acting in parallel combinations. Journal of Morphology 180: 243–252

Richardson C, Jull G, Hodges P, Hides J 1999 Therapeutic exercise for spinal stabilization in low back pain. Churchill Livingstone, Edinburgh

Shultz A, Andersson G B J, Ortengren R et al 1982 Analysis and quantitative myoelectric measurements of loads on the lumbar spine when holding weights in standing postures. Spine 7: 390–397

Sturrock R D, Wojtulewski J A, Dudley Hart F 1973 Spondylometry in a normal population and in ankylosing spondylitis. Rheumatology and Rehabilitation 12: 135–142

Troke M, Moore A P, Maillardet F J, Hough A, Cheek E 2001 A new, comprehensive normative database of lumbar spine ranges of motion. Clinical Rehabilitation [in press]

Twomey L T, Taylor J R 1983 Sagittal movements of the human lumbar vertebral column: a quantitative study of the role of the posterior vertebral elements. Archives of Physical Medicine and Rehabilitation 64: 322–325

Tyrell A R, Reilly T, Troup J D G 1985 Circadian variation stature and the effects of spinal loading. Spine 10: 161–164

Valencia F P, Munro R R 1985 An electromyographic study of the lumbar multifidus in man. Electromyography and Clinical Neurophysiology 25: 205–221

Van Herp G, Rowe P J, Salter P M 2000 Range of motion in the lumbar spine and the effects of age and gender. Physiotherapy 86(2): 42

CHAPTER CONTENTS

Introduction   225

Definitions   226

'Normal' posture   226
The ideal static standing posture   227
The ideal lying posture   227
The ideal static sitting posture   229

The importance of balance and posture   229

Balancing mechanisms to maintain posture   231
Pressure receptors in the feet   231
Vestibular system   232
Tonic neck reflexes   232
The visual system   232
Interaction of postural information to maintain
balance   233

**Factors that contribute to poor or altered
posture   233**

Deviations from the ideal posture   234
Scoliosis   235
Kyphosis   235
Lordotic (hollow back) posture   235
Kypholordotic posture   236
The sway back posture   236
The flat back posture   237

Retraining posture and balance   237

Summary   238

Acknowledgement   238

13

Posture and balance

T. Howe   J. Oldham

OBJECTIVES

At the end of this chapter you will be able to:

1. **Define posture and balance**

2. **Describe the ideal posture in lying, sitting and standing**

3. **Discuss the importance of balance and posture and the mechanisms of their interaction**

4. **Discuss the control of balance and posture**

5. **Describe abnormalities of posture and balance**

6. **Discuss the re-education of posture and balance.**

INTRODUCTION

The evolutionary process has resulted in modern man (homo sapiens). One of the early phases of human evolution was the adoption of an erect posture, allowing the development of bipedal gait and freeing the arms for other uses, e.g. tool making. Modern man is designed for mobility: muscles generate forces that are exerted about their attachments to bone, resulting in movement. However, compared to their four-legged counterparts, humans are precariously balanced animals. Four-legged animals are quite stable and difficult to unbalance when pushed. On the other hand, two-legged animals (humans) easily fall over. Two major factors account for this instability: the small contact surface area of the feet relative to the rest of the body, and a high position of centre of gravity relative to the ground.

Gravity is constantly pulling the body towards the ground. This force has to be counteracted by the muscles exerting a continuous pull on the skeleton in the opposite direction to these forces (Thibodeau & Patton 1993). The role the muscles play in this respect cannot be overestimated. In addition, the bones of the skeleton are too irregularly shaped to stand upon each other and maintain an upright position alone (Thibodeau & Patton 1993). The presence of ligaments surrounding joints is still insufficient to afford stability. Therefore, a passive stability is insufficient and active mechanisms must be employed to maintain balance and posture. These mechanisms do not operate when a person is asleep, hence the inability to sleep unsupported or standing up.

The ability of the muscles to counteract gravity by graded levels of contraction is carefully controlled by the nervous system. The mechanisms by which this is achieved will be described in detail below. Many other systems contribute to the ability of muscles to maintain posture. These include the respiratory, digestive, circulatory, excretory and endocrine systems (Thibodeau & Patton 1993). These will not be considered further in this chapter but the important contribution of other body systems must not be forgotten.

DEFINITIONS

Before proceeding any further, balance and posture need to be defined. The two concepts cannot be considered in isolation as they are interdependent. The term *posture* means simply position or alignment of body parts (Thibodeau & Patton 1993). It is usually thought of in terms of the spine, but it should be remembered that all body parts have a role to play in postural alignment. Furthermore, posture cannot be separated from movement, but should be regarded as 'temporarily arrested movement' as it is in a constant state of change (Bobath 1978), as anyone trying to stay still for any length of time will know.

Defining 'good' posture is less easy, however, and it can refer to a position that requires the least effort to maintain, puts the least strain on ligaments, bones and joints or maintains the centre of mass over the base of support (Thibodeau & Patton 1993).

Balance, on the other hand, can be defined as 'a state in which the body is in equilibrium' (Galley & Forster 1987). This concept refers to the series of physiological mechanisms that exist to inform the body that a compromise in posture has taken place and undesired movement will occur, and the resulting mechanisms then restore that posture and prevent the undesired movement. Posture is a result of balancing each body part with respect to the other body parts.

'NORMAL' POSTURE

Normal posture is difficult to define as every person has a unique anthropometric and physiological profile. Morphological body types (somatotypes) may be classified according to three extremes: ectomorphs (long and thin), endomorphs (short and fat) and mesomorphs (athletic and muscular) (Carter et al 1983). Most people are a combination of all three extremes. These anatomical differences, particularly the inborn length of the ligaments, account for many of the greatest differences in posture. People with loose ligaments tend to stand with hyperextended knees and hips (resting on their iliofemoral ligaments) and with flexible, exaggerated curves of the spine that are much greater than those seen in people with tighter ligaments (Larson & Gould 1974). Furthermore, the majority of the population rarely adopt good posture, with slouching being particularly prevalent. In addition, posture may alter throughout the day and may be related to fatigue and emotional state. The number of postural variations makes it difficult to define what constitutes normal posture, particularly in a population that rarely adopts a good one. An ideal posture tends only to be observed in trained individuals and the therapist must aim for a posture that suits the circumstance, i.e. body shape and interaction with the environment, rather than a typical posture.

The ideal static standing posture

When assessing posture, observations should be undertaken with the subject barefooted as pressure distribution over the feet will differ depending on whether or not shoes are worn (Galley & Forster 1987). The ideal erect posture should be assessed in three dimensions, i.e. laterally, anteriorly and posteriorly, by comparing parts of the body with a plumb or imaginary vertical line. When viewing an ideal posture from the lateral aspect, this standard reference line should pass just anteriorly to the lateral malleolus of the ankle, immediately anterior to the midline of the knee and then directly through the greater trochanter, bodies of the lumbar vertebrae, shoulder joints, bodies of the cervical vertebrae and lobe of the ear (Kendall et al 1993) (Fig. 13.1).

The head should be erect and well balanced on the neck and not held too far anteriorly (poking chin) or posteriorly (Galley & Forster 1987).

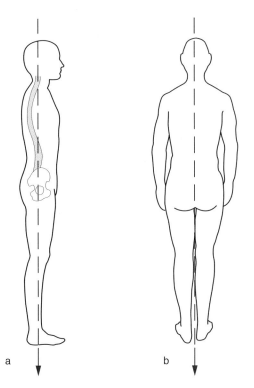

a   b

Figure 13.1 A well aligned standing posture: (a) lateral view; (b) posterior view.

Incorrect positioning of the head may lead to neck and eye pain and associated headaches. The chest should be erect without tension or over-expansion, and the abdomen should be flat and relaxed without sagging or retraction (Galley & Forster 1987).

Finally, the lumbar area of the back should be slightly hollow (slight lumbar lordosis) (Norris 1994). When viewed from the front, the bare feet should be placed approximately 8 cm apart and the line should bisect the body into two equal halves. Body weight should be evenly distributed between the two halves (Galley & Forster 1987). In this position the pubic symphysis, anterior superior iliac spines and the point of the shoulders should be on the same level in the horizontal plane (Galley & Forster 1987, Kendall et al 1993). When observing the posterior view, other anatomical landmarks including the knee and buttock creases, iliac crests, dimples over the sacroiliac joints, inferior angle of the scapulae, acromion processes, ears and external occipital protuberance can also be used for horizontal alignment (Norris 1995). See Table 13.1 for a posture checklist.

Task 13.1 Postural assessment

Assess the posture of some of your fellow students. Select a sample of males and females and try to include different extremes of somatotypes. Use the posture check-list to help you assess their standing posture. They will not be exactly 'normal' for the reasons discussed previously. Note the differences in posture between males and females.

The ideal lying posture

So far the discussion in this chapter has related to the standing position. However, the strict definition of posture also relates to other body positions. A lying position is known as a *recumbent posture*. If this position is face down, it is referred to as a *prone posture* and if face up, a *supine posture*. In these cases, the pull of gravity is not through the longitudinal axis of the body but through each segment of the body that is in contact with the supporting surface (Larson &

Table 13.1 Posture checklist

Anatomical landmark	Description
Anterior view	
Head alignment	central/L or R lateral tilt/L or R rotation
Shoulders	level/L or R elevation/L or R protracted/L or R retracted
Waist skin creases	equal/L or R side flexion
Pelvis ASIS	level/L or R elevation
Patellae	level/L or R medially positioned/L or R laterally positioned/L or R elevated
Feet	neutral/L or R laterally positioned/L or R medially positioned/L or R flat
Posterior view	
Head alignment	central/L or R lateral tilt/L or R rotation
Acromion processes	level/L or R elevation/L or R protracted/L or R retracted
Inferior angle of scapulae	level/L or R elevation/L or R abduction/L or R adduction/L or R winging
Thoracic spine	neutral/L or R scoliosis/kyphosis
Lumbar spine	neutral/L or R scoliosis
Waist skin creases	equal/L or R side flexion
Iliac crests	level/L or R elevation
S-1 joint dimples	level/L or R elevation
Buttock creases	level/L or R elevation
Knee creases	level/L or R elevation
Knee position	L or R extension/L or R hyperextension/L or R flexion
Feet (weight bearing)	equal/L or R diminished
Lateral view	
Head alignment	neutral/anterior poking/extended
Shoulders	level/L or R elevation/L or R protracted/L or R retracted
Thoracic spine	normal/kyphosis/flattened
Lumbar spine	normal/increased lordosis/flattened
Pelvis	neutral/anterior tilt/posterior tilt
Hip position	neutral/L or R extended/L or R flexed
Knee position	L or R extension/L or R hyperextension/L or R flexion

Gould 1974). Lying is the least energy consuming of all positions. Whatever the lying position adopted, localised pressure points develop and the position has to be adapted constantly. This is all too obvious when lying on a very hard surface, e.g. the floor. The development of pressure points is a particular problem in people with altered skin sensation, e.g. following spinal injury or peripheral nerve lesions, as they are unable to detect their development and skin breakdown may result. Such individuals must be made aware of the dangers of assuming the same posture for long periods of time and special mattresses to reduce the risk may be provided.

The ideal lying position is one in which rigid body segments sink down just enough to allow remaining segments to accept support from the mattress and essentially maintain the same body alignment as in standing (Larson & Gould 1974).

The condition of the mattress is very important. A soft mattress offers little support: when lying supine, the lumbar spine is in a position of flexion and when lying prone, the lumbar spine is forced into an exaggerated lordosis or hyperextension. In side lying in particular, the head will also need to be supported by a pillow to retain its line with the body (Galley & Forster 1987). The number of pillows used and their type also influence posture. Too many pillows or very firm pillows force the head into flexion when supine, and side flexion when side lying. Sleeping posture is important in people who have neck and back injuries as poor posture may aggravate their symptoms. Recently, special pillows and mattresses have become available that offer a more ideal position for the head and neck and afford greater support for the lumbar spine during lying.

The ideal static sitting posture

The sitting posture is more relaxing than that of standing. This position provides a greater supporting surface and allows relaxation of the muscles of the lower limb (Galley & Forster 1987). In the correct sitting position, the centre of mass should extend through the ischial tuberosities and just in front of the eleventh thoracic vertebra (Larson & Gould 1974). Without the additional support to the thighs and back common to most chairs, this is a highly unstable position.

The ideal sitting posture is achieved when:

- the ischial tuberosities provide the major base of support
- the upper thighs add to the sitting base without placing undue pressure on the back of the knee joint
- the lumbar spine is in mid-flexion
- the entire spine is supported via a backrest with a slight backward inclination from the perpendicular
- the weight of the legs is transferred to the supporting surface of the floor by the feet (Larson & Gould 1974).

Unfortunately, this position is practically impossible to attain with many modern seating arrangements. Seats are often too soft and deep, short or long and have too much of a backward slope. Furthermore, it is very common for individuals to slide their pelvis forwards (slouch) resulting in a centre of mass behind the ischial tuberosities. This results in a convex curvature of the lumbar spine (loss of the lumbar lordosis) (Larson & Gould 1974) and concave curvature of the thoracic spine, the former placing excessive strain on the posterior spinal ligaments and causing posterior bulging of the intervertebral discs. Different sitting postures are also achieved depending on whether the subject is sitting on a chair or the floor (Fig. 13.2).

THE IMPORTANCE OF BALANCE AND POSTURE

The importance of balance and posture cannot be overemphasised as demonstrated in the following quote by Carpenter (1984): 'Movement begins and ends in posture and for the most time the motor system is not in fact concerned with moving the body at all but rather with keeping it still.' This definition is, however, a gross over-simplification with postural adjustment (i.e. maintenance of balance) playing a fundamental role throughout the performance of a movement (Bobath 1969, Peterkin 1969). Indeed, movement occurs against a pliable postural tone adjusted to maintain the equilibrium of the person (Peterkin 1969, Willard 1992).

In the standing position and throughout a movement, humans are in dynamic rather than static equilibrium (Green 1978). Gravity is continuously trying to pull us towards the ground (Thibodeau & Patton 1993). Any slight deviation from the upright posture must be counterbalanced to maintain that position. A number of complex mechanisms are involved in this process. These range from those systems that tell us when our posture has been compromised and we are in danger of falling to those mechanisms that restore our equilibrium. This chapter focuses on these two mechanisms and describes how through balancing mechanisms we can maintain posture.

Balance is essential for every activity carried out during waking hours and skilled movements are dependent upon the ability to maintain equilibrium in a variety of positions and under many conditions (Davies 1985). The lower limbs must be able to support the body on its base of support and withstand any unexpected perturbations (Stein 1982). Muscles make continual adjustments to maintain balance and equilibrium. This requires contraction of the flexors and extensors synergistically and with precise timing. Thus, it can be seen that balance and posture are intimately related. Posture may be seen as the starting point and the end point of movement.

Bobath (1978) has developed the concept of the normal postural reflex mechanism (NPRM) providing the background for all skilled movements (it should be noted that this concept presupposes an intact adult brain). The NPRM is dependent upon three factors: normal muscle tone, reciprocal innervation and inhibition, and

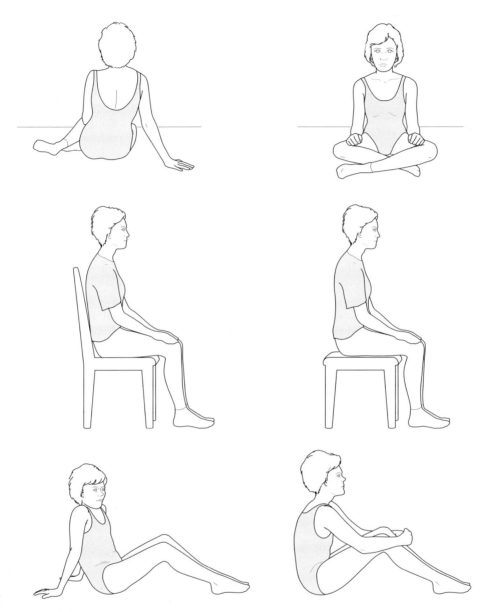

Figure 13.2 Different sitting positions.

automatic movement patterns. Normal muscle tone must be sufficiently high to support the body against gravity and to initiate and control movement, but not so high that it impedes movement. Reciprocal innervation and inhibition allow stabilisation of certain body parts while allowing selective, coordinated and controlled movement of others. Automatic movement patterns include the righting and equilibrium reactions that provide the background for all voluntary movements. These reactions range from very small changes in muscle tone that are not visible to the naked eye to gross movements of the limbs and trunk (Davies 1985).

Task 13.2 Effects on balance

Stand on a wobble board with your feet approximately 10 cm apart then with your feet together. Then try standing barefoot on a large medicine ball. How do these alterations in base of support alter your ability to balance?

Stand with the aid of elbow or axillary crutches so that your feet and the crutches are in a straight line. Attempt to maintain your balance while a fellow student pushes you in anterior and posterior directions. Now place the crutches slightly in front of you so that you form an approximate triangle with the crutches and your feet. What difference does this make to your ability to balance?

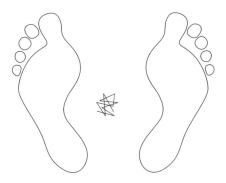

Figure 13.3 The oscillating path of the body's centre of mass during standing.

BALANCING MECHANISMS TO MAINTAIN POSTURE

Three major physiological mechanisms exist to inform the body that a compromise in posture has taken place and to elicit a series of balancing reactions to restore that posture. These are: the vestibular system, the visual system and pressure receptors in the feet. In addition, neck righting reactions have a role to play. These systems do not operate in isolation but offer an integrated approach to maintenance of posture involving the entire nervous, muscular and skeletal systems.

Pressure receptors in the feet

Pressure receptors in the feet provide the body with information about the distribution of body support. Difference in pressure at different points on the sole of the foot tell us the position of the vertical projection of the centre of mass relative to body supports (Carpenter 1984). This is very important, for in order for the body to remain upright, its centre of mass must always pass through its base of support, i.e. the feet in the upright position. When the line of gravity falls outside of this position the body will fall over (Norris 1993). To prevent such a catastrophe, the position of the body must change to restore the status quo (Carpenter 1984).

If position is shifted from an equal pressure distribution under both feet to an increased pressure under one foot, the body responds by increasing the tone of the extensor muscles in that limb with a corresponding increase in the flexor muscles in the opposite limb (Green 1978). As a result, the body is prevented from falling over and an upright posture is maintained (Carpenter 1984). These reactions are seen in a more dramatic form if the body is pushed from side to side. The body has to constantly maintain an upright position by reversing its reactions in response to the direction of force. These mechanisms form the *postural sway reaction*. These reactions are not solely related to external force but also apply in normal standing when the body is never completely still but swaying constantly (Fig. 13.3).

The postural sway reaction assumes that some support is already present. Other movements may be required, however, if the position of the centre of mass of the body extends outside its base of support. These include *stepping reactions* where two feet are involved and *hopping reactions* where there is only one foot involved. In cases where postural support is required, but not present, *placing reactions* are employed.

Proprioceptive input from the skin, and pressure and joint receptors of the foot, have been observed to play a significant role in minor perturbations of the supporting surface, but are of minor importance during rapid displacements of the supporting surface (Deiner et al 1984). It should be noted that a complete loss of proprioceptive input from the lower limbs results in a severe loss of postural stability and a pathognomonic body tremor (Deiner et al 1984). Pressure receptors are to be found not only in the feet but also throughout the body. These receptors contribute to the total knowledge of body position but for simplicity are not considered in detail here.

Vestibular system

The vestibular system provides the body with two sets of information. Rotation of the head activates sensory receptors of the:

- semicircular canals to provide information regarding the angular acceleration of the head (Berne & Levy 1993)
- otolith organs to provide information about the effective direction of gravity.

Stimulation of the semicircular canal system provides information about the rate rather than direction of movement (Seeley et al 1992). Such information results in postural adjustments mediated by commands transmitted through the spinal cord via the lateral and medial vestibulospinal tracts and reticulospinal tracts (Berne & Levy 1993, Rutishauser 1994). The lateral vestibulospinal tract activates the extensor muscles throughout the body that control posture. The medial vestibulospinal tract causes contraction of neck muscles that counteract the movement of the head (Berne & Levy 1993). If the head is moved to the right, increased postural tone on the right side prevents falling in that direction.

The otolith organs are the only organs that provide information about the absolute position of the head in space. These organs include the utricle and saccule; their prime function is to keep the head upright despite changes in the position of the body. This is achieved through changes in tone of the neck muscles via mechanisms known as the *head righting reflexes* (Carpenter 1984). These mechanisms restore the position of the head to its neutral balanced position (Seeley et al 1992).

The vestibular system is poorly developed in humans and balancing in daytime is mainly carried out via impulses from the eyes (Green 1978). In people with visual impairments, however, balance has to be maintained by the pressure of the feet and the vestibular mechanisms described above.

Tonic neck reflexes

Changes in neck muscle tone are not only mediated in response to information received via the vestibular system but from the muscle spindles of the neck itself. One of the largest concentrations of muscle spindles exists in the neck (Berne & Levy 1993). Stimulation of these spindles evokes tonic neck reflexes. Bending the head to the left will result in the contraction of the extensor limbs on the left side and relaxation of the flexor limbs on the right (Berne & Levy 1993).

The visual system

Other receptors in the head that assist in the maintenance of posture by providing information about the position of the head are those of the retina (Carpenter 1984). The visual system tells us that the image of an object has moved relative to the retina. The ability of this system to distinguish between an object moving, the eye moving relative to the head, or the head and eye moving together is of paramount importance to the maintenance of posture. How this is achieved, however, is still subject to debate, though the end point of the reflex results in contraction of the neck muscles to right the head (Keel & Neil 1966).

The important role of the eyes in the maintenance of balance, however, can be illustrated by asking a person to stand on one leg initially with the eyes open and then closed. Once the eyes are closed, the person tends to fall over as the visual reference point for maintaining that position is lost. In addition, the visual system enables the precise timing and control of a movement in relation to the environment (Galley & Forster 1987),

---

Task 13.3 Factors affecting balance

Find a partner and ask him/her to time how long you are able to stand on your non-dominant leg while barefoot and with your eyes open. Repeat this procedure with your eyes closed. Note the differences in your ability to balance.

With your eyes closed spin yourself around in a circle several times then try and stand still. What factors are contributing to your altered ability to balance?

for example the foot striking a step when alighting a bus.

Interaction of postural information to maintain balance

The various postural reactions described above in the normal person are coordinated in definite cortically controlled patterns common to everyone (Bobath 1969). These reactions are automatic and involve predictable changes in muscle tone according to the position of a person's head in relation to the trunk. This results in a corresponding increase in flexor or extensor activity to restore balance. These *automatic postural reaction patterns* form the background against which automatic and voluntary movement patterns are based (Bobath 1969). Figure 13.4 illustrates the interrelations between the various mechanisms involved in the maintenance of posture.

FACTORS THAT CONTRIBUTE TO POOR OR ALTERED POSTURE

There are many factors that contribute to poor posture. These include: pain, decreased range of movement and flexibility, muscle imbalances, altered joint biomechanics, pathological conditions, joint hypermobility and ligament laxity, altered sensation and proprioception, psychological state, adaptations to the environment, and finally and more commonly persistent adoption of poor posture (habituation). Poor posture puts abnormal strains on muscles, bones, joints and ligaments. In some cases this may lead to deformity which may interfere with various bodily

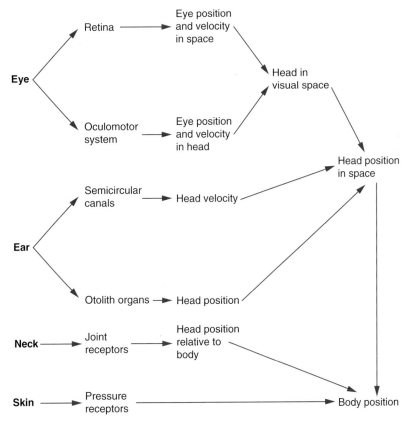

Figure 13.4 The interrelations between the various mechanisms involved in the maintenance of posture. (Reproduced with permission from Carpenter 1984.)

functions, such as respiration, digestion, circulation (Thibodeau & Patton 1993) and mobility.

Pain causes reflex contraction (spasm) of the muscles surrounding the source of the pain. This is the body's mechanism of restricting movement (splinting) of the injured body part to protect it from further damage. Obviously this causes an alteration in posture. For example, following an injury to the hand, a natural response is to hold the arm close to the body and, usually, the other arm is wrapped around it for added protection. Patients who have a prolapsed intervertebral disc in the lumbar region often present with muscle spasm in their paravertebral muscles. This is often unilateral and causes a lateral tilt of the pelvis. This altered posture disappears when the cause of their pain is resolved.

Decreased range of movement occurs for the following reasons: decreased flexibility of the muscles or ligaments surrounding a joint or altered joint biomechanics following trauma, pathology or congenital malformation. Muscle tightness occurs following muscle imbalances where one muscle group is stronger than another. Excessive strengthening of a muscle group leads to hypertrophy (enlargement) of the muscle fibres, but this could lead to increased soft tissue apposition and a decreased range of movement results. Weakness in the antagonist muscle group (muscles working in opposition) means that they are unable to resist the action of the stronger muscles that are causing an alteration in posture. It is, therefore, important to incorporate flexibility exercises into muscle strengthening regimens and that care is taken to avoid creating muscle imbalances between muscle groups (agonists and antagonists). Injury to bones or joints that causes a mechanical or bony restriction to movement may also result in altered posture due to an altered alignment of body parts.

Task 13.4 Altered posture

Get your partner to simulate a leg length discrepancy by getting him to place one foot on a book approximately 3–4 cm high. Note the differences this makes to his standing posture.

Laxity of ligaments surrounding joints allows the movement of the joints beyond normal limits; this is known as *hypermobility*. This causes an alteration in posture as the end of joint range is increased. This can be seen in female gymnasts who are able to hyperextend their lumbar spine. The length of ligaments is predetermined at birth but they may also become elongated by persistent overstretching and may become lax following injury.

Alterations in sensation and proprioception mean that awareness of the position of a body part in space and its relationship with a supporting surface are diminished. This may affect posture as individuals are unable to determine the position of their body parts with respect to others.

Psychological state has a large influence on posture (Morris 1982). Compare, for example, the postures adopted by: a footballer who has just scored a goal and the players on the opposite team; a parent scolding a child and the child being scolded; a person who has just had an important honour bestowed on him and a person who is feeling depressed or anxious. Therapists should be aware of how feelings of anger, fear, elation, depression, anxiety, submission and power can alter the posture of an individual. Many people have to adapt their posture to meet the needs of their environment. This is especially true in the work place. For example, people working at a word processor spend much of their time looking at a VDU. If the position and height of the VDU are incorrect, unnecessary strain may be placed on the muscles and ligaments of the neck and back due to this habitual altered posture. A factory worker may spend all day in a position that facilitates the task undertaken while leaning over a production line. If this adoption of an abnormal posture is a regular occurrence, anatomical structures may become overstretched and pain and long-term damage may result.

DEVIATIONS FROM THE IDEAL POSTURE

The major posture types that will be considered in this section are: scoliotic, kyphotic, lordotic, kypholordotic, sway back and flat back. These posture types will be considered with respect to the body segment alignment, and those muscles that are elongated and weak or short and strong respectively.

Scoliosis

Scoliosis is a lateral curvature of the lumbar and/or thoracic spine and may be either mobile or fixed (Fig. 13.5). Mobile scoliotic postures may result from:

- persistent adoption of such a posture
- a painful pathology, e.g. a prolapsed lumbar vertebral disc
- a compensation for lower limb problems, e.g. leg length discrepancy or abnormal pelvic tilt
- reduced muscle strength or altered muscle tone of the paraspinal muscles unilaterally, e.g. following head injury or CVA (stroke).

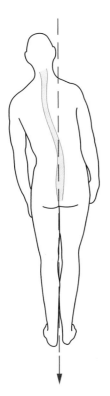

Figure 13.5 Posterior view of a subject with a thoracolumbar scoliosis.

A fixed (structural) scoliosis does not disappear with alterations in posture. The vertebral bodies rotate towards the convexity and the spinous processes towards the concavity of the curve. Secondary curves develop to counteract the effects of the initial scoliosis but these often become fixed later (Apley & Solomon 1982).

Kyphosis

Kyphosis is an increase in the convexity of the thoracic spine when viewed laterally. A kyphosis may be either mobile or fixed (Apley & Solomon 1982). Mobile kyphosis may be the result of:

- persistently adopting such a posture, e.g. in obese individuals or during pregnancy and immediately following childbirth
- association with other postural defects, e.g. flat feet
- weak erector spinae muscles
- a compensation to hip deformity, e.g. fixed flexion or congenital dislocation of the hip.

Fixed kyphosis occurs in patients with ankylosing spondylitis and Scheuermann's disease and senile kyphosis exists in the elderly as a consequence of intervertebral disc degeneration.

Lordotic (hollow back) posture

In normal posture the lumbar spine should be slightly hollow. This hollowing (the lumbar lordosis) is influenced by the tilt of the pelvis. The pelvis balances on the hip joints like a see-saw. Control of this see-saw is maintained by the abdominal, spinal and hip muscles and the surrounding ligaments (Norris 1994). The abdominal, gluteal and hamstring muscles work together to tilt the pelvis backwards and flatten the lumbar spine. At the same time the hip flexors and spinal extensors increase the lumbar curve by tilting the pelvis forwards (Norris 1994). If an imbalance in these muscles results in excessive lengthening and weakness of the abdominal and gluteal muscles and tightening of the iliopsoas and spinal extensor muscles, the person assumes a 'pot belly' type posture (Norris 1994). The pelvis is tipped forwards and increases the curvature of the lumbar spine (Fig. 13.6a). This muscle imbalance is known as the *pelvic crossed syndrome* (Norris 1994). In addition to the problems described above, the hamstrings attempt to compensate for the weakened gluteal muscles during walking. Since the hamstrings are not as strong as the gluteals, hip extension is weaker. The body tries to compensate for this by extending the lumbar spine, resulting in further undue stress in this area (Norris 1994).

Kypholordotic posture

The body segment alignment of individuals with a kypholordotic posture will be altered in the following way (Fig. 13.6b). The head will be the most anteriorly placed body segment. It will be held forwards but the cervical spine will be extended, i.e. they will have a 'poking chin'. The scapulae may be abducted. They will have an increased thoracic kyphosis with an increased lumbar lordosis and the pelvis will be tilted anteriorly. They will stand with their hips flexed but

their knees will be hyperextended. They will have elongated and weak neck flexors, with weakness also in the upper portion of erector spinae and the external oblique. Conversely, the neck extensors and hip flexors will be short and strong. If the scapulae are abducted, there will be weakness of the middle and lower fibres of the trapezius but the serratus anterior, pectoralis major and/or minor and upper fibres of trapezius will be short and strong.

The sway back posture

The body segment alignment of an individual with a typical sway back posture is altered in the following way (Fig. 13.6c). The pelvis is positioned in neutral or often is tilted posteriorly and is positioned to be the most anterior of the subject's body segments. Subjects have a kyphosis of the thoracic region with a flattening of the lumbar lordosis. This results in the hip joints being positioned in front of the standard posture line with observable hyperextension of the hip

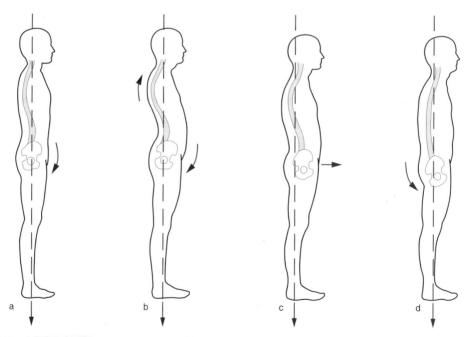

Figure 13.6 Lateral views of different posture types: (a) lordotic; (b) kyphotic; (c) sway back; (d) flat back. (Adapted with permission from Kendall F P et al 1993 Muscle testing and function, 3rd edn. © Williams and Wilkins.)

and knees. Where the subject stands predominantly on one leg, the pelvis will be tilted down to the non-favoured side. This gives the appearance of a longer favoured leg but this is only evident in the standing position.

Individuals with a sway back posture will have weak and elongated hip flexors with short and strong hamstrings due to standing with hyperextended hips. If one leg is favoured, the gluteus medius (especially posterior fibres) will be weak and elongated, the tensor fascia lata will be strong and the iliotibial band will be tight on the favoured side. The external oblique, upper back extensors and neck flexors will be elongated and weak whereas the upper fibres of internal oblique and low back musculature will be short but not strong.

The flat back posture

The altered body segment alignment of individuals with a flat back posture is as follows (Fig. 13.6d). They will have a posterior tilt of the pelvis and a loss or flattening of the lumbar lordosis. They will stand with hyperextended hip and knee joints and the head will be positioned anteriorly, resulting in increased flexion of the upper thoracic spine. They will have elongated and weak hip flexors with short and strong hamstrings. The erector spinae (back muscles) may be slightly elongated and weak but the abdominal muscles may be strong.

RETRAINING POSTURE AND BALANCE

As we have seen, there are many factors that contribute to poor posture. Therapists should identify whether there are any pathological or biomechanical abnormalities and whether any anatomical structures are tight or weak. They should then initiate a programme of stretching for tight structures and strengthening for those muscle groups that are weak. This should be monitored to avoid developing a further muscle imbalance or instability. Pathological or biomechanical abnormalities will require further investigation and may necessitate involvement from orthotists or surgeons.

Many patients are unaware that their posture is incorrect and may in fact be contributing to their physical symptoms. For the correction of habitual posture it is essential that the patient is aware of what is correct and what is bad and has become 'habit'. It is only then that correction may begin to take place: patient education is, therefore, essential. This may include advice on the height of furniture and work surfaces, types of mattresses, pillows, etc. and lifting and handling techniques.

Full length mirrors are frequently used in physiotherapy departments to make patients more aware of their static posture either in sitting or standing and dynamic posture during movement. Mirrors are also employed in gait retraining, for example following the provision of a prosthesis after lower limb amputation.

A further method of posture retraining is biofeedback. This is a technique involving the use of biological signals. Electromyographic activity (EMG) is produced by muscles when they are active. These signals may be detected by an electronic device. Any muscle contraction results in an increase in electrical activity, i.e. an increase in the amplitude of the EMG signal. EMG may be used to detect when unwanted movements or positions are occurring and these may be identified to the patient by the sounding of an alarm or by the illumination of a light switch. The miniaturisation of such devices allows them to be worn by subjects in their normal environments while performing normal activity. This is especially useful in occupational health, where habitual adoption of a bad posture may cause injury. The identification of an incorrect posture or unwanted muscle activity allows subjects to reassess their posture and, if appropriate, alter it.

Patterns of muscle activity (dynamic posture and balance) may also be retrained using visual feedback by interfacing the EMG with a computer and appropriate computer software. Patients may be able to play games by using the intensity of muscle contraction or using activity in different muscle groups. This technique is especially useful in posture and balance education in children.

Balance may be affected by a person's ability to move quickly from one position to another. Several factors may have an influence on this: pain, musculoskeletal pathology, muscle weakness, biomechanical abnormalities, proprioceptive loss, reduced neuromuscular control and age. *Static balance* refers to a person's ability to maintain balance when in a specific posture and *dynamic balance* refers to keeping the body's segments under control during movement to prevent falling. Obviously, both types of balance are important and may require retraining. Static balance is perhaps the easiest to retrain as it involves maintaining the body's equilibrium in a particular posture. This may be achieved by starting with a large base of support or by increasing the amount of support above normal levels. As balance improves this additional support may be gradually reduced. For example, in standing extra support may be achieved by holding on to a rigid support, e.g. wall bars, with the arms. A larger base of support is achieved by standing with the legs wide apart; a smaller base of support is obtained by standing with the feet together.

Dynamic balance may be facilitated by using moveable supports instead of rigid ones, e.g. gymnastic balls instead of wall bars, or by using more unstable bases of support, e.g. wobble boards. Advanced training may involve a person standing on a wobble board and attempting to maintain balance while throwing and catching a medicine ball. More functional tasks may include walking over an uneven surface, turning round corners and negotiating obstacles. As mentioned earlier, methods of biofeedback may also be useful.

SUMMARY

Balance and posture are interrelated and a series of physiological mechanisms exist to inform the body if posture has been compromised and the body is in danger of falling. The body responds by altering its posture (moving) in an attempt to maintain or regain its balance. These mechanisms form a feedback loop and are constantly informing the body of changes in position and pressure distribution. Normal static posture is difficult to define as every person has a unique anthropometric and physiological profile. However, there are some common types of deviations from the normal. Some examples of these different types of posture have been described and methods for retraining balance and posture have been introduced. It should be remembered that balance and posture are vital for everyday activities and it is often not until a failure of one or more components of these complex systems that we realise how sensitive the system is. The physiotherapist plays a major role in posture education and the retraining of balance and posture following pathology or injury.

Task 13.5

Answer the following questions:
1. What are the main physiological systems involved in balance?
2. What factors contribute to poor posture?
3. What are the common types of poor habitual posture?
4. What methods may be used to retrain posture?
5. What factors should be taken into account in patients who have sensory impairments?
5. What implications do visual impairments have during recovery from injury?
7. What advice may you offer patients when teaching them to use crutches or walking sticks?
8. What methods may be used to retrain balance?

ACKNOWLEDGEMENT

The authors would like to thank Mr Chris Norris for his contribution to this chapter.

REFERENCES

Apley A G, Solomon L 1982 Apley's system of orthopaedics and fractures, 6th edn. Butterworths, London

Berne R M, Levy M N 1993 Physiology, 3rd edn. C V Mosby, St Louis

Bobath B 1969 The treatment of neuromuscular disorders by improving patterns of co-ordination. Physiotherapy 55: 18–22

Bobath B 1978 Adult hemiplegia: evaluation and treatment, 2nd edn. William Heinemann Medical Books, London

Carpenter R H S 1984 Neurophysiology, 1st edn. Edward Arnold, London

Carter J E L, Ross W D, Duqet W, Aubry S P 1983 Advances in somatotype methodology and analysis. Year Book of Physical Anthropology 26: 193–213

Davies P M 1985 Steps to follow. Springer-Verlag, Berlin

Deiner H C, Dichgans B, Guschlabauer B, Mau H 1984 The significance of proprioception on postural stabilisation as assessed by ischemia. Brain Research 296: 103–109

Galley P M, Forster A L 1987 Human movement: an introductory text for physiotherapy students, 2nd edn. Churchill Livingstone, Edinburgh

Green J H 1978 An introduction to human physiology, 4th edn. Oxford University Press, Oxford

Keel C A, Neil E 1966 Samson Wright's applied physiology, 11th edn. Oxford University Press, London

Kendall F P, McCreary E K, Provance P G 1993 Muscle testing and function, 4th edn. Williams and Wilkins, Baltimore

Larson C B, Gould M 1974 Orthopaedic Nursing, 8th edn. C V Mosby, St Louis

Morris D 1982 The pocket guide to manwatching. Triad/Granada, London

Norris C M 1993 Weight training principles and practice, 1st edn. A & C Black, London

Norris C M 1994 Flexibility principles and practice, 1st edn. A & C Black, London

Norris C M 1995 Spinal stabilisation 4: muscle imbalance and the low back. Physiotherapy 81: 20–31

Peterkin H W 1969 The neuromuscular system and re-education of movement. Physiotherapy 55: 145–153

Rutishauser S 1994 Physiology and anatomy: a basis for nursing and health care, 1st edn. Churchill Livingstone, Edinburgh

Seeley R R, Stephens T D, Tate P 1992 Anatomy and physiology, 2nd edn. Mosby Year Book, St Louis

Stein J F 1982 An introduction to neurophysiology. Blackwell Scientific Publications, Oxford

Thibodeau G A, Patton K T 1993 Anatomy and physiology, 2nd edn. C V Mosby, St Louis

Willard F H 1992 Medical neuroanatomy. J B Lippincott, Philadelphia

CHAPTER CONTENTS

Introduction   241

Normal levels of arousal   242

Physiology of stress and relaxation   243

When stress becomes abnormal   243
Pattern of stress   244

Relaxation therapy   245
General and local relaxation   246
Developing self-awareness   246
Preparing for relaxation   247

Specific relaxation techniques   247
Contract-hold-relax or contrast method   248
The physiological or Mitchell's technique   248
Visualisation or the suggestion method   249
Sedative massage   249
EMG biofeedback   249
Low frequency breathing exercises   250
Pendular exercises   250
Rhythmical passive movements   251
Physical activity   251

14

Tension and relaxation

M. Trew

OBJECTIVES

When you have completed this chapter you should be able to:

1. **Understand the difference between positive and negative stress**

2. **Understand the basic physiological changes in tension and relaxation**

3. **Recognise the common changes in movement patterns or posture that occur in situations of tension**

4. **Describe several different methods of inducing relaxation.**

INTRODUCTION

Often minor degrees of stress or tension can affect normal posture and patterns of movement, and where levels of tension are very high, human movement will be noticeably disrupted. This chapter considers stress or tension in general terms and how it may affect movement. The chapter concludes by considering several different relaxation techniques and emphasises the importance of the individual taking 'ownership' of the relaxation process rather than being a passive participant.

Though the general population is familiar with the words 'tension' and 'relaxation', a surprisingly large number of people are unable to recognise these two states in themselves. This may be partially because well developed physical self-awareness is not common, probably because

Table 14.1 Definitions of stress, tension and relaxation

Stress	Tension	Relaxation
Strain	Strain	Looseness
Pressure	Rigidity	Becoming less tense
Force	Barely suppressed emotion	Becoming less rigid
Response to adverse stimulus	Conflict	Passivity
Constraining influence	Anxiety	Being at rest
Disruption of homeostasis	Tautness	Diminished awareness

there is a tendency to regard the body as something to be accepted until it starts to go noticeably wrong. It may also be because concepts like stress, tension and relaxation are not easy to define precisely (Table 14.1). Despite this, everyone has the potential to know what tension and relaxation are, though some people may need guidance to recognise these states in themselves. When people are able to monitor their own levels of tension and relaxation, they have taken the first step in being able to control and modify their reactions to stress.

NORMAL LEVELS OF AROUSAL

It is quite normal to vary between periods of stress when arousal is high and periods of low arousal and relaxation. In fact, these differences in the level of arousal are essential for efficient activity. When action is needed, the arousal level is high, the level of muscle tone is raised and non-essential systems become relatively inactive. When there is no call for high levels of mental and physical activity, then it is appropriate for the general level of arousal to be reduced so that energy may be conserved and depleted energy stores may be replenished.

In addition, all individuals have natural periods of greater or lesser mental and physical arousal throughout each day. The most obvious example is the wake/sleep cycle. At a more detailed level this basic rhythm is also evident in the various functions of the body: the rhythmical contraction and relaxation of the heart, the inspiratory and expiratory phases of the breathing cycle, and in movement, where one muscle group contracts whilst the antagonists relax to allow the movement to take place. These alter-

nating rhythms can be speeded up or slowed down in response to both internal and external stimuli, depending on the needs and demands of the particular situation.

Relaxation requires a de-emphasis of arousal states and, in particular, a reduction in muscular activity but, because the mind and the body are inextricably linked, there may also be a reduction in mental activity. Mental states such as anxiety, emotional tension and fear can all have a deleterious effect on tension and it is not possible when considering relaxation to divorce emotional states from physical states (Elton 1993). The body/mind effect reflects the links between the autonomic nervous system and the cerebral cortex of the brain and when trying to induce relaxation it is essential to be aware of this association.

When the natural balance between tension and relaxation is disrupted it can lead to an excessively high level of mental and physical arousal during which the muscular, respiratory and cardiovascular systems start to exhibit inappropriate activity. This is variously described as stress, tension, anxiety or an inability to relax and it leads to feelings of mental and physical tiredness, headaches, abnormal joint postures and a loss of the fine control of movement (Basmajian & Wolf 1990). In severe cases, other systemic manifestations such as dizziness, dysfunction of the digestive system, shortness of breath and disruption of the immunological response may occur (Baker 1987). Stress is defined by Selye (1984) as the non-specific result of any demand upon the body. This result can be mental, somatic or both. The physiological responses to stress are controlled by the autonomic nervous system and the psychological responses are thought to be controlled from the hypothalamus and the limbic lobe of the cerebral cortex.

PHYSIOLOGY OF STRESS AND RELAXATION

The autonomic nervous system is divided into two separate systems, the sympathetic and the parasympathetic, and they control the viscera. Afferent impulses from the viscera are integrated either at spinal level or within the reticular formation of the pons, medulla and midbrain. The two systems frequently act in a complementary manner affected by the quantity and type of synapse transmitter. The sympathetic system releases noradrenaline and the parasympathetic nerve endings release acetylcholine. Noradrenaline is also released as a hormone by the adrenal gland thus enhancing the effect of the sympathetic system.

The cardiovascular centres of the pons are responsible for the regulation of blood pressure. The dorsal vagal nuclei contain the parasympathetic preganglionic cell bodies of the vagus nerve which is responsible for the control of the viscera of the thorax and upper abdomen. The Edinger-Westphal nuclei of the midbrain control the reflex changes of the eye. These nuclei receive input from the reticular formation and other sensory inputs, particularly from the hypothalamus (Moffett et al 1993).

It is the sympathetic system that is activated in times of stress, initiating the 'fight or flight' response. The body becomes ready for action: there are chemical changes in skeletal muscle which result in the development of tension in the contractile components; in the eyes the pupils dilate and there is vasoconstriction of the salivary glands leading to a dry mouth. There is an inhibition of gastric and digestive secretions and a constriction of the sphincters with an increase in sweating. There is also an increase in the rate and force of heart contractions delivering more blood and, therefore, more oxygen to the tissues that need them. Cardiac output is increased and the distribution of blood is adjusted through constrictions of the small blood vessels in the skin and abdominal viscera, so that blood is not directed to non-essential tissues. In addition to all this there is a bronchodilatation in the lungs and a general increase in metabolism.

These are natural responses to stress and they only become inappropriate and possibly pathological when the original reason for stress is removed and the responses remain. Because so many systems are affected by the normal stress response, it is not surprising that in individuals who have abnormal levels of tension there may be symptoms involving a vast range of body systems. For example, experimental work has shown that abnormally high and prolonged levels of adrenaline and noradrenaline in animals lead to hyperactivity and enlargement of the adrenal cortex, and atrophy of the thymus and lymph nodes (Selye 1984). It has also been shown that prolonged and excessive stress weakens the effectiveness of the immune response and therefore increases vulnerability to disease. At a subjective level, anyone who has experienced high levels of stress will have noticed the general feeling of tiredness which results from sustained high levels of muscular activity.

Relaxation produces the opposite situation and, amongst other things, results in a noticeable reduction in blood pressure and heart and respiratory rates. There is also a reduction in blood cholesterol and blood glucose levels and the activity of the sympathetic nervous system is diminished (Everett et al 1995). Muscle tension is no longer generated and the elastic components of the muscles cause the fibres to return to their resting length; this is muscle relaxation (Astrand & Rodahl 1987). In complete muscle relaxation there is little or no apparent activity in the contractile components, although the presence of elastic components in muscle means that there is always a small degree of muscle tone.

WHEN STRESS BECOMES ABNORMAL

At times of either personal or environmental stress there will be challenges and difficulties to face. These lead to a rise in the level of arousal in the brain and the wide range of physical responses discussed earlier. This normal stress response, which is often experienced by the population at large, is usually followed by fatigue, a reduction in the level of arousal and eventually sleep. Selye (1984) defined this form of stress as positive because it is clear that a certain level of arousal is necessary to meet the challenges of life and living efficiently. Problems arise only when the response to stress becomes excessive and out of control, in which circumstances stress can be described as negative or distressful.

The capacity to cope with stressful events varies from person to person. Some people have the ability to recognise excessive stress and deal with these situations or prevent them occurring (Baker 1987). Others fail to recognise excessive stress or are unable to take avoiding action, which inevitably leads to the development of stress symptoms. At a gross level these symptoms include fatigue, loss of sleep and work inefficiency, which lead to further muscle tension, causing even greater fatigue. Individuals will often attempt to make up for the loss of efficiency by trying to increase their level of arousal, but this is self-defeating as it leads to more physical and emotional tension. If this situation is allowed to continue, a self-perpetuating cycle becomes established which can lead to depression and ill health.

There is no clear dividing point between the experience of positive stress and the change into a clinically recognised anxiety disorder because the duration of stress symptoms varies greatly as does an individual's ability to cope. However, there is no doubt that stress is a major problem which can affect any member of the population and this is evidenced by a review by Durham & Allan (1993) which indicated that at least 30% of the population may be driven to seek professional help for stress related problems.

Pattern of stress

The physical symptoms of stress which are easily recognised are often reflected in over-activity of the general body musculature. This excessive muscular tension forms well recognised patterns. An individual may demonstrate inappropriate muscular tension in any of the major muscle groups, but usually one or two muscle groups may be particularly affected. Because the pattern of tension may manifest itself in a variety of ways, it is important to observe the whole body when looking for signs.

The facial muscles often show abnormal tone; corrugator and frontalis, when not relaxed, will produce vertical and horizontal lines on the forehead. Tension headaches may develop if there is excessive tone in the occipitofrontalis and the suboccipital muscle groups. Inappropriate muscle activity in orbicularis oculi and muscles of the eyelids can either result in the eyes being narrowed or held widely open or in ticks, particularly on the inferior surface. Very frequently the masseter muscle responds to stress by contracting to hold the jaws tightly together; on careful observation of the lateral aspect of the cheeks it is often possible to see the muscle twitching. For some people, tension in the muscles of the jaw may also manifest itself in grinding of teeth during sleep. The tongue may be held rigidly on the roof of the mouth and the muscles of the throat may contract abnormally, making speech rather harsh and lacking in fluency of pronunciation. There may also be a click as the tongue unsticks itself from the roof of the mouth at the start of each sentence.

The posture of the head at times of stress varies between individuals, but common to all is elevation of the shoulder girdle as a result of abnormal tension in the upper fibres of the trapezius. This is easily recognised because the neck appears shortened and the normally sloping contour of the neck/shoulder region becomes more angular. The upper limbs are often held quite rigidly close to the chest with the elbows flexed. The trunk is generally held stiff and, because of tension in the abdominal musculature, diaphragmatic respiration can be inhibited so that the individual has to breathe using the intercostal and accessory muscles of respiration. In these cases, upper chest movement is observable and the accessory muscles in the neck can be seen contracting.

In general, repeated movements such as finger tapping or swinging the knees from flexion to extension when sitting can be indicators of abnormal muscle tone. Classically, it is also expected that adduction/flexion patterns are symptomatic of stress. This may be seen in a seated subject who is tense and will sit rigidly on the edge of the chair with their lower limbs adducted and flexed, while in a standing subject the arms may be folded tightly and the legs crossed at the ankle.

Though there are many ways in which stress or tension can be manifested, it is rare for one person to demonstrate all these symptoms simultaneously and it may be necessary to use careful observation in order to identify the signs. In addition, some people have learned to hide the signs of tension and in consequence will make an effort to slump back in their chair or to stand in a relaxed manner. Despite these efforts it is hard to control tension indicators and an experienced observer will usually be able to notice some abnormal movements or postures.

Apart from postural symptoms and general feelings of fatigue, increased stress can show in other ways. There may be an increase in adrenaline production which will result in an increase in heart and respiratory rate. There may also be changes in blood and digestive chemistry which become abnormal if maintained for any length of time (Astrand & Rodahl 1987). Skilled performance of motor tasks is usually decreased, with a higher incidence of anxiety-induced errors in people who are tense than in people who are more appropriately relaxed (Basmajian & Wolf 1990). This is probably caused by a combination of reduced muscle control in those muscles with abnormal tone and a disruption of concentration. Tension can also lead to emotional changes which may vary from anger to despair; intellectual performance may also suffer in these circumstances.

Many students suffer from increased tension, which can interfere with their performance. The stress of study, fear of failure, desire to succeed and pace of work, as well as poor environmental conditions and financial worries, may all contribute to this condition.

Task 14.1

Make a list of the symptoms that you manifest when tense. Watch other people carefully and see if you can notice examples of tension in the way in which they move or in their general posture.

RELAXATION THERAPY

There are a number of specific techniques that can be used to encourage relaxation but it is clear that treating the symptoms alone is not enough and the underlying cause must also be addressed. It is important to seek a solution for the causes of tension as well as learning methods to remove the symptoms. Relaxation techniques can be either physical or behavioural in approach, but there is controversy over which might be the most successful. Elton (1993) suggests that a combination of physical and behavioural techniques is most successful and that it may therefore be necessary for the patient with severe, chronic symptoms to seek help from those versed in both physical and psychological therapy. There is further evidence of the specificity of effectiveness of relaxation techniques. This means that a cognitive treatment approach will have mainly cognitive effects whereas if a physiological approach is used, most benefits will be seen in the reduction of the physical manifestations of tension (Lehrer et al 1994). If an individual has a generalised response to stress, then a mixed approach to relaxation may be the most appropriate treatment.

In physiotherapy the goal of relaxation therapy is primarily to encourage patients to gain physical control so that their response to stress is appropriate rather than destructive. This should then lead to the adoption of normal body posture and normal patterns of movement which will be more energy efficient and will, in turn, lead to a reduction in the feelings of fatigue. Some relaxation techniques require the patient to be rather passive: for example a sedative massage or a session in a flotation tank may be enjoyable and temporarily effective but overall the improvements are less likely to be long lasting than when a technique is used which encourages self-control (Elton 1993). For treatment to be effective patients have to recognise tension in themselves and understand its causes and effects. Once this is achieved and they are aware of their abnormal responses to stress, they can be taught to adopt strategies which will lead to more normal reactions and an immediate improvement in physiological function (Elton 1993).

General and local relaxation

Methods of relaxation may involve either learning to relax generally or developing the ability to recognise tension in specific parts of the body and then targeting individual muscles.

General relaxation can be used either as a treatment in its own right or as part of a more extensive treatment plan. Sometimes patients are very tense due to psychological or physical stress, and treatment of a totally unrelated condition may be impossible until general relaxation is gained; in this case relaxation will be preparatory to the main programme.

At other times general relaxation is not appropriate and the treatment objective may be to teach control of abnormal tension in specific muscles. This is often the case where fear of pain leads to protective muscle spasm round a particular joint and in this case local relaxation is often used in conjunction with pain-relieving treatments.

Case Study 14.1

An executive secretary in her mid-thirties was referred for treatment for unspecified low back pain. On arrival it was noticed that she sat very upright in the chair with her legs tightly wound round each other. Her arms were folded and her shoulder girdle was noticeably elevated. Initially it was thought that she was probably nervous about the impending treatment and that once she realised that the session would be neither painful nor unpleasant, she would relax. This did not happen and it became evident that even undertaking an assessment of her back problem was going to be difficult because of the degree of tension she exhibited. The remainder of the session was spent making her aware of her tension levels and giving her strategies for relaxation. For the next few weeks treatment focused primarily on relaxation and as she became more adept at reducing tension she was able to report a marked reduction in her back problem, a reduction in the incidence of headaches and an increase in general wellbeing. She now continues the relaxation on her own at home and has not required further treatment.

Developing self-awareness

Whatever technique is used, whether for local or general relaxation, the first step is to gain the patients' cooperation and develop their self-awareness. Until patients can recognise the feeling of abnormal muscular activity they will not be effective in trying to reach a more normal level. They must also learn to recognise the 'feel' of being relaxed so that they can monitor their level of success (Madders 1988). Developing self-awareness can be done by using a variety of biofeedback mechanisms. A mirror is an effective means of demonstrating abnormal posture and the success of attempts to reduce increased tone is immediately apparent. Videotape can also be used to record the patient's posture and movement patterns and it can then be viewed and discussed. Repeat filming will demonstrate the success of the intervention process. Patients can also be made aware of the level of activity in their muscles by using electromyography (EMG). Simple EMG biofeedback machines will indicate the level of electrical activity in those muscles underlying the electrodes. Patients are encouraged to try and relax while using the EMG output to measure the degree of success. Electronic blood pressure and pulse rate monitors can also be used as effective biofeedback mechanisms and at a simpler level patients can take their own pulse or count their own respiratory rate. With the information gained they can impose conscious control over cardiac or respiratory rate.

The overriding aim is that patients come to recognise the feeling of relaxation and that they know what activities will cause a reduction in the symptoms of stress. Emphasis is placed on teaching them to discriminate between abnormal and normal tension so that they can recognise when they have been successful in achieving a relaxed state and are able to produce relaxation at will. The skills of monitoring muscle activity, joint position, respiratory and heart rates have to be learned and this demands regular practice and concentration.

Associated with the development of self-awareness must be the acceptance that relaxation has to be self directed. Often when people are stressed and may be upset or frightened by the symptoms produced by their condition, they want to hand over control to the therapist. If relaxation is to be successful in the long term, patients have to take back control and learn to relax independent of their therapist. It is essential that at the start of the relaxation sessions the therapist agrees with the patients that they must gradually take over the responsibility for the relaxation process. Once they can do this, they are likely to be able to control the manifestations of stress regardless of their environment.

Preparing for relaxation

When teaching the patient total body relaxation it is advisable in the early stages to work in a fairly quiet, pleasantly warm environment where the patient can concentrate on the task in hand (Mitchell 1990). The choice of starting position should be left to the patient but it must be one of comfort and full support. Side, supine or prone lying with pillows and blankets for support and comfort are the most likely to be successful but should never be imposed upon the patient. Often during the process of relaxation therapy the initial starting position may become inappropriate and patients should be reassured that they may change position at any time.

As the ability to relax develops, different positions should be adopted and the environment should be made less protective until the patient is able to relax under any circumstances. It is essential that the treatment sessions proceed beyond the application of a technique and the therapist's goal should be to help patients develop strategies which will allow them to relax in situations which have previously generated stress (Crist & Rickard 1993).

The words used in the treatment session are important. Instructions should be brief, to the point and spoken in a calm, quiet manner so that they give a mental concept of what is required. The same phrases and commands should be used repeatedly so that the words themselves may become a trigger for relaxation. Harsh sounding words should be avoided and where a command to relax is given the tone of the voice should reflect the meaning. The therapist should conceal his own personality so that the focus of the session is on the task and not on the individuals involved. Timing is also important. Patients must be given ample time to assimilate the instructions and monitor their responses, in particular whether they have achieved a release of tension. In the introductory sessions this may take considerably longer than might be expected.

SPECIFIC RELAXATION TECHNIQUES

Apart from teaching patients to develop an increased self-awareness and, through that, a measure of personal control therapists may also use specific relaxation techniques. There are two main approaches: progressive muscle relaxation, which is based on work reported by Jacobsen in 1929, and cognitive or imaginal techniques.

Progressive muscle relaxation depends on the contraction of a muscle or muscle groups followed by a period of relaxation. Jacobsen was clear that there was a link between mental and physical tension and that if the physiology of the muscles could be altered by reducing tone, there would be a concurrent positive effect on the mind (Everett et al 1995). Whilst Jacobsen advocated contracting the major muscle groups which demonstrated tension, Laura Mitchell, some thirty years later, advised contracting the muscles antagonistic to those in tension. She worked on the principle that it would be better to avoid increasing the tension in an already tense muscle and that by contracting the antagonist, reciprocal inhibition of the tense muscle would occur. An alternative approach has been advocated by Carlson in the last two decades. Carlson, like Mitchell, considers that a muscle that is already demonstrating inappropriate tone might get worse if required to contract. Instead it is proposed that the muscles affected by tension should be stretched rather than be required to contract (Carlson et al 1996). This stretching is done utilising the effects of gravity, so for example the patient might allow the head to 'loll' to one side or another so that the neck muscles are fully stretched. The stretches are held for 10–30 seconds until the full benefit of the manoeuvre is felt.

Cognitive or imaginal techniques require the focusing of thoughts on an activity or place or on a repetitive sound or movement. There are several approaches to these techniques. The individual can practise visualisation, where the stressful situation is imagined as being non-stressful or non-threatening, and this is a technique often used in sport or by business people. In guided imagery the patients think about pleasant experiences and by so doing try to distance themselves from stressful situations. The direction of their thoughts can be towards real events which they found pleasant and are happy to think about, or they can be guided to imagine a perfect situation in which they feel little or no stress.

Whilst there is no clear evidence as to which approach is most effective or whether personality type might affect the choice of procedure (Crist & Rickard 1993), the best technique for specific patients may be that which targets their main manifestations of stress (Lehrer et al 1994). In any event, the therapist needs to be flexible when choosing the relaxation technique and must be prepared to change the approach if success is not being achieved.

Contract-hold-relax or contrast method (Gardiner 1981, Ricketts & Cross 1985, Hollis 1988)

Fox (1996) cites work undertaken by Sherrington in the early part of the twentieth century which suggested that a maximal relaxation follows a maximal muscle contraction. This mechanism is mediated through the golgi tendon organ. When a muscle contracts hard, considerable tension is placed on the golgi tendon organs in that muscle and this stimulates the inverse stretch reflex. Impulses from the golgi tendon organs in the contracting muscle pass to the spinal cord and synapse through to alpha motor neurones which transmit the impulses to the same muscle. These are inhibitory impulses and, if the original contraction was strong enough, will result in inhibition of contraction and therefore relaxation (Fox 1996). It is possible that this reflex is utilised in some relaxation techniques.

The contract-hold-relax relaxation technique requires the patient to undertake, in sequence, strong isometric contractions of all major muscle groups and in particular those which are manifesting abnormal tone. The contraction is held and it is then followed by a period of relaxation which should be at least as long as the contraction. The patient should be asked to concentrate on the feeling of relaxation in order to learn to reproduce it. It is usual to work distal to proximal and to begin with one limb and teach contraction of each individual muscle group. When each major muscle group in a limb has been taken through this process, a total limb isometric contraction is undertaken before the process is repeated on the next limb. This process is repeated for all four limbs and the trunk and face. Interspersed at regular intervals through the session should be relaxed diaphragmatic breathing with the emphasis on the expiratory phase.

Commands:

- Tighten (a muscle) — hold — let go
- Breathe deeply in — hold — let the air sigh out of your mouth.

The speed of progression through this technique depends on the patient. It may be necessary to repeat each of the stages many times before relaxation is obtained and it may take many weeks before the whole body is involved.

The physiological or Mitchell's technique (Gardiner 1981, Hollis 1988, Mitchell 1990)

The patient is required to contract the muscles antagonistic to those in tension. This moves the nearby joints out of the position of tension and simultaneously induces reciprocal relaxation in the previously tense muscle groups. After each contraction the patient should be made to concentrate on the feeling of the new, relaxed position.

It is thought that this technique utilises the mechanism of reciprocal innervation. As a muscle contracts, impulses from the muscle spindle will pass via the spinal cord to the antagonistic muscle group causing inhibition (Kandel et al 1991). For example, if the trapezius muscle is exhibiting abnormal tone, the patient will be encouraged to contract the shoulder girdle depressor muscles to cause reciprocal inhibition of trapezius.

It is usual to work proximal to distal and to start with the upper limbs followed by the lower limbs, trunk and finally the head. Relaxed diaphragmatic breathing exercises are interspersed throughout the programme. As with the previous technique, groups of muscles are worked individually after which these movements are summated before moving on to the next limb. The starting position is not important as it will change as the patient relaxes.

Commands:

- Move in a given direction — stop — let go
- Feel the new position
- Breathe deeply in — hold — let the air sigh out of your mouth.

Visualisation or the suggestion method (Hollis 1988)

The aim of this method is to encourage the patient not to think of things that worry them but to concentrate on something that is non-threatening and pleasurable. It is a form of auto hypnosis and rather similar to techniques used in certain types of mediation. Whereas the previous two techniques concentrated on reducing muscle tone with the presumption that mental relaxation would follow, this technique tries to reduce the mental activity and replace worrying thoughts with something pleasant. If the technique works, then a reduction in muscle tone should follow automatically. Ricketts and Cross (1985) suggest that this method is most successful with individuals who may be able to relax physically but find it difficult to stop thinking.

The room must be quiet and warm and the patient comfortable and well supported. It may help to cover them with a blanket. In hypnotic tones the physiotherapist guides the patient to think about pleasurable, non-threatening experiences or objects. Patients are encouraged to absorb themselves in what is being said, fully concentrating on the word picture being painted by the physiotherapist. The physiotherapist should persuade the patient to think about repetitive movements or sounds such as waves gently lapping on the shore or the gentle rustle of a breeze in the trees. The physiotherapist should speak slowly and in low tones. No harsh sounding words should be used and long vowel sounds should be drawn out.

Interspersed in this technique can be the suggestion that the patient's limbs feel heavy or that they feel to be gently floating. As before, this technique is improved by the inclusion of deep, relaxed breathing exercises.

Before starting this technique it is important to explore the types of experiences that have given the patient pleasure or the nature of the object on which they wish to focus. In this way the technique will be appropriate and meaningful. Individuals who find this technique particularly helpful can learn to trigger relaxation when alone by thinking about their chosen subject. It is also helpful to concentrate on repetitive sounds or actions such as breathing.

Sedative massage (Madders 1988)

Slow, rhythmical stroking, effleurage and kneading can be very relaxing and are a valuable way of introducing the patient to the concept of relaxation. It is essential that the physiotherapist's hands are relaxed and remain so throughout the treatment. The strokes should initially be light but the depth can be increased as the patient adapts to the feel of the massage. For some people being asked to undress or being touched can be stressful and where this is the case it is possible to allow the patient to remain clothed. Once patients are suitably positioned for the massage a large blanket is tucked firmly round them and stroking is applied through the material. As the aim of all relaxation therapies is to enable patients to take control over their own body, massage should only be seen as an interim step; as soon as possible the patient should be introduced to more active methods.

EMG biofeedback (Basmajian & Wolf 1990, Elton 1993)

This method has been shown to be most successful when used in conjunction with other approaches (Elton 1993). Biofeedback gives specific information about the state of tension in individual muscle groups, enabling patients to take control of the reduction of tone in their muscles with confidence. There is instant feedback of success and the impartiality of the machine's response is often seen as reassuring.

The electrodes are attached over muscle groups which are known to be in tension and the patient is placed in a variety of starting positions and encouraged to reduce the electrical activity in the muscles. Once sufficient self-awareness has been developed, the patient is able to reduce inappropriate muscle tone without the help of the machine. Nigl and Fischer-Williams (1980) reported several cases of low back pain associated with abnormal muscle activity which were greatly improved by using EMG to teach specific muscle relaxation. Where there is a generalised response to stress, the electrodes are often placed over the frontalis muscle and patients can be taught to control their stress using input from this muscle.

Low frequency breathing exercises
(Madders 1988, Leuner 1991)

Low frequency diaphragmatic breathing exercises induce relaxation and can be used alone or in conjunction with other techniques. In order to breathe diaphragmatically, the abdominal muscles must relax to let the diaphragm descend. In the expiratory phase a sighing action is encouraged so that the air is expired through elastic recoil of soft tissue whilst the respiratory muscles and muscles of the throat and mouth relax. The frequency of respiration should be low in order to avoid hyperventilation. As the patient is resting whilst being asked to undertake deep breathing, it is necessary to reduce the respiratory rate to less than the normal resting rate in order not to disrupt the normal blood chemistry. Eight or ten breaths a minute is often successful and pauses may be incorporated at the end of both the inspiratory and the expiratory phases. This technique results in a reduction in muscle tone as well as a reduction in blood pressure, heart rate and electrical activity in the brain

---

Case Study 14.2

Mrs V was an asthmatic patient with serious social problems. Her husband was in prison and she was trying to bring up three teenaged children in a small flat on the thirteenth floor of an ageing tower block. She was unable to work and had to cope on a very limited income. She was deeply concerned that her children should not follow the example of her husband and turn to crime, but she found it very hard to exert control over them. A major problem was that the lift in the block of flats was frequently out of action and her asthma made it impossible for her to tackle the stairs. Consequently, she felt a prisoner in her home and her children were aware that she had no control over them once they were out of the flat. She was experiencing frequent, serious asthma attacks which were resulting in repeated periods of hospitalisation. It was decided to try low frequency breathing exercises and general relaxation with this patient and the results were quite dramatic. The incidence of asthma attacks serious enough to warrant hospitalisation dropped to approximately one per year and with the improvement in her health she felt slightly more able to cope with her life in general.

(Leuner 1991). The mental relaxation which most patients feel from this method results from both the physiological changes and the concentration needed to maintain a low frequency respiratory pattern. This is a repetitive, non-stressful activity which leads to mental relaxation in much the same way as some meditative techniques.

Pendular exercises (Hollis 1988)

Relaxed swinging of a limb is a repetitive rhythmical movement which probably causes relaxation through two mechanisms. Firstly, it raises the threshold of transmission of impulses from sensory receptors in the moving joint and surrounding soft tissues, leading to a reciprocal inhibition of the afferent impulses from the same spinal segment and a reduction in local muscle tone. Secondly, the repetitive nature of the movement tends to reduce mental tension. Any starting position which allows a limb to swing with a minimal amount of muscular effort can be used. Pendular exercises in suspension are particularly effective, but whatever position is chosen, the exercise should start with small range movements and never move beyond what is comfortable.

Rhythmical passive movements

These are similar to pendular exercises in that the limb is subjected to gentle repetitive movements until the threshold of sensory receptors is raised. In this technique the patient should attempt to relax whilst the physiotherapist moves the limb. It is important to undertake this technique with constant velocity and range of movement of the joints as any variation in these factors will disrupt the rhythmicity of the procedure.

Physical activity

Several authors have shown that physical activity reduces stress levels and a thorough review of the current state of knowledge has been presented by Paluska and Schwenk (2000). It has also been shown that when a relatively high level of physical fitness is developed, the responses to acute stress are improved (Wilfley & Kunce 1986, Roth & Holmes 1987, Brandon & Loftin 1991). It does not appear that the form of the physical activity is crucial to the technique and swimming, running, ball sports and fast walking have all been shown to be successful. There is no evidence as to whether aerobic exercise or anaerobic exercise is the most effective. Exactly how physical activity can have a beneficial effect on anxiety is not known as there are a number of hypotheses, none of which have been satisfactorily proved. It is possible that exercise may provide a distraction from the sources of stress or, on the other hand, it may improve the individual's feelings of self-efficacy so that confidence increases and feelings of anxiety decrease. Many physical activities can be quite challenging, both in the physical demands they make and also in the level of skill required to perform the activity well. If stress has arisen through feelings of lack of confidence, then success in a non-threatening physical activity may help to restore the patient's feelings of self worth and control. There is also conflicting evidence about the possible physiological benefits of exercise on tension. A well popularised theory is that exercise increases the production of endorphins and that these endorphins can induce feelings of mild euphoria which will lead to a positively altered mood state. It has also been suggested that exercise improves brain synaptic transmission which, it is hypothesised, can be impaired in stress situations (Paluska & Schwenk 2000).

Despite the conflicting and often poor quality evidence to support exercise as a means of relaxation, the balance of research indicates that exercise will have a positive effect. A note of caution has to be sounded as there is also evidence that physical activity is only effective if undertaken in moderation and that if it is taken to extreme levels then the activity in itself will induce stress. The individual who becomes fixated on the need to exercise and who pushes his or her body to the limit will have gone beyond the beneficial effects of exercise and will have reintroduced stress with all its unwanted side effects.

Although it is possible to teach relaxation, the causes leading to excessive tension should not be ignored and the patient should be encouraged to seek solutions for the original cause of stress. This is likely to involve other members of the health care team or the social or welfare services. While the original cause of stress continues, the ability to move with an economy of effort and therefore less fatigue will be reduced.

REFERENCES

Astrand P O, Rodahl K 1987 Textbook of work physiology, 3rd edn. McGraw-Hill, New York

Baker G H 1987 Psychological factors and immunity. Journal of Psychosomatic Research 31: 1–10

Basmajian J V, Wolf S L 1990 Therapeutic exercise, 5th edn. Williams and Wilkins, Baltimore

Brandon J E, Loftin M J 1991 The role of fitness in mediating stress: a correlational exploration of stress reactivity. Perceptual and Motor Skills 73: 1171–1180

Carlson C R, Collins F L, Nitz A J, Sturges E T, Rogers J L 1996 Muscle stretching as an alternative relaxation training procedure. Journal of Behaviour Therapy & Experimental Psychiatry 21(1): 29–38

Crist D A, Rickard H C 1993 A fair comparison of progressive and imaginal relaxation. Perceptual and Motor Skills 76: 691–700

Durham R C, Allan T 1993 Psychological treatment of generalised anxiety disorder: a review of the clinical significance of results in outcome studies since 1980. British Journal of Psychiatry 163: 19–26

Elton D 1993 Combined use of hyposis and EMG biofeedback in the treatment of stress-induced conditions. Stress Medicine 9: 25–35

Everett T, Dennis M, Rickett E 1995 Physiotherapy in mental health; a practical approach. Butterworth-Heinemann, Oxford

Fox S I 1996 Human physiology, 5th edn. W C Brown, Boston

Gardiner M D 1981 The principles of exercise therapy, 4th edn. Bell & Hyman, London

Hollis M 1988 Practical exercise therapy, 3rd edn. Blackwell Scientific Publications, Oxford

Jacobsen E 1929 Progressive relaxation. University of Chicago Press, Chicago

Kandel E R, Schwartz J H, Jessell T M 1991 Principles of neural science, 3rd edn. Elsevier Science Publishing, New York

Lehrer P, Carr R, Sargunaraj D, Woolfolk R L 1994 Stress management techniques: are they all equivalent, or do they have specific effects? Biofeedback and Self Regulation 19: 353–401

Leuner H 1991 Ein neuer weg sur tiefenentspannung: das respiratorisch feedback. Kranken Gymnastik 43: 246–253

Madders J 1988 Stress and relaxation. Macdonald & Co, London

Mitchell L 1990 Simple relaxation: the physiological method for relieving tension. John Murray, London

Moffett D F, Moffett S B, Schauf C L 1993 Human physiology and foundation frontiers. Mosby Year Book, St Louis

Nigl A J, Fischer-Williams W 1980 Treatment of low back strain with electromyographic biofeedback and relaxation training. Psychosomatics 21: 495–499

Paluska A A, Schwenk T L 2000 Physical activity and mental health, current concepts. Sports Medicine 29(3): 167–180

Ricketts E, Cross E 1985 The Whitchurch method of stress management by relaxation exercises. Physiotherapy 71: 262–264

Roth D L, Holmes D S 1987 Influence of aerobic exercise training and relaxation training on physical and psychological health following stressful life events. Psychosomatic Medicine 49: 357–365

Selye H 1984 The stress of life. McGraw-Hill, New York

Wilfley D, Kunce J 1986 Differential physical and psychological effects of exercise. Journal of Counselling Psychology 33: 337–342

CHAPTER CONTENTS

Introduction   253

The fetus and neonate   254
Reflex activity   255

Developing mature movement patterns   256
The development of hand control   256
The development of walking ability   256

Adolescence onwards   256

The transition into old age   257

Physiological changes associated with
ageing   259
Cardiovascular changes   259
Respiratory system changes   259
Muscle changes   260
Neurological changes   261
Skeletal changes   261
Postural changes with age   262
Gait changes with age   263

Improving movement and function in older
people   264
The fear of falling   267

15

Human movement through the life span

M. Trew

OBJECTIVES

When you have completed this chapter you should:

1. **Understand how human movement changes from birth to extreme old age**

2. **Be aware of the importance of reflexes in developing controlled movement capabilities**

3. **Have a basic knowledge of the stages involved in developing hand control and walking**

4. **Understand why physical ability may deteriorate with increasing years**

5. **Understand the basic physiological changes that can occur with age**

6. **Recognise age induced changes in posture and gait**

7. **Understand the importance of recognising that some age changes are reversible**

8. **Understand the concept of the threshold of ability.**

INTRODUCTION

This chapter is about the changes that occur in human movement throughout the life span. Whilst it is appropriate to consider people as individuals, most of us follow a common pattern as we develop movement abilities in childhood, and again follow an equally common pattern as we age. Newborn children are helpless and totally dependent on others until they have developed the basic skills and quality of movement needed to cope with normal life. There is rapid acquisition of motor skills in the first few years of life, after which the developmental process slows down. During late teens and until late middle age there is a period of stability where changes in human movement ability are not specifically noticeable and then from the sixth decade onwards there is measurable change which, sadly, is towards a decline in ability. The age at which different motor skills are acquired in childhood is remarkably similar between children, most children developing the same skills within one or two months of each other. At the other end of the life span, the onset of deterioration of certain skills and abilities varies greatly between individuals, mostly because loss of ability is dependent on variables such as lifestyle, disease, trauma and personality. The similarity in the developmental sequence in children has made it possible to identify milestones of achievement and to provide guides to the approximate age at which these milestones are likely to occur. Delay or failure in achieving a number of these milestones may be indicative of abnormality but such information must be treated with great caution as there are many examples of children who followed an atypical development sequence and went on to be exceptional achievers as adults.

Task 15.1

If you know someone with a baby, ask if you may go and observe. When the baby is awake and moving, compare what you see with the suggested milestones given in the first three tables in this chapter. If you don't know anyone with a baby, ask your parents or someone you know who has had a child if they can remember when the major milestones occurred. Most parents will remember when their baby first stood and walked. Compare what you find out with the suggested average milestones in the tables.

THE FETUS AND NEONATE

In the uterus the fetus starts to make jerky movements from the age of about 3 months when it is approximately 3 cm long. The tiny size of the fetus and the fact that these movements mainly involve the mouth and fingers mean that the mother is not aware of the activity. By the start of the fifth month the fetus is about 20–26 cm long and fully formed, it moves frequently and it is at this time that the mother becomes aware of what is happening. Movements become less jerky as the months pass but at this stage they are not apparently purposeful and are probably stimulated by reflex activity. The increase in fetal activity does not continue in a linear manner and at about the sixth month there is a quiescent period when not much movement occurs. Why this should be is not clear; however, it is known that at this time the higher centres in the brain are developing and as they are responsible for control of purposeful movement, the quiet period may represent a transition between primitive and more purposeful activity. In the eighth and ninth months of pregnancy the fetus is very active. Although the space in the uterus is cramped and the fetus is becoming quite large, about 48–53 cm long, it moves frequently, turning and changing position and 'kicking' and 'punching' with its arm and legs (Cole & Cole 1993, Gallahue & Ozmun 1998).

The reasons for fetal movement are not clear. Some animal studies have led to the belief that movement in the uterus is necessary if normal development of bones, joints, muscles and the peripheral nervous system is to occur, but the evidence to support this in humans does not exist. It is clear that some fetal activity is a response to external stimuli and it has been shown that a loud noise outside the uterus will stimulate the fetus to move. It is also speculated that the increasing levels of activity are part of the preparation for life after birth. The movements in the uterus may be establishing motor pathways and developing some level of coordination in preparation for the neonatal period. They may also be having a strengthening effect on the muscles.

The full term neonate has a predominantly flexed posture, has few movement skills and is helpless when considered alongside most other newborn animals. In the early days of life most movements are under the influence of reflexes although infants also demonstrate some purposeful activity. At birth children can hear and see and can turn their heads to follow sounds or the shape of a face, but many of the other movements they make at this stage are clearly the result of primitive reflexes (Illingworth 1990).

Reflex activity

A reflex can be defined as a prompt, stereotyped reaction to a stimulus and in the early days of life most of the movements made by children are reflex responses to stimulus. The reflexes can be divided into categories: some of them are protective; some are for survival; but others appear to have the role of establishing the movement patterns needed in later months. Thus the rooting reflex is an example of a survival reflex as it helps the infant find the nipple and nourishment, whereas the blink and cough reflexes have obvious protective functions. The walking reflex is thought to play a part in establishing the patterns needed for true walking (Gallahue & Ozmun 1998).

Table 15.1 lists some of the primitive reflexes which are commonly seen or which may have value in the development of mature human movement patterns. Many of these reflexes are present at birth and then fade after a few months: for example the grasp reflex usually disappears at about 4 months. It has been speculated that the ability to grasp strongly may be protective as it enables the infant to grasp an adult's hair or clothes when being carried or picked up. The grasp reflex is so strong that children have been seen to hold their whole body weight with one hand. It is important that this reflex does not persist beyond a few months as it would be undesirable to grip everything that touched the palm of the hand. Other reflexes, such as the labyrinthine righting reflex, appear later; in this case at about 2 months after birth. This reflex causes the infant to position the head with the vertex uppermost and the plane of the face vertical. Thus, when the infant is placed in prone or supine the reflex will cause the head to lift and this is the foundation stage in developing the movement patterns to sit upright, stand or walk.

During the normal developmental process most of the primitive reflexes seen in the young child are suppressed or modified as movement maturity develops (Gallahue & Ozmun 1998).

Table 15.1 Some primitive and developmental reflexes seen in the first year of life (After Illingworth 1990, Bee 1999)

Reflex	Stimulus	Response
Rooting	Light touch on the cheek or corner of lip	Head turns to stimulus, tongue moves towards stimulus
Grasp	Pressure on the ulnar side of the palm	Strong finger flexion to make a grip
Moro	Either a sudden noise or allowing the baby's head to drop slightly when held in supine	Abduction and elevation of the upper limbs with abduction and some extension of the fingers. This is followed by a flexion pattern of upper limb movement
Placing	Touch on the anterior tibia or dorsum of the foot	Flexion of the hips, knees and dorsiflexion, as if to move the limb so the foot can be placed on the object it touched
Walking	When held upright – pressure on the soles of the feet	Reciprocal flexion and extension of the lower limbs in a pseudo-walking pattern
Leg extension	Pressure on the sole of the foot	Extension of the trunk, hips and knees
Asymmetrical tonic neck	Rotation of the head to one side	Ipsilateral shoulder abduction and elbow extension. Response is often mild and may only show as an increase in muscle tone
Symmetrical tonic neck	a) Flexion of the neck	An increase in flexor tone in the trunk, upper and lower limbs which may result in movement
	b) Extension of the neck	An increase in extensor tone in the trunk, upper and lower limbs which may result in movement
Righting reflexes (labyrinthine, neck and body)	Rotation of the head in relation to the trunk	Repositioning of the head or trunk either to maintain the correct relationship of the head with the trunk or to position the head correctly in relation to gravity

However, these reflexes are never totally lost and may be seen again under conditions of stress or following brain damage.

DEVELOPING MATURE MOVEMENT PATTERNS

The amount of physical, cognitive and social development that occurs in the first two years of life is phenomenal. As part of the process of physical development, the infant has to learn to overcome most of the dominant primitive reflexes and to gain voluntary control of movement. Whilst it is necessary to retain those reflexes that enable the child to maintain posture and to cope with the effects of gravity and disturbance of balance, there must also be ability to override some of the primitive reflexes. If this does not happen, movement cannot become individualised and specialised and cannot adapt to a variety of different situations. There are many excellent textbooks that deal in detail with all aspects of the development of the infant and child and it is beyond the remit of this chapter to consider how all the body systems mature. In this book examples have been used of how the infant develops hand control, learns to move purposefully, sits, stands and walks, in order to convey a flavour of the early age-related changes in human movement.

The development of hand control

For the human being the ability to use the hand is very important. Approximately six months before birth the fetus is able to move its fingers and a month later can open and close its hand, but by the time the child is born little further progression in hand ability has been achieved and the hand is relatively useless (Rosenbaum 1991). At this stage the grasp reflex predominates and for most of the time the hand is held closed. It takes approximately six years for good hand control to be developed and children continue to learn new skills and to develop greater speed and precision in increasingly complex hand activities throughout their school days. Table 15.2 shows the main milestones of the development of hand control.

The development of walking ability

In order to be able to walk the infant first needs to achieve a number of related physical milestones. These start with the development of trunk and head control; it would be difficult to walk if it were not possible to maintain a stable relationship between the trunk and the head or between the trunk and the lower limbs. Secondly, the child normally has to be able to crawl before walking can occur; though there are some children who never crawl but shuffle on their bottoms before they stand and walk. Children then have to be able to get into standing and balance unaided before they can finally and successfully walk. The achievement of walking occurs around one year after birth though at this stage it is not performed in a skilful manner. It takes several more years before walking and running can be seen to be developing fluency and precision. Table 15.3 shows the major milestones leading to the ability to walk well.

ADOLESCENCE ONWARDS

By adolescence motor ability is very well developed, to the extent that 'children' in their teens are able to compete, and win in international sporting events such as gymnastics. Improvement in motor ability continues to be seen and as children move through adolescence to adulthood they show improvements in their balance, strength and speed (Gallahue & Ozmun 1998). Skill in performing complex, precision tasks such as playing a violin also continues into adult life, providing sufficient practice is undertaken. However, for many young adults, their performance in motor skills levels off fairly quickly, and then starts a gradual decline into middle age and a more rapid decline in the sixth or seventh decade.

THE TRANSITION INTO OLD AGE

The loss of the ability to move easily and freely can start to become a problem at any time from middle age onwards, but is most commonly associated with old age. The onset is often insidious and it is sometimes difficult to decide whether a reduction in movement ability is

Table 15.2 Milestones in the development of manipulative skills (After Illingworth 1990, Holt 1991, Rosenbaum 1991, Brierley 1993, Bee 1999)

Age	Skill acquisition
Birth	Grasp reflex dominant. Hands mostly held closed
3 months	The grasp reflex is almost gone and the hands are usually held open. Can hold an object between both hands. May try to hit objects
4 months	Reaches for objects. Plays with objects held in both hands. Grasps at many things but has no precision or eye/hand coordination
5 months	Can grasp objects voluntarily in one or both hands, but the object is held on the ulnar side of the hand in a crude grip and the thumb is not involved. Starts to show the ability to estimate where to position the hand in order to intercept a moving object
7–9 months	Passes object from one hand to the other and holds the object on the radial side of the hand. Towards the end of this period may demonstrate the beginnings of a precision grip. May be able to hold and eat a biscuit. Points. Voluntarily lets go and can place objects in containers
9–12 months	Is able to grip between the pads of the fingers and thumb but the grip is not strong and can not be sustained. Holds a spoon in a primitive grip. Has limited precision but can hold objects as small as a pea. Waves
15 months	Has the precision to place one cube on top of another and can, rather clumsily, drink from a cup. Can remove shoes
18 months	Eye/hand coordination improving but can't turn over individual pages of a book. Can scribble with a pencil and may be able to imitate simple shapes. Can build a cube tower of three cubes. Removes gloves or socks and unzips clothes. Handedness becomes apparent
2 years	Can put on shoes and socks. Can unscrew a lid. Starts to use scissors. Has the precision to draw a circle. Copies activities of parents and other children
$2\frac{1}{2}$ years	Can build a tower of 8 cubes. Has more precision in using a pencil and can draw horizontal and vertical lines
3 years	Can undertake most dressing tasks except buttons and laces. Can draw a man. Can catch a large ball between arms and body
4 years	Can manage buttons. Can draw a square
5 years	Can tie shoelaces. Drawings are neater, more controlled
6 years	Can draw a diamond. Is able to undertake hand activities quickly. Has a fairly mature throwing and catching pattern. Can manipulate a needle and thread
7 years and beyond	All the basic motor skills for the upper limb have been developed and from now on, the child and adult learns new and more complex skills or develops greater precision in existing skills

---

Task 15.2

Before reading the next section of this chapter, make a list to describe what you think an elderly person in their eighth or ninth decade would be like. Use the headings of 'appearance', 'functional abilities', 'physical abilities' and 'mental capacities' to help you. Make a second list using the same headings but now applying the criteria to someone in their 30s.

Compare your thoughts with other students to see if you are in agreement and then keep a note of the results of this task. When you have reached the end of this chapter, return to this task and see if you have altered your opinions in any way.

---

caused by age induced changes and disease, or whether it is a consequence of an increasingly sedentary lifestyle.

There are many reasons why older people are usually less active than their younger counterparts. Elderly people tend to avoid or have no need to undertake activities that require strength, speed or extreme ranges of joint movement. Older women, in particular, spend increasing periods of time in sedentary pursuits that make no major physical demands and they are therefore vulnerable to the adverse effects of disuse atrophy (Fiatarone 1990). Added to this, cultural expectations tend to constrain physical activity in the later years of life. In a number of cultures there is an expectation that life should slow down with the passage of years and that old people deserve to take life easy. Where these social expectations exist it is almost inevitable

Table 15.3 Milestones in the development of sitting, standing and walking (After Illingworth 1990, Holt 1991, Brierley 1993, Bee 1999)

Age	Skill acquisition
Birth	No head control, hips and knees flexed in lying, unable to extend spine at all. Walking reflex present in supported standing
3 months	Head control developing, able to raise head against gravity. In prone lying can take weight on forearms. When supported in sitting, is able to keep head up, though not able to hold it still. Rapidly developing control of the head on trunk movement. Walking reflex has disappeared and the baby is unable to bear weight when held in standing
5 months	Head no longer wobbles when held in sitting and control of the head position in relationship to the moving trunk is quite good. Is able to hold the spine in extension when placed in sitting or supported standing. Can bear weight in standing, when supported by an adult
7–9 months	In prone, can take weight on one or both hands. Can sit supported in a chair and briefly sit unsupported. Can roll from supine to prone and prone to supine. Has sufficient trunk control to hold the spine straight when reaching for objects. Develops ability to pull into standing. When held in standing, likes to bounce
9–12 months	Now crawling, initially by pulling body forwards with arms. Has sufficient trunk control to sit unaided without losing balance. Able to stand holding on to furniture, progresses to lifting one leg and then walking whilst holding on. Is not able to sit down with any control
12 months	Crawling has developed so that weight is borne on feet rather than knees. When sitting, can rotate trunk or head to look round. Walks holding the hand of an adult
13 months	Walks unaided, but with a wide base and has little control
15 months	Climbs stairs on hands and knees. Walking improving but unable to stop or turn with control
18 months	Can carry object whilst walking. May be able to run. Can get on to a chair. Ascends and descends stairs providing there is a handrail. Jumps from both feet
2 years	Can walk backwards. Is able to run and kick with limited control. Can manage stairs unaided but places both feet on each step
$2\frac{1}{2}$ years	May be able to walk on tiptoes
3 years	Can balance briefly on one leg. Goes up stairs normally but finds stair descent difficult. Can jump off a low step
4 years	Goes down stairs normally
5 years	Can skip normally
6 years and beyond	Development now takes the form of increases in speed and strength and the ability to combine movements in complex patterns. By 8 years should be able to ride a bicycle

that many older people's lifestyles will become increasingly sedentary and the development of disuse atrophy will eventually contribute to physical deterioration. Not only will a sedentary lifestyle result in a gradual decline in physiological function, but it can also have an adverse effect on psychological function. The combination of a sedentary lifestyle with those physical changes that are an inevitable consequence of ageing will eventually result in a reduced ability to perform even the most basic physical and cognitive tasks associated with activities of daily living. These circumstances lead inexorably to a reduction in quality of life and a substantial dependence on carers.

Although the general population usually accepts a slower pace of life and a loss of ability with the passage of years, the changes caused by inactivity are both preventable and reversible (Raab et al 1988, Fiatarone 1990). Good health education and health promotion schemes that explain the importance of maintaining a reasonably active lifestyle in the middle and later years are clearly important. Elderly individuals who exercise regularly are less likely to suffer from movement problems and those who take up exercise late in life benefit from an improvement in function in a number of body systems (Aniansson et al 1984, Meusel 1984, Grimby 1988, McArdle et al 1996, Pereira et al 1998, Cress et al 1999). Being old chronologically is not necessarily the same as being old physically. A seventy-year-old with good health, the right temperament and social opportunities can demonstrate better motor skills and abilities than a sedentary 30-year-old. However, a reduction in movement capability and the ability to perform functional activities will have a catastrophic effect on the quality of life. It is therefore essential not to lose sight of the fact that a number of physical changes associated with growing old can be prevented, slowed down or even reversed. The remainder of this chapter considers how ageing can have a direct effect on movement and the ability to undertake everyday activities. Age-induced changes in posture and gait are used as examples, and the final part of this chapter explores how exercise can benefit older people who wish to remain fully active and self sufficient.

PHYSIOLOGICAL CHANGES ASSOCIATED WITH AGEING

Human movement in elderly people can be compromised in three main ways:

1. Through structural changes which are a direct result of the ageing process. This might include changes in the structure of the eye leading to deteriorating vision; or the loss of muscle fibres leading to reduced strength and endurance.

2. Changes related to the effects of disease or trauma which may or may not be associated with growing old. In this category can be found disease such as osteoarthritis or osteoporosis. The most common trauma associated with the ageing process is a fractured neck of femur following a fall.

3. As a consequence of the effects of inactivity.

Cardiovascular changes

The function of the cardiovascular system is significantly reduced in older people and this has a negative effect on both the intensity and duration of physical activity. Resting heart rate changes little with age, but the maximum heart rate attainable on activity drops significantly, causing a concurrent reduction in exercise tolerance. The expected maximum heart rate for older people can be obtained by using the formula: 220 minus the age in years = maximum heart rate. This is an approximate guide that must be used with caution as actual values vary greatly between individuals.

By the age of 85, resting stroke volume is reduced by about 30% and the myocardium is noticeably hypertrophied. Also, at this age, resting cardiac output may be less than half the value it was in the third decade (Fitzgerald 1985).

These changes impair the ability of the heart to deliver blood to the tissues; oxygen uptake in the muscles is also reduced, not because of a loss of muscle oxidative enzymes but as a consequence of the actual loss of muscle fibres. It seems likely that the oxidative enzymes are little affected by age, though there may be a reduction in the resynthesis of ATP due to a reduction in phosphogens (Grimby 1986). With both a reduced delivery of blood to the muscles and a reduction in the number of muscle fibres available to utilise oxygen, there is a general reduction in movement capacity, particularly in endurance activities. A further adverse effect of ageing on the cardiovascular system is the loss of elasticity in the arterial walls. This leads to an undesirable increase in blood pressure on strenuous activity due to the arteries' inability to accommodate the increase in blood flow.

These cardiovascular changes make activity more difficult with advancing years but in themselves do not have too serious an effect on the ability to perform normal, everyday functions. However, if the natural age changes are combined with a long-term loss of fitness due to an increasingly sedentary lifestyle, then the consequences may start to become serious and essential functional activities may require so much energy that they take an unacceptable length of time to complete or become impossible.

Respiratory system changes

Increasing age may result in degenerative changes in the costovertebral and costosternal joints and may be combined with calcification of the costal cartilages. Eventually these changes will lead to a reduction in thoracic mobility in both the anteroposterior and lateral directions. Elastic recoil of the chest wall, which is necessary for expiration, becomes reduced as a consequence of generalised loss of elastic tissue and this puts major emphasis on movements of the diaphragm as a means of changing thoracic diameter and lung capacity. All these changes mean that a disproportionate amount of effort is needed for the process of respiration during strenuous activity and these age changes can eventually lead to a 20% increase in respiratory energy requirements (Fitzgerald 1985). By the age of 70, vital capacity can also have decreased by 50% yet, despite all these changes, it appears that a decrease in respiratory function is not a major factor in the limitation of exercise tolerance in elderly people, particularly if they have habitually maintained a fairly active lifestyle. The changes in the heart, the peripheral circulation and the muscles appear to be far more significant in reducing movement capabilities than age-related changes in the respiratory system.

Muscle changes

With increasing age there is a reduction in both aerobic and anaerobic capacity affecting the endurance, strength and speed attributes of muscle. As with the other body systems the most marked changes occur in extreme old age, particularly after the eighth decade (Grimby 1986, Young 1986, Fiatarone 1990). The rate of loss of strength has been extensively studied but the results are inconclusive. It appears that age-related loss of strength may be dependent on the genetic makeup of the individual but it also varies between muscles, some appearing to be more affected than others. Gender is also a factor with the menopause being responsible for a marked loss of strength in women (Grabiner & Enoka 1995).

In elderly people beyond their eighth or ninth decade the reduction in muscle bulk has occurred to such an extent that it can easily be noted on visual examination. This reduction in muscle mass is mainly a consequence of loss of muscle fibres, though there may also be a reduction in size of the Type II fibres (fast twitch), the latter probably caused by disuse atrophy. Although the visible signs of loss of muscle bulk are not always appar-

ent until old age, computer tomography shows that muscle fibres are being lost from at least the age of 30 when they start to be replaced with intramuscular fat. The fat masks visual signs of muscle fibre loss until a substantial number of fibres have disappeared (Fiatarone 1990).

Despite the significant loss of muscle fibres, there is normally sufficient spare capacity for this not to be a major constraint on function until extreme old age is reached. Once again it is the combination of age changes and disuse atrophy that is likely to be the cause of the 'weakness' exhibited by many old people.

Task 15.3

Start observing children, young adults, middle-aged and elderly people. Watch the speed with which they tackle everyday tasks and the ranges of joint movement that they employ. Are you able to note any differences between these age groups?

The lifestyles of many middle-aged and elderly individuals put little demand on the Type II fibres which are responsible for power and speed activities and this inevitably leads to disuse atrophy. Fitness training programmes for middle-aged and older people also tend to concentrate on activities which will not stimulate Type II muscle fibre activity. Rapid muscle contractions, in particular, are rarely included in therapeutic or recreational activity sessions.

Interestingly, the pattern of atrophy of Type II fibres is not constant throughout all regions of the body. The quadriceps appear to be more subject to atrophy than muscle groups in the upper limb, though this may be a reflection of a reduction in lower limb activities rather than an age-induced change in muscle structure (Grimby 1988). It is hypothesised that the muscles of the upper limb remain in constant use, even when the individual has lost the ability to walk, and are often used in fairly rapid movements. This continued use probably contributes to the retention of a greater proportion of Type II fibres in upper limb muscle groups when compared with lower limb muscles.

Most authorities feel that the decrease in muscle function and muscle mass is mainly due to the loss of muscle fibres and a reduction in oxygen delivery. Whilst there may be a reduction in the enzymic capacity of muscle, this is not a necessary consequence of old age and therefore can be slowed down by the use of exercise (Fitzgerald 1985, Grimby 1986, McArdle et al 1996). An individual muscle fibre in an elderly person is structurally and functionally similar to one in a young person and will therefore respond to physical demands and training in the same way. It is the reduction in number of fibres and the reduced delivery of oxygen which reduces the overall power and endurance capacity of the muscle, not age changes affecting the structure of the muscle fibre itself (Young 1986).

Neurological changes

The neurological system is not protected against age-induced changes although in the absence of disease or trauma it can, in some individuals, continue to function remarkably well into extreme old age. Commonly, ageing can cause a reduction in the effectiveness of the neurotransmitters, a change in nerve cells, especially in the number and effectiveness of synaptic connections, and a reduction in the number of nerve cells (Pickles et al 1995). Reaction times are significantly increased with age, probably due to the reduction in nerve conduction velocity which can be altered by up to 15% (Fitzgerald 1985). The number of motor units decreases so that activation of muscle becomes more difficult. There will eventually be a reduction in sensory capacity as the number of sensory nerve endings declines and thresholds for transmission of sensory information increase. All these factors may lead to the control and quality of performance of human movement being reduced (Fitzgerald 1985, Grimby 1986).

Skeletal changes

With increasing age there is often a significant loss of bone mass, particularly in elderly women, which may be due to the ageing process or caused by disease. The situation can be exacerbated by lack of exercise, a reduction in dietary calcium, poor diet and also genetic factors (Pickles et al

1995). This osteoporosis and the increased incidence of falls in older people make them particularly vulnerable to fractures. Skeletal changes usually manifest in alterations in posture, particularly in the development of thoracic kyphosis, which is very common in older people. Skeletal changes in the hands and feet are also noticeable in most elderly people and may eventually lead to a reduction in functional ability.

Reduced range or quality of movement in joints is a common problem associated with age. In older people connective tissue and muscle become less elastic, altering the quality of joint movement. Individuals who adopt a sedentary lifestyle are vulnerable to soft tissue contractures. Any loss of range of movement in the major joints will inevitably reduce the ability to move normally and undertake functional activities with the same efficiency as a younger person. Arthritis starts to develop from an early age and after the sixth decade it is a common cause of movement problems. Research indicates that there is a gender effect on the incidence of musculoskeletal disorders, with women being more likely to have joint problems than men (Arber & Ginn 1994). This, coupled with the fact that in most countries women live longer than men, inevitably leads to musculoskeletal problems being a significant factor in reducing movement capabilities in older people. Joint disease, combined with a reduction in function of other body systems, greatly reduces the functional ability of older people and has an adverse effect on their quality of life. Providing there are no serious degenerative changes, appropriate exercise can increase the range of movement and a small improvement in joint range may cause a disproportionately large functional improvement (Fitzgerald 1985).

Task 15.4

Look through your grandparents' photograph album. Can you identify the physical changes that are occurring through their life? Can you suggest the reasons for these changes?

Ask your grandparents about the lifestyle they were leading when the photographs were taken and evaluate whether their answers support the theories of ageing discussed in this chapter.

Postural changes with age

With increasing years most elderly people show some common deviations from normal posture. These deviations occur at different times for different people but are most usual in the eighth and ninth decades. Static standing posture shows typical changes that probably originate in the spine.

These cause an alteration in the resting position of the centre of gravity leading to other body segments readjusting to compensate (Fig. 15.1). In many elderly people there is an increase in the thoracic kyphosis and either a flattening of the lumbar curve with posterior pelvic tilt or a compensatory increase in lumbar lordosis. Many older people, when standing, adopt a posture of hip and knee joint flexion and ankle joint dorsiflexion. This is in contrast to the more extended joint positions seen in younger adults. With the thoracic spine in a position of kyphosis, the upper limbs will no longer rest by the sides but hang in front of the body when the individual is relaxed. This displaces the centre of gravity even further anteriorly and can stretch the individual's balance ability to the limit. To compensate, the older person may extend both shoulder joints in order to position the upper limbs posteriorly

in relation to the trunk. This has the effect of favourably readjusting the centre of gravity in relation to the base of support, making the maintenance of equilibrium less of a challenge. A negative effect of holding the upper limbs posteriorly is that shoulder joint muscles have to contract to maintain this position and this inevitably increases energy expenditure and leads to sensations of fatigue. In order to reduce the energy requirements of this upper limb posture the older person may clasp fingers behind the back.

There are a number of reasons why postural changes occur in older people. In the spine it is common to find degenerative changes in the intervertebral discs, osteoporosis of the vertebrae and trunk muscle weakness. Structural changes in the discs and vertebral bodies lead to an increasingly flexed posture which weak trunk musculature and poor postural habits fail to correct. The changes in the lower limb alignment in standing may be a compensatory mechanism for the alteration in spinal posture and the alteration in position of the centre of gravity (Kauffman 1987, Pickles et al 1995). They are also likely to be associated with shortening of the soft tissues anterior to the hip joint, which makes the achievement of full hip extension impossible. If the hip cannot fully extend in standing, then

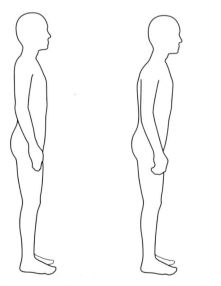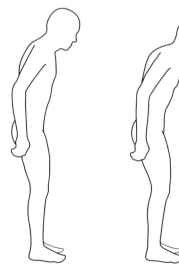

Figure 15.1 Typical postural changes associated with ageing.

compensatory repositioning of the knee and ankle joints is necessary if a relatively upright posture is to be maintained. The abnormal pattern of flexion in the lower limbs in standing may also be a reaction to the deterioration in balance ability seen in older people. By adopting a flexed posture of the hip and knee joints in standing the overall length of the lower limbs is reduced, thus lowering the centre of gravity in relation to the base and somewhat increasing stability.

Gait changes with age

It is easy to observe the differences in gait between old and young people but in line with other age changes, the age at which they occur varies between individuals. Gait in itself is highly variable, but despite this as people get older a typical pattern of gait changes can be seen. The gait pattern is not grossly different from the gait of younger people, but most aspects show modifications.

All studies investigating age-related changes in gait have reported that preferred walking velocity drops with age (Finley et al 1969, Murray et al 1969, Hageman & Blanke 1986). Walking velocity is dependent on stride length and cadence, both of which are also reduced in older people, though the main difference occurs in stride length. Murray et al (1969) found that the mean stride length of young men was 89% of their height, and that it reduced to 79% of body height in men over 80 years; a similar reduction was also found in women. Minor hip flexion contractures have been found in many elderly people and these appear to affect gait adversely by reducing the stride length and through that reducing walking velocity (Kerrigan et al 1998). The reductions in cadence are not found to be as great as in stride length and have variously been reported as reducing by only one or two steps per minute.

It is well documented that balance ability reduces as people grow older and it is therefore logical to expect increases in stride width and foot angle in order to provide a larger base of support. Murray et al (1969) found a small increase of about 2 cm in the stride width of elderly men and an increase in foot angle from an average of 8° in men under 25 years to 13° in men over 80 years. Double stance is the most stable phase of the gait cycle and in older people approximately 10% more time is spent in this phase than in younger people. The swing phase, which is a time of great vulnerability when only one foot is in contact with the ground, is reciprocally shortened. If the swing phase is reduced in time and the cadence is barely increased then it is inevitable that the stride length will be reduced. As mentioned earlier, there is usually a loss in spinal rotation and arm swing. This contributes to the reduction in walking velocity as it causes a reduction in step length and, in some cases, a reduction in the cadence.

As joint range has been shown to diminish in older people it has led some scientists to study the range of movement of dorsiflexion during gait. A reduction of 5°–10° in ankle joint excursion in older women has been identified in the early swing phase (Finley et al 1969, Hageman & Blanke 1986) and this might be a contributing factor to falls in this age group. If the older person is not able fully to dorsiflex the foot at the start of the swing phase then there is an increased risk of catching the toe on the floor and stumbling. To compensate, there is a slight increase in flexion at the hip and knee joints which shortens the swing limb during the swing phase. In the younger age range minimum toe clearance during the swing phase is about 1 cm but in men over 80 it has been shown to be 2.6 cm.

The ground reaction forces generated in the gait of older people have also been studied and a reduction in the propulsive force generated at the push off phase has been identified (Murray et al 1969, Winter et al 1990, Whittle 1991, Kerrigan et al 1998). Weakness of the plantar flexors in older people would lead to a reduction in the ability to propel the body forwards and it is likely that this would be another factor contributing to a reduction in walking velocity. The main changes in gait of older people are given in Table 15.4.

When gait changes associated with age are considered as a whole it can be seen that they are all interrelated and it is difficult to identify which

Table 15.4 Age-related changes in gait

Factor	Effect of ageing
Step length	Decreases
Stride length	Decreases
Stride width	Increases
Cadence (steps/mn)	Little change or a decrease
Single stance period	Decreases
Double stance period	Increases
Velocity	Decreases
Trunk rotation	Decreases
Anterior/posterior pelvic tilt	Decreases
Range of ankle movement	Decreases
Hip lateral rotation	Increases
Toe clearance	Decreases

factors have caused gait changes and which are responsive to gait changes. On the whole, changes in gait are probably due to: altered posture; a reduction in joint and, in particular, spinal movement; muscle weakness; and a loss in balance ability which is rooted in neurological changes (Winter et al 1990, Pickles et al 1995).

IMPROVING MOVEMENT AND FUNCTION IN OLDER PEOPLE

It is far more worthwhile that people approach old age with a good level of physical fitness and an expectation that they will continue to be physically active than that they slide into such an inactive lifestyle that they eventually need intervention from a therapist. To a certain extent an individual's expectations of old age will be based on cultural norms and financial constraints. All cultures ascribe certain roles to old people and in many cases these carry expectations of a reduction in involvement in society and a general reduction in activity levels. If changes in society's expectations are to take place, then they will have to occur from childhood onwards. There is a tendency for it to be thought unusual for an elderly person to be active and adventurous and such individuals are often labelled as 'super gran' or 'super grandad'. There needs to be a change in society so that younger people are brought up recognising that it is normal for their grandparents to be active and take a full and interested part in life. Good health education can establish and reinforce these expectations, which can then be carried throughout the life span. If expectations can be changed then there may be a greater likelihood of older people maintaining physical wellbeing and, hopefully, a concurrent good quality of life.

Financial constraints also influence lifestyle and those with low incomes are more likely to have poor diets and less access to a range of enjoyable physical activities than those who are affluent. In the major industrialised countries women are more likely to have an income near to the level of the poverty line than men and also a greater level of physical impairment (Arber & Ginn 1994). As women live longer than men these factors are clearly significant, but the solution is not easy to find and changes in society may be necessary.

For those individuals who reach old age in poor physical condition and who live a sedentary lifestyle, intervention from the health care team is likely to be necessary. The combination of inactivity and ageing has been shown to lead to poor balance, a loss of muscle mass, poor exercise tolerance and some limitation in joint movement. If the worst circumstances prevail, then by the eighth decade many sedentary people may be so frail that the limit of their physical ability is reached simply by the performance of normal activities of daily living. This leaves them with little or no physical capacity in reserve and it takes only the slightest deterioration for their level of ability to drop below the requirements of daily life. Such a drop, which can be caused by a minor illness requiring a few days bedrest, often proves catastrophic and results in loss of independence. Young (1986) describes a threshold of ability which is necessary for the performance of activities of daily living; if an individual falls below that threshold then self-care becomes impossible. Many very old people live on the border of that threshold because of the debilitating effects of age changes, disease and inactivity. For them, generating sufficient torque in their quadriceps and hip extensor muscles in order to rise from a low chair or toilet may be the equivalent of a 1 RM (repetition maximum) load, and getting dressed may well cause the heart rate to rise to its age-predicted maximum. Under these circumstances it is no wonder that frail elderly people find the simplest activities difficult and take an inordinately long time to complete even the most basic of daily tasks.

Eventually some old people reach the stage when the simple and essential activities of everyday life require maximum ability; their frailty usually results in increasing dependency on the help of others and also a greater likelihood of accidents. The quality of life for these frail old people is often poor, and their dependency places a consequent strain on their relatives and carers (Fiatarone 1990).

For their own self-respect and for the benefit of their carers, elderly people need to be able to undertake, at the very least, the basic activities of daily living. They need the physical attributes to be able to move around their living area unassisted and to attend to their eating and toileting needs.

There is evidence that even at an extreme age training can induce positive changes and a small strength gain may represent a very large improvement in the quality of life. The beneficial effects of exercise for young people are well known and it is generally accepted that older people can experience the same positive changes. Effective exercise programmes given to people in the older age range will, at the very least, maintain their existing condition, if not improve the function of all major body systems. This should include the heart, lungs, musculoskeletal, metabolic and central and peripheral nervous systems. Some authors have additionally noted that the progress of vascular disease, diabetes, hypertension, chronic obstructive airways disease, osteoporosis and arthritic conditions is retarded in subjects who undertake exercise programmes (Fitzgerald 1985, Thompson et al 1988, Fisher & Pendergast 1995).

Unfortunately, conclusive proof that exercise for old people is beneficial is lacking. Some authors have shown benefits: Aniansson et al (1984) found that training elderly people two times a week for 10 weeks using a strength training programme produced up to 13% increase in quadriceps strength and a general feeling of wellbeing. Conversely, other authors have not been able to show improvement. Thompson et al (1988) exercised a small group of elderly subjects for 16 weeks at a level which should have induced a training effect. At the end of the exercise programme, however, no significant improvement had been shown. Whether statistically significant improvement equates well with functional improvement is not known. If the subjects were near that all important threshold of ability, then a small improvement might not be statistically significant but might make a large difference in the ability to undertake activities of daily living and to the quality of life. Consensus of opinion suggests that exercise is beneficial to older people and that the very least effect that can be expected following a programme of exercise is an increased feeling of wellbeing and an enthusiasm for maintaining an adequate level of physical activity (Meusel 1984, Fitzgerald 1985, Thompson et al 1988, McArdle et al 1996, Hurley & Hagberg 1998).

Endurance exercises have been shown to increase the maximum oxygen uptake and reduce the heart rate, blood pressure and blood lactate in elderly people (Fitzgerald 1985, Hurley & Hagberg 1998). With appropriate long duration training, muscle strength and endurance can increase with the same order of magnitude as that seen in younger people on an identical training programme. Obviously no amount of exercise can replace lost muscle fibres, but for those that remain it is possible to induce hypertrophy, better recruitment of motor units and improved delivery and uptake of oxygen (Grimby 1986).

A major concern is that if frail or very old people are to see a substantial improvement in their physical capacity, they may need exercises of an intensity which they are unable to tolerate. The physiotherapist has to achieve a balance between exercise and activity which is so gentle as to be ineffective and exercise which might be effective but which will place a dangerous stress on the heart (Shephard 1984). Some studies have recently shown that providing there are no disease processes which would contraindicate exercise, resistance training is both safe, desirable

---

Task 15.5

Go to your library and obtain a journal or magazine which publishes the results of athletics meetings. Look at the results for the veterans and note their ages. These athletes don't fall into the stereotyped category of old people and are able to perform to high levels and obtain great satisfaction.

As not all people enjoy competitive sport, it is necessary to be aware of other sorts of activities which could maintain or increase levels of physical ability. Talk to a range of middle-aged and older people about what sort of activities they might find enjoyable and list the results of your discussions. Consider whether the activities you have listed are likely to have a beneficial effect.

---

and effective (Pickles et al 1995). Careful monitoring and a gradual build-up of the intensity of exercise should be sufficient to ensure the safety of the patient and there are many examples of elderly people achieving activity levels well above those of younger members of the population (McArdle et al 1996).

Ideally, as people age they should be encouraged to develop the habit of exercise so that the age changes which might reduce their ability to perform everyday activities may be avoided or delayed. Unfortunately, this does not happen in many cases and the physiotherapist may have no contact with patients until they become dependent following a long period of inactivity. Under these circumstances, motivation to exercise is often difficult but if the exercise programme is specifically planned for the individual's needs and if achievable goals are set, significant improvements may be seen. Patients should be made aware of the treatment goals and should, where possible, take an active part in their setting. They should be taught how to monitor their own progress and records should be kept so that improvements can be seen and can be used as motivators.

Exercises for very frail people who have a history of falls or who have significant lower limb problems may initially have to be non-weight bearing and chair based, but the principles of exercise are the same whether for young people, fit elderly people or people who are old and frail. The exercise programme should include exercises which will increase:

- joint range
- muscle strength
- muscle endurance
- heart and respiratory rate
- the ability to move groups of muscles and joints quickly
- coordination
- balance
- the ability to perform functional activities.

For those elderly people who are more fit, encouragement to take part in any physical activity is important: brisk walking, jogging and dancing are excellent methods of undertaking weight bearing exercise. In all three examples the participants will be using major muscle groups and joints and there will be some beneficial stress placed on their balance mechanisms and their cardiovascular and respiratory systems. Swimming utilises major muscle groups in both the upper and lower limbs, moves the joints through a wide range of movement and stresses the heart and lungs satisfactorily, but it is non-weight bearing. Non-weight bearing activity can be beneficial if the individual has joint pain but swimming does not require or stimulate balance reactions and the effects of weight bearing through the spine and long bones are lost. As such it should be seen as an adjunct and not an alternative to other weight bearing activities.

Very little research has been undertaken into the most effective duration of exercise programmes for elderly people. Presumptions must be made that the rules that apply to the design of exercise programmes for the young population will be appropriate across the age range. Exercises should be undertaken not less than two times a week. Initially, the duration of the exercises will depend on the ability of the individual who may have to start at a very low level of perhaps a few minutes per day. The exercises, whether for the power or endurance capacity of muscle, should show progression and, if possible, the level of endurance exercises should take the heart rate into the cardiac training zone (60–80% of the predicted maximum heart rate for the individual). Exercise programmes to improve the development of strength in older people should follow the same rules as for younger people and the load should aim to be between 6 and 10 RM (repetition maximum) for each individual. Providing there are no pathological reasons why an older person should not work at this level, it is essential to ensure that the principle of 'overload' is followed.

The fear of falling

In addition to those factors already considered in this chapter, it is necessary to address the effect of the fear of falling on human movement and the ability to perform functional activities. With ageing can come an increase in falling frequency and this phenomenon presents a major problem to the patients, their carers and the rehabilitation team. With every fall is the possibility of musculoskeletal damage and this may lead to the faller being placed on bedrest. For those people with an already reduced threshold of physical ability, any period of inactivity can prove very serious and may lead to dependency. Falling also leads to a loss of confidence when undertaking weight bearing activities and this in turn leads to a reduction in those activities. Currently there is no consensus on why elderly people fall, but it is

likely that it is a consequence of a number of factors, some of which are intrinsic to the individuals and some of which are related to their environment (Pickles et al 1995). A thorough assessment of the individuals and their environment may reveal potential contributing factors on which a rehabilitation programme may be built. If not, then a programme which improves lower limb joint range and muscle function, especially around the ankle joint, combined with exercises to improve postural stability, may be successful.

The future for old people, in terms of their ability to move and function normally, can be excellent. The maintenance of a reasonable level of physical activity into old age is important and, where fitness levels have dropped significantly, hope should not be given up because there is always capacity for improvement.

Task 15.6

Look again at your description and attitudes towards older people. Having read the chapter, have your opinions and expectations changed? Are your thoughts towards ageing more positive or more negative?

REFERENCES

Aniansson A, Ljungberg P, Rundgren A, Wetterqvist H 1984 Effect of a training programme for pensioners on condition and muscular strength. Archives of Gerontology and Geriatrics 3: 229–241

Arber S, Ginn J 1994 Women and aging. Reviews in Clinical Gerontology 4: 349–358

Bee H 1999 The growing child, an applied approach, 2nd edn. Longman, New York

Brierley J 1993 Growth in children. Cassell Education, London

Cole M, Cole S R 1993 The development of children, 2nd edn. Scientific American Books, New York

Cress M E, Buchner D M, Questad K A, Esselman P C, deLateur B J, Schwartz R S 1999 Exercise: effects on physical functional performance in independent older adults. Journals of Gerontology. Series A, Biological Sciences and Medical Sciences 54(5): 242–248

Fiatarone M A 1990 Exercise in the oldest old. Topics in Geriatric Rehabilitation 5(2): 63–77

Finley F R, Cody K A, Finizie R V 1969 Locomotion patterns in elderly women. Archives of Physical Medicine 50: 140–146

Fisher N M, Pendergast D R 1995 Application of quantitative and progressive exercise rehabilitation to patients with osteoarthritis of the knee. Journal of Back and Musculoskeletal Rehabilitation 5: 33–53

Fitzgerald P L 1985 Exercise for the elderly. Medical Clinics of North America 69: 189–196

Gallahue D L, Ozmun J C 1998 Understanding motor development. Infants, children, adolescents, adults, 4th edn. McGraw-Hill, Boston

Grabiner M D, Enoka R M 1995 Changes in movement capabilities with aging. In: Holloszy J O (ed) Exercise and sport sciences reviews. Williams and Wilkins, Baltimore, ch 3, p 67

Grimby G 1986 Physical activity and muscle training in the elderly. Acta Medica Scandinavica, Supplement 711: 233–237

Grimby G 1988 Physical activity and effects of muscle training in the elderly. Annals of Clinical Research 20: 62–66

Hageman P A, Blanke D J 1986 Comparison of gait of young women and elderly women. Physical Therapy 66(9): 1382–1387

Holt K S 1991 Child development. Diagnosis and assessment. Butterworth-Heinemann, Oxford

Hurley B F, Hagberg J M 1998 Optimising health in older persons: aerobic or strength training? Exercise and Sport Sciences Reviews 26: 61–89

Illingworth R S 1990 The development of the infant and young child, normal and abnormal, 9th edn. Churchill Livingstone, Edinburgh

Kauffman T 1987 Posture and age. Topics in Geriatric Rehabilitation 2: 13–28

Kerrigan D C, Todd M K, Della Croce U, Lipsitz L A, Collins J J 1998 Biomechanical gait alterations independent of speed in the healthy elderly: evidence for specific limiting impairments. Archives of Physical Medicine and Rehabilitation 79(3): 317–322

McArdle W D, Katch F I, Katch V L 1996 Exercise physiology, energy, nutrition and human performance, 4th edn. Lea & Febiger, Philadelphia

Meusel H 1984 Developing physical fitness for the elderly through sport and exercise. British Journal of Sports Medicine 18: 4–12

Murray M P, Kory R C, Clarkson B H 1969 Walking patterns in healthy old men. Journal of Gerontology 24: 169–178

Pereira M A, Kriska A M, Dat R D, Cauley J A, LaPorte R E, Kuller L H 1998 A randomised walking trial in post menopausal women. Archives of International Medicine 158: 1695–1701

Pickles B, Compton A, Cott C, Simpson J, Vandervoort A 1995 Physiotherapy with older people. W B Saunders, London

Raab D M, Agree J C, McAdam M, Smith E L 1988 Light resistance and stretching exercise in elderly women: effect upon flexibility. Archives of Physical Medicine and Rehabilitation 69: 268–272

Rosenbaum D A 1991 Human motor control. Harcourt Brace, San Diego

Shephard R J 1984 Management of exercise in the elderly. Canadian Journal of Applied Sport Science 9: 109–120

Thompson R F, Crist D M, Marsh M, Rosenthal M 1988 Effects of physical exercise for elderly patients with physical impairments. Journal of the American Geriatrics Society 36: 130–135

Whittle M 1991 Gait analysis, an introduction. Butterworth-Heinemann, Oxford

Winter D A, Patla A E, Frank J S, Walt S E 1990 Biomechanical walking pattern changes in the fit and healthy elderly. Physical Therapy 70: 340–347

Young A 1986 Exercise physiology in geriatric practice. Acta Medica Scandinavica, Supplement 711: 227–232

Index

Page numbers in **bold** refer to tables or figures.

A

A band, **10**
Abdominals (anterior abdominal wall muscles), 29, 30, 215
Abduction, **23**
Acceleration, 48–49
  angular, 49–50
  definition, 48
  in kinematic analysis, 146
  law of, 39
  swing phase of walking, 178, 182
Accessory movements, 86, 88, 100–101
Acetylcholine, 243
Achilles tendon, 60
Acromioclavicular joint, 31, 200
Actin filaments, 8, 9, 10, 11
Action potentials, muscle, 17, 156
Action/reaction, law of, 39, 43
Active assisted exercise, 102, 124–125
Active exercise, free, 102
Active insufficiency, 22
Active movements, 93, 102–103
  pendular, 102
  rhythmical, 102
  single or patterned, 102
Activities of daily living, ability to perform, 264–265
Activities of daily living (ADL) scales, 164–166
  Barthel index, 163, 165–166
  extended scale (Nottingham), 164, 166, **167**
Adduction, **23**
Adipose tissue, 212–213
Adolescence, 107, 256–257
Adrenaline, 245
Aerobic metabolism, 109–110
Age
  range of movement and, 93
  stress/strain responses and, 100
Ageing, 259–264
  cardiovascular changes, 259
  gait changes, 263–264
  loss of strength, 107–108, 260
  muscle changes, 260–261
  neurological changes, 261
  physiological limits, 110
  postural changes, 262–263
  respiratory system changes, 259–260
  skeletal changes, 261
  see also Elderly
Agonists, 21
Alpha motor neurones, 17, 72, 73
American College of Sports Medicine guidelines, 117
Amphiarthroses, 86
Anaerobic metabolism, 117
Anatomical basis of human movement, 2, 23–34

Angular motion, 49–50
  combined with linear, 50
  moment of inertia and, 50
Ankle
  dorsiflexors (anterior tibial muscles), 28–29, 184
  ligaments, 28
  sprained, 29
Ankle joint, 28–29
  activity in walking, 179–182
  age-related changes, 263
  functional anatomy, 28–29
  movement analysis, 56–60
  movements, 28
  in rising from a chair, 189, 190
Annulus fibrosus, 207, **208**
Antagonists, 21–22
Anterior cruciate ligament, stress/strain curve, **98**
Anterior tibial muscles (ankle dorsiflexors), 28–29, 184
Antigravity muscles, 73, 76, 226
Anxiety, 242
  disorder, 244
Aponeurotic attachments, 24
'Arches', hand, 197, **198**
Archimedes' principle, 65
Area under force-curve, 55
Arm
  function, 199–200
  see also Upper limb
Armrests, 190
Arousal, normal levels, 242–243
Arteries, age-related changes, 259
Arthritis, 261
Arthrokinematics, 88
Articular cartilage see Hyaline (articular) cartilage
Articular processes, **205**, 210
Articular surface contact, 90
Assistant movers, 21
Assisted exercise
  active, 102, 124–125
  auto-, 102
  manual, 102, 125–126
  mechanical, 102
Asymmetrical tonic neck reflex, **255**
Ataxia, 81
Athletes, **108**, 112
Atlantoaxial joint, 204, 217, 218
Atlanto-occipital joint, 204, 217, 218
Attention, diversion, 138
Auditory cortex, 78
Autogenic inhibition, 74
Automatic postural reaction patterns, 230, 233
Autonomic nervous system, 243
Axes of movement, 86, **87**

B

Balance, 4, 52–53, 225–239
  age-related changes, 263

definition, 226
dynamic, 238
importance, 229–230
mechanisms, 231–233
retraining, 237–238
spinal movements and, 221
static, 238
walking up and down stairs, 187
Ballistic movements, 81
Ballistic stretching, 100
Barthel activities of daily living (ADL) index, 163, 165–166
Basal ganglia, 70, 76–77, 78, 79
Base of support (BOS), 52, **53**
  stability and, 53
Basilar artery, 213, **214**
Bending, **62**
Biceps muscle, 33
  long head, 32
Biofeedback, 237, 246
  EMG, 237, 246, 249–250
Biomechanics, 37–68
  basic concepts, 38–39
  centre of gravity and base of support, 50–53
  definition, 37
  deformation of materials, 61–64
  fluids, 64–68
  force see Force
  movement analysis, 55–61
  work, power, energy and momentum, 53–55
Blood pressure, 243, 246, 259
Body segments, 85–86
  centre of mass (COM), 50, **51**
  description of movements, 86–88
  mass, **51**
Body types (somatotypes), 108–109, 226
Body weight (mass), 107, 108
Bone, 23–24
  age-related changes, 261
  destructive disease, 91
  muscle attachments, 21, 24
  stress-strain curves, 98
Brachialis muscle, 33
Brain stem, 70, 76–77, 79
  bulbofacilitatory area, 72–73
Breaking strength, 97
Breathing exercises, low frequency, 250
Buoyancy, 65
  centre of, 65
  moment of, 66, **67**

C

Cadence, 179
  age-related changes, 263
  kinematic analysis, 146–147
Calcium, 9
Calf muscles
  activity in walking, 181
  stretch–shortening cycle, 14, **15**

Calorimetry
    direct, 159
    indirect, 159
Capillaries, muscle, 8, 118
Cardiac muscle, 118
Cardiorespiratory fitness, maintaining, 117, 174
Cardiovascular system, age-related changes, 259
Carpals, 196
Cartesian coordinate system, 87–88
Cartilage, hyaline *see* Hyaline (articular) cartilage
Cauda equina, 211–212
Caudate nucleus, 77
Ceiling effects, measurement scales, 165
Central nervous system (CNS), control of movement, 69–83, 131
Central pattern generators, 72, 77
Centre of gravity (COG), 50–53
    age-related changes, 262
    body, 50–52
    in kinematic analysis, 146
    in rising from a chair, 188, 189, 190
    stability and, 53
    in walking, 177, **178**
Centre of mass (COM), 50
Centre of pressure (COP), 52, **53**
    stability and, 53
Centrifugal force, 44
Centripetal force, 43–44
Cerebellum, 70, 78, 79–81
    anatomical and functional divisions, 79, **80**
    functions in motor control, 79–81
Cerebral cortex, 70, 77–79
Cervical spine, **205**
    intervertebral disc, 210
    intervertebral foramina, 213
    movements, 30, 216, 217, 218
    in rising from a chair, 189, 190
Cervicothoracic junction, 218
Chair
    getting out of, 187–190
    height, 189, 190
    motorised seat lift/spring assisted, 190
Children, strength, 107
Cine film, for kinematic analysis, 144–148
Circuit training, 118
Circumduction, 24, 31
Clavicle, 31
Closed chain movements, 195, 200, 201
Close pack position, 24, 88
Clothing, 125
Coccyx, 205
Cognitive information processing model, 130
Cognitive techniques, relaxation, 247–248
Collagen, 90
    changes in, 94, 99–100

intervertebral disc, 207, 208
    stretching, 98, 100
Communication, role of hand, 198
Compression, **63**
    linear, 61, **62**
Compression-torsion, **62**
Computers
    for EMG processing, 157, 158
    for kinematic analysis, 146–148, 151
Concentric contractions, 13, 14
    force:velocity relationship, 14–15
Contract-hold-relax method, 248
Contractures, prevention, 94
Contrast relaxation method, 248
Corticospinal pathway, 78
Cosine, 38
Costovertebral joints, 210, 259
Counternutation, 221
Crawling, 256, **258**
Creep, 64
Cross bridges, 10, 11
Cross-sectional area (CSA), muscle, 19–20, 107
    anatomical (ACSA), 108, **109**
    measurement, 108–109
    physiological (PCSA), 108, **109**
Cross transfer, 122
Crutch walking, 195, 201
Cultural expectations, older people, 264
Curvilinear movement, 47

D

Damping, 98
Dancing, 266
Deceleration, 48–49
    definition, 48
    spinal function, 222
    swing phase of walking, 178–179, 182
Deep flexors, foot, 28
Deep vein thrombosis, prophylaxis, 94–95
Deformation (of materials), 61–64
    definition, 61
Degrees of freedom, 86–87
    freezing, 135
    spinal motion segment, 218, **219**
Delorme programme, 116
Deltoid muscle, 32, 33, 200
Density
    fluid, 65
    relative, 65
Development
    infant, 256, **257**, **258**
    upper limb, 193–194
Diaphragm, 30
Diarthroses *see* Synovial joints
Digitisation, in kinematic analysis, 146
Disability, 162
    rising from a chair and, 190
    see also Functional status

Displacement, 48
    angular, 49
    linear, 48
Distance, 48
Distraction, cognitive, 138
Disuse atrophy, 257–258, 260
Double stance, 178, 263
Drop foot, 29
Drugs, effects on stress/strain responses, 100
Ductility, 64, 98
Dynamics, inverse, 55–56
Dynamic tripod grip, 197
Dynamometers, 113, 114
    isokinetic, 114, 152
Dynamometry, isokinetic, 152–153

E

Eccentric contractions, 13–14
    force:velocity relationship, 15–16
    for strength training, 115
Ectomorphs, **108**, 226
Eddy currents, 66, **67**
Elasticity, 96
Elastic limit, 64, 97
Elastic materials, 64, 96–98
Elastic range, 64, 97
Elastin, 98, 99
Elbow joint, 33, 199–200
    functional anatomy, 33
    movements, 33
Elderly, 256–267
    fear of falling, 267
    improving movement and function, 264–267
    physiological changes, 259–264
    rising from a chair, 190
    strength training, 107–108, 265, 266–267
    transitional change, 256–259
    see also Ageing
Electrogoniometers, 148–150
Electromyography (EMG), 156–159
    basis, 156
    biofeedback, 237, 246, 249–250
    clinical value, 158
    force production and, 158–159
    isometric tension and, 159
    isotonic tension and, 159
    phasic muscle activity and, 158
    processing, 157–158
    raw trace, 157–158
    recording, 156–157
    types of electrodes, 156
    in walking, 179, **181**
EMG *see* Electromyography
'End-feel', joint, 91
Endomorphs, **108**, 226
Endorphins, 251
End plates, spinal, 207
Endurance, 106, 110–111
    indices, 153

limitations, 110
  measurement, 110–111
Endurance training, 117–118
  changes during, 118
  for elderly, 265, 266–267
  principles, 111, 112
Energy, 53, 54
  conservation, 54
  costs, muscle contraction type and, **13**, 14
  elastic (strain), 54
  expenditure
    analysis, 159
    in gait, 175, 183
    walking up and down stairs, 187
  heat, 54
  kinetic, 54
  mechanical, 54
  metabolic, 54
  potential (gravitational), 54
Engram, 134
Environment
  influence on movement, 2, 3
  postural effects, 234
  stable, 138
  therapeutic exercise and, 121
  unstable, 138
ε, 61
Equilibrium, 52–53
  dynamic, 53
  in movement analysis, 57–58
  reaction, 230
  static, 52–53, 57–58
Erector spinae muscles, 29, 30, 215
Exercise
  age-related limitations, 259, 260
  assisted *see* Assisted exercise
  effects, 103
  to increase strength and performance, 114–115
  older people, 257–259, 261
  therapeutic, 118–127
    assessment before, 118–119
    body positioning, 120–122
    causes of problems, 126–127
    choice of activity, 120–122
    cross transfer, 122
    early re-education of movement, 124–126
    for elderly, 265–267
    finishing position, 123
    irradiation, 122
    later stages, 126
    maintenance, 126
    muscle imbalance, 123
    overflow, 122
    patterns of movement, 122
    preparation for, 120
    review and progression, 124
    selection and use, 119–120
    starting position, 123
    teaching and learning, 124
    trick movements, 122–123
  see also Physical activity; Training

Experience, knowledge through, 4
Extended activities of daily living scale (Nottingham), 164, 166, **167**
Extension, **23**
  in rising from a chair, 190
Extensor carpi muscles, 33
Extensor digitorum muscles, 33
External abdominal oblique muscle, 30
Eyes, in postural maintenance, 232–233

F

Facet joint, *see* Zygapophyseal (facet) joint
Failure, 64, 97
Falls, fear of, 267
Fatigue, 110–111
  central, 110–111
  measurement, 111
  peripheral, 110
  resistance, 19, 110
  stress-related, 243, 244
Fat pads, 86, 212
Fatty tissue, 212–213
Feedback, proprioceptive, 133–134
Feed forward, 134
Femoral neck fractures, 259
Fetal movements, 254–256
Fibrous tissue, 92
'Fight or flight' response, 243
Film
  for kinematic analysis, 144–148
  for relaxation therapy, 246
Filtering process, 132
Final common pathway, 130
Financial constraints, older people, 264
Fixators, 21
Fixed muscle attachments, 21
Flat back posture, **236**, 237
Flexibility, 234
Flexion, **23**
Flexor carpi muscles, 33
Flexor digitorum muscles, 33
Flexor withdrawal reflex, 74, **75**, 79
Floor effects, measurement scales, 165
Flow, 66, **67**
  laminar (streamlined), 66, **67**
  turbulent, 66, **67**
Fluids, 64–68
  density, 65
  flow, 66, **67**
  movement through, 66–68
  pressure, 65
  relative density/specific gravity, 65
  stability in, 65–66
Foot, 29
  functional anatomy, 29
  initial floor contact, 177
  movements, 29
  pressure receptors, 231–232

Foot angle, **176**, 179
  age-related changes, 263
Foot flat, **176**, 177
  joint and muscle activity, 181
Foramen transversaria, 213
Force, 24, 37, 39–50
  advantage, 46–47
  analysis, 40–43
  causing deformation, 61–64
  centripetal, 43–44
  couple, 40
  definition, 39–40, 106
  description, 40
  effects, 47–50
  equation, 40
  external, 44
  frictional *see* Friction
  generation by muscle, 107
    contraction type and, 13–14
    determinants, 19–20
    EMG assessment, 158–159
    factors affecting, 11–17
    frequency of stimulation and, 16–17
    gradation, 17–18
    muscle length and, 11–13
    power and, 16
    velocity of contraction and, 14–16
  ground reaction *see* Ground reaction force
  horizontal, 58
  internal, 44
  measurements, 153–156
  moment of *see* Moment(s), of force
  net joint, 55–56, 57, 58
  normal, 44
  plate, 154, **155**
  resolution, 40–42
  resultant, 40, 42–43
  summation, 16, 40
  systems, 40
    3–dimensional, 40
    colinear, 40, **41**
    concurrent, 40, **42**
    co-planar, 40, **41**
    orthogonal, 40, **41**
    parallel, 40, **41**
  types, 43–44
  velocity relationship, 14, **15**
  vertical, 58
Force-curve, area under, 55
Forearm, function, 199–200
Foreign bodies, intra-articular, 92
Fractures
  limiting movement, 92
  older people, 259, 261
Frail elderly, 264–265
  exercise programmes, 265–266
Frame rate, in kinematic analysis, 147
Free body diagram (FBD), 56
  foot, 57, 58
  lower leg, 61
Freezing degrees of freedom, 135

Friction, 3, 44
  coefficient of (μ), 44
  dynamic or kinetic, 44
  static, 44
Frontal axis, 86
Frontal plane, **23**, 86, **87**
Functional status
  definition, 164
  measurement scales, 164–166
  older people, 264–265
Fusiform muscles, 19
Fusion frequency, 16, 17

G

Gait, 174
  age-related changes, 263–264
  cycle, 176–177
  energy expenditure, 175, 183
  ground reaction forces, 182–183
  high stepping, 184
  kinematic analysis, 146–147
  movement analysis, 56–61
  pelvic movements, 221
  spatial components, 175–176
  temporal components, 175–176
  terminology, 175–177
  Trendelenburg, 184
  upper body movement, 182
  see also Stance phase; Swing phase;
    Walking
Gamma motor neurones, 17, 72–73
Gastrocnemius muscle, 28, 184
Gender differences
  arthritis, 261
  income in old age, 264
  muscle strength, 107–109, 260
  range of movement, 93
Gestures, hand, 198
Glasgow assessment scale for head
  injuries, 162
Glenohumeral joint
  functional anatomy, 32–33
  limitation of movement, 91, 92
  movements, 31–32, 200
Glenoid labrum, 90
Glide, 88, **89**
Globus pallidus, 77
Gluteus muscles, **26**
Golgi tendon organs, 72, 73–74
  dynamic response, 73
  relaxation therapy, 248
  static response, 73
  v muscle spindle, 74
Goniometers
  electrogoniometers, 148–150
  hand-held, 148
  polarised light, 150–151
Goniometry, 89
Grasp reflex, 194, 255, 256
Gravity, 3, 43
  centre of see Centre of gravity
  line of (LOG), 52, 53

in movement analysis, 57
muscles supporting body against,
    73, 76, 226
Grip, 196–197
  dynamic tripod, 197
  lateral pinch, 197
  power, 197
  span, 197
  tip, 197
Ground reaction force, 43
  centre of pressure, 52, **53**
  in gait, 182–183
  measurement, 153–154, **155**
  in movement analysis, 57, 58
  in running, 184
Guided imagery, 248

H

Hamstring muscles, 27, 185
Hand, 33–34
  'arches', 197, **198**
  closed chain movements, 195, 200,
    201
  control, development, 256, **257**
  function, 196–198
  functional anatomy, 34
  gestures, 198
  movements, 33
  open chain movements, 195,
    199–200, 201
  sensory function, 198–199
Handicap, 162
Head
  control, development, 256, **258**
  righting reflexes, 232
  support, 204–211
Hearing, movement to enhance, 221
Heart rate (pulse rate)
  biofeedback, 246
  maximum, 117, 259
  in stress, 243, 245
Heat
  energy, 54
  production, 96–97
Heel off, 177–178
  joint and muscle activity, 181–182
Heel strike, **176**, 177
  joint and muscle activity, 179–180,
    181
Height, diurnal change, 208
Hip
  abductors, 25, 26, 184
  adductors, 25
  extensors, 25, 26
  flexors, 25–26
Hip joint, 24–26
  activity in walking, 179–182
  age-related changes, 262–263
  functional anatomy, 25–26
  movements, 24–25
  in rising from a chair, 189, 190
Hollow back posture, 235–236

Hopping reactions, 231
Human movement
  anatomical basis, 23–34
  forces and stresses, 24
  lifespan approach, 253–268
  measuring and evaluating, 143–160
  study of, 1–4
Hurdling, 221
Hyaline (articular) cartilage, 86, 90
  destruction, 91
  nutrition, 95, 101
  spine, 207
  viscoelastic properties, 99
Hydrodynamics, 64–66
Hydrostatic pressure, 65
  intervertebral disc, 208, **209**
Hydrostatics, 64–66
Hydrotherapy pools, 64
Hypermobility, joint, 92, 234
Hypothenar eminence, 33
Hysteresis, 96–97, 98, 150

I

I band, **10**
Ilia, 211
Illustrations, as learning aids, 124
Imaginal techniques, relaxation,
    247–248
Immobilisation, 92, 99–100
  VO_{2max} and, 110
Immune response, effect of stress, 243
Impulse, 55
Inertia
  definition, 40
  law of, 39, 40
  moment of, 50
  role in walking, 175
Infant development, 256, **257**, **258**
Information processing model, 130,
    131–135
Infraspinatus muscle, 32
Injury, limiting movement, 92
Insertion, muscle, 21
Instability, 225–226
Internal abdominal oblique muscle,
    30, 215
Interneurones, spinal cord, 71
Interossei muscles of hand, 33
Interphalangeal (IP) joints, 196
Interspinales muscle, 214
Interspinous ligament, 210, **211**
Intertransversarii muscle, 214
Interval scales, 163
Intervertebral disc, 29, 30, 204, 206–210
  age-related changes, 262
  effect of movement, 216
  nutrition, 208–210
Intervertebral foramina, 212–213
Interviews, 163
Intra-articular discs, 86
Inverse dynamics, 55–56
Inverse stretch reflex, 73–74, 248

Irradiation, 122
Isokinetic contractions (exercise), 14, **114**
Isokinetic dynamometer, 114, 152
Isokinetic dynamometry, 152–153
Isokinetic systems
   assisted exercise, 102
   strength training, 113, 115
Isometric contractions (exercise), 13, 14, 113–114
Isometric tension, EMG and, 159
Isotonic contractions (exercise), 14, **114**
Isotonic systems, for strength training, 113, 115
Isotonic tension, EMG and, 159

J

Jogging, 266
Joint(s), 2
   accessory movements, 86, 88
   active movements, 93, 102–103
   activity in walking, 179–182
   angles, 146
   axes of movement, 86, **87**
   capsule, 86, 90
   cartilagenous, 86
   classification, 86
   degrees of freedom, 86–87
   describing movements, 86–88
   'end-feel', 91
   fibrous (fixed), 86
   hypermobility, 92, 234
   mobility, 85–104
   passive movements, 93, 94–102
   physiological movements, 86, 88
   planes of movement, 86, **87**
   range of movement (ROM), *see*
     Range of movement
   synovial *see* Synovial joints
   types of movement, 93
Joule, 53, 106

K

Kinaesthetic awareness, 95
Kinematics, 37, 144–151
   spatial reference system, 144, **145**
   use of film, 144–148
     qualitative and quantitative, 145–148
   use of goniometers, 148–151
Kinetics, 37, 151–153
Knee joint, 26–28
   activity in walking, 179–182
   functional anatomy, 27–28
   movement analysis, 61
   movements, 26–27
   in rising from a chair, 189, 190
Knowledge of performance, 132
Kypholordotic posture, 236

Kyphosis, 235, **236**
   thoracic, in older people, 261, 262

L

Labra, intra-articular, 86
Labyrinthine righting reflex, 255
Lactic acid, 110
Lateral inhibition, 71–72
Lateral peroneus muscle, 28
Latissimus dorsi muscle, 31, 32, 201, 215
Laws of motion, 39
Learned movements, 130
Learning
   motor *see* Motor learning
   therapeutic exercise, 124
   training and, 112
Least packed position, 24
Leg extension reflex, **255**
Length:tension relationship, 11–13
Length specificity, strength training, 115–116
Levator scapulae muscle, 31, 215
Levers, 45–46
   first order, 46
   mechanical advantage, 46–47
   second order, 46
   third order, 46
Lifespan approach, 253–268
Lifestyle
   older people, 264
   sedentary, 257–258, 261, 264
Lifting, 30–31, 215
Ligaments, 86, 90
   laxity, 226, 234
   limits of flexibility, 90–91
   spinal, 210, **211**
   viscoelastic properties, **98**, 99
Ligamentum flavum, 29, 90, **98**, 210, **211**
Limb circumference, 108–109
Linear motion, 47–49
   combined with angular, 50
Line of gravity (LOG), 52, 53
Link-segment model, 56, **57**
Liquids, 64–65
Loading, 61
   linear, 61–64
   paths, 96–98
   phase *see* Foot flat
   rotational, **62**
Locomotion, 174
Loose bodies, 101
Loose pack position, 24, 88
Lordosis, lumbar, 29, 215, 235
Lordotic posture, 235–236
Lower limb
   function, 173–191
   movement analysis, 56–60
   spinal functions, 215, 221
Lumbar spine, **205**
   functional anatomy, 30–31
   movements, 29–30, 217, 219–220

Lumbricals muscle, 33
Lying posture, 227–228

M

MacQueen training programmes, 116
Manipulation, 101–102
Markers, skin, 146, 147–148, 151
Maslow's hierarchy of needs, 199
Mass, centre of (COM), 50
Massage, sedative, 249
Mattress, 228
Maturation approach, 135
Maximal oxygen consumption (VO_{2max}), 110
Maximal velocity of shortening (Vmax), 15, 21
Measurement, 4, 5, 143–160
   electromyography, 156–159
   energy expenditure, 159
   force and pressure, 153–156
   kinematic, 144–148
   kinetic, 151–153
Measurement scales, 161–172
   data collection methods, 163
   functional status, 164–166
   general principles, 162–163
   quality of life, 167–171
   reliability, 162
   scoring methods, 162–163
   validity, 162
Mechanical advantage, 46–47
Mechanical approach, 2
Medulla oblongata, 76
Memory, 136–137
   long-term, 132, 136–137
   short-term, 136
Menisci, 86, 90
Meniscoid inclusions, 210
Menopause, 107, 260
Mesencephalon, 76
Mesomorphs, **108**, 226
Metacarpals, 196
Metacarpophalangeal joint (MCP), 196
Metacentre, 66
Metatarsophalangeal joints, 180
Midbrain, 76
Middle age, 257
Mid-stance, **176**, 177
   joint and muscle activity, 181
Mid-swing, **176**, 178, 182
Milestones, developmental, **257**, **258**
Mirrors, 237, 246
Mitchell's relaxation technique, 248–249
Mitochondria, muscle cells, 8, 118
Moment(s)
   arm, 45, **46**
   of buoyancy, 66, **67**
   external, 45
   of force, 44–47
     effects, 47–50
   of inertia, 50

Moment(s) (*contd*)
  internal, 45
  net joint *see* Net joint moments
  turning, 25
Momentum, 55
  role in walking, 175
Moro reflex, **255**
Motion
  angular *see* Angular motion
  laws of, 39
  linear, 47–49
  linear and angular combined, 50
Motivation, 112, 121
Motor association area, 70, 77–78
Motor control, 131–137
  accuracy, 135
  assessment, 143–144
  consistency, 135
  efficiency, 135
  limitations, 134
  schema theory, 131–135
Motor cortex, 70, 77–78, 81
  organisation, 78
  primary, 78
Motor engram, 82, 134
Motor learning, 2–3, 129–141
  definition, 129–130
  historical perspective, 130
  maturation approach, 135
  memory and, 136–137
  motor control and, 131–137
  perceptual cognitive approach, 136
  in rehabilitation setting, 137
  skills, 135, 137–140
  in strength training, 116
  training and, 112
  variable practice and, 137
Motor neurones
  alpha, 17, 72, 73
  gamma, 17, 72–73
  spinal cord, 71
Motor skills *see* Skills
Motor system
  lateral descending pathway, 77
  medial descending pathways, 76–77
Motor unit, 17–18
  rate coding, 17–18
  recruitment, 17, **18**
Movement
  learned, 130
  neural control, 69–83, 131
  reflex, 130
  through fluids, 66–68
  types, 130
Movement analysis, 55–61
  higher up leg, 60–61
  lower leg, 56–60
Moving muscle attachments, 21
Multidimensional approach, 2
Multifidus muscle, 214
Muscle(s), 2, 7–10
  action potentials, 17, 156
  active insufficiency, 22
  activity in walking, 179–182

age-related changes, 260–261
antigravity, 73, 76, 226
atrophy, 92
  age-related, 260–261
  disuse, 257–258, 260
attachments, 21, 24
contraction, 11–17
  dynamic, 13
  factors affecting force generation, 11–13
  force, 107
  frequency of stimulation, 16–17
  power output, 16
  static, 13
  types, 13–14
  velocity, 14–16, 107
contractures, 94
cross-sectional area *see* Cross-sectional area (CSA), muscle
elasticity, 94
fascicles, **8**, 19
force generation, *see* Force, generation by muscle
fusiform, 19
hyperplasia, 116–117
hypertrophy, 92, 116–117, 234
imbalance, 123, 234
length, 11–13, 21
limit of extensibility, 91
passive insufficiency, 22–23
pennate, 19, 20
phasic activity, 158
power, 16, 21, 55
progressive relaxation, 247
range of movement, 22–23, 89
  inner, 22
  middle, 22
  outer, 22
relaxation, 243
roles, 21–22
sensory receptors, 72–74
strap, 19
strength *see* Strength
in stress, 244
structure, 8–10, 19–21
tension, 11–13, 243
  active, 11–12, 99
  EMG assessment, 159
  passive, 12, 99
  relaxation therapy, 246
  total, 12–13
tone, 230
training *see* Training
triangular, **19**
viscoelastic properties, 99
work, 13–14, 54
Muscle fibres, 8–9
  age-related loss, 260–261
  alignment within muscle, 19
  type I, 18, 19
  type IIa, **18**, 19
  type IIb, 18–19
  type IIc, 18, 19
  types, 18–19

Muscle spindles, 72–73
  neck, 232
  primary and secondary endings, 72
  role in voluntary movement, 72–73
  static and dynamic response, 72
  v golgi tendon organs, 74
Musculoskeletal system, 2, 7–35, 86
Musgrave footprint pressure plate, 154, **155**
Musical instrument, playing, 201–202
Myofibrils, **8**, 9
Myofilaments, **8**
Myoglobin, 17
Myosin filaments, 8, 9, 10, 11
Myotactic reflex, *see* Stretch reflex

N

Neck, tonic reflexes, 232, **255**
Necking, 97
Needle electrodes, 156
Needs, Maslow's hierarchy of, 199
Negative transfer, motor skills, 139
Neonate, 254–256
  reflex activity, 255–256
Nerve roots, 70–71, 212
Nervous system
  age-related changes, 261
  control of movement, 69–83, 131
Net joint forces, 55–56
  calculation, 57, 58
Net joint moments, 55–56
  calculation, 57, 58–59, 147
Neurological impairment, 92
Newton, Sir Isaac, 39
Newtons (N), 40, 106
Noise, electromyography, 156, 157
Nominal scales, 163
Noradrenaline, 243
Normal postural reflex mechanism (NPRM), 229–230
Nottingham extended activities of daily living scale, 164, 166, **167**
Nottingham health profile, 168, 170–171
Nucleus pulposus, 207–208, 210, 216
Nutation, 221
Nutrition
  articular cartilage, 95, 101
  intervertebral disc, 208–210
  role of movement, 101

O

Observation, 163
  for evaluating movement, 144
  skills, 4, 5
Old age
  transition into, 256–259
  see also Elderly
Open chain movements, 195, 199–200, 201

Optoelectronic devices, 150–151
Ordinal scales, 163
Organs, protection of vital, 211–213
Origin, muscle, 21
Osteoarthritis, 91, 259
Osteoporosis, 259, 261, 262
Otolith organs, 232
Overflow, 122
Overload, 111–112
Oxford programme, 116
Oxygen consumption, maximal
    (VO2max), 110

P

Pain, 92, 95, 234
Parallel, motor learning in, 132
Parasympathetic nervous system, 243
Parkinson's disease: disability index,
    162
Pascals, 44, 65
Pascal's law, 65
Passive insufficiency, 22–23
Passive movements, 93, 94–102
    auto-relaxed, 95
    continuous (CPM), 96
    relaxed, 94–96
        contraindications, 95
        effects, 94–95
        indications, 94, 124–125
        manual, 94
        mechanical, 96
        principles of application, 95
    rhythmical, 251
    see also Stretching
Patella, 27
Pattern generators, central, 72, 77
Pattern recognition, 132
Patterns of movement, 4
    kinematic analysis, 146
    maintaining functional, 95, 122
Pectoral girdle, see Shoulder girdle
Pectoralis major muscle, 32, 201
Pelvic crossed syndrome, 236
Pelvic girdle support, 211
Pelvis, muscle function, 215
Pendular exercises, 250
Pennate muscles, 19, 20
Perception-action coupling, 133
Perceptual cognitive approach, 136
Performance
    exercise to increase, 114–115
    knowledge of, 132
    strength and, 108
    in stress, 245
Peroneus muscles, 28, 29
Phalanges, 196
Photographs
    for kinematic analysis, 145
    as learning aids, 124
Physical ability see Functional status
Physical activity
    age-related limitations, 259, 260

decrease in normal, 100
older people, 256–259, 261, 265–267
for relaxation, 251
see also Exercise; Training
Physiological approach, 2
Physiological movements, 86, 88
Physiological relaxation technique,
    248–249
Pillow, 228
Pinch grip, 197
Piriformis muscle, 215
Placing reactions, 231
Placing reflex, **255**
Planes of movement, 86, **87**
Planning faults, exercise therapy, 126
Plantar flexors, 28, 29
Plastic change, 64
Plastic flow, 64
Plastic range, 97
Plyometric testing, 5
Pons, 76
Popliteus muscle, 28
Positioning
    correcting poor body, 120
    finishing, 123
    starting, 123, 125
Positive transfer, motor skills, 139
Postural reflex mechanism, normal
    (NPRM), 229–230
Postural sway reaction, 231
Posture, 225–239
    age-related changes, 262–263
    causes of poor/altered, 233–234
    definition, 226
    deviations from ideal, 234–237
    'good', 226
    importance, 229–230
    lying, ideal, 227–228
    mechanisms maintaining, 231–233
    neural control, 70, 76–77
    'normal', 226–229
    retraining, 237–238
    sitting, ideal static, 229
    spinal function, 222
    standing, ideal static, 227, **228**
    in stress, 244–245
'Pot belly' posture, 235–236
Power, 53, 54–55
    definition, 106
    grip, 197
    measurements, 152–153
    muscle, 16, 21, 55
    muscle strength and, 107
    training for, 117, 266–267
Practice, variable, 137
Premotor area, 78
Pressure, 44
    centre of (COP), 52, **53**
    definition, 44
    in fluids, 65
    intervertebral disc, 208, **209**
    measurements, 153–156
    plates, 154–155
    points, 228

receptors, foot, 231–232
in-shoe measuring devices, 154,
    155–156
Primary motor area, 78
Prime movers, 21
Problem-solving approach, 120, **121**
Progressive muscle relaxation, 247
Progressive rate training (PRT), 116
Progressive resistance exercises (PRE),
    116
Prone posture, 226
Proprioception, 231–232, 234
Proprioceptive feedback, 133–134
Proprioceptive neuromuscular
    facilitation (PNF), 122
Propriospinal fibres, spinal cord, 72
Propulsive phase, 177–178
Proteoglycan gel, 208
Psoas major muscle, 215
Psychological approach, 2
Psychological factors
    in posture, 234
    therapeutic exercise, 120–121, 126
Psychological problems, 92
'Pull up' phase, 184–185
Pulse rate see Heart rate
Purkinje cell, 79
Push off, **176**, 177–178
    joint and muscle activity, 181–182
Putamen, 77
Pythagoras' theorem, 38

Q

Quadriceps lag, 28
Quadriceps muscle, 27
Quality of life
    definition, 167–168
    disease specific, 168
    generic health profiles, 168
    measurement scales, 167–171
Quality of movement, assessment,
    143–144

R

Radians, 49
Radioulnar joint
    inferior, 33, 199
    superior, 33
Range of movement (ROM), 88–89
    abnormal limitation/restriction,
        91–93
        causes, 234
        treatment, 93
    facilitation, 90
    full, 88
    maintaining, 94
    measurement, 89
    normal limitation/restriction, 90–91
    see also Muscle(s), range of
        movement

Rate coding, 17–18
Ratio scales, 163
Reaching activities, 221
Reaction times, 133, 135
    age-related increase, 261
Reciprocal inhibition, 74, 230
Reciprocal innervation, 74, 79, 230, 248
Rectification, 158
Rectilinear movement, 47
Rectus abdominis muscle, 30, 31
Recumbent posture, 226
Recurrent inhibition, 71–72
Re-education, movement, 124–126
Reflexes, 130
    definition, 255
    primitive and developmental,
        255–256
    spinal cord, 72
Refractory period, 134–135
Rehabilitation
    motor learning, 137
    multidisciplinary, 119
Relative density, 65
Relaxation, 241–252
    definition, **242**
    physiology, 243
    therapy, 245–251
        developing self-awareness,
            246–247
        general and local, 246
        methods, 247–251
        preparation for, 247
Reliability, measurement scales, 162
Renshaw cell, 71
Repetition Maximum (RM), 109, 116
Repetitions
    for motor learning, 138
    for training, 116, 124
Resilience, 98
Resistance exercises, 113, 124
    see also Strength training
Resistive forces, 125
Respiratory rate, 243, 245
Respiratory system, age-related
    changes, 259–260
Response
    programming, 131, 133–134
    selection, 131, 133
Reticular formation, 76, 243
Reticulospinal pathways, 76
Rheumatoid arthritis, 91
Rhomboid muscles, 31, 32–33, 215
Rhythmical passive movements, 251
Ribs, 210–211
Righting reaction, 230
Righting reflexes, 255
Robinson-Bashall functional
    assessment for arthritis
    patients, 162
Roll, 88, **89**
Rooting reflex, 255
Rotation, **23**, 39, 49–50
    external, **23**
    internal, **23**
    negative, 39
    positive, 39
Rotator cuff muscles, 32, 200
Rotatores muscle, 214
Rubrospinal pathway, 78
Running, 183–184

S

Saccule, 232
Sacroiliac joints, 211, 220–221
Sacrum, 204–205, 211
Sagittal axis, 86
Sagittal plane, **23**, 86
Sarcomeres, **8**, 9–10
    length:tension relationship, **12**
    in parallel, 19–20
    in series, 20–21
Sarcoplasmic reticulum (SR), 9
Scalar quantities, 39
Scales, measurement see Measurement
    scales
Scapula, 31, 200–201
Scar tissue, 92
Schema theory, 131–135
Scoliosis, 235
Seated phase, **188**, 189
Sedative massage, 249
Sedentary lifestyle, 257–258, 261, 264
Segments, body see Body segments
Self-awareness, 4, 5, 246–247
Self-rating scales, 163, 168
Semicircular canals, 232
Sensitivity, measurement scales, 162,
    165
Sensory association areas, 70
Sensory cortex, 70, 82
Sensory engram, 82
Sensory feedback control, 82
Sensory function
    age-related changes, 261
    hand, 198–199
Sensory inputs
    cortical processing, 78
    spinal cord, 70–71
Sensory neurones, spinal cord, 71
Sensory receptors
    muscle, 72–74
    vestibular system, 232
Series, motor learning in, 132
Serratus anterior muscle, 31, 32–33,
    215
SF36 (Short Form 36), 168, 169–170
Sharpey's fibres, 207
Shear, 61–62, **63**
    modulus, 62
    sacroiliac joints, 221
    strain, angle of, 62
Shock absorber, spine as, 221–222
Short Form 36 (SF36), 168, 169–170
Shoulder complex, 31–33
    functional anatomy, 32–33
    movements, 31–32
Shoulder girdle
    function, 200–201
    movement during walking, 182
Shutter speed, in kinematic analysis, 147
Sign language, 198
Sine, 38
Sitting
    position, 229, **230**
    spinal muscle activity, 215
    standing from, 187–190
SI units, 38
Size principle, motor unit recruitment,
    17
Skeleton, 23
    age-related changes, 261
Skills, 135, 137–140
    acquisition, 138–140
    closed, 137–138
    construction, 138–139
    differentiation, 139–140
    negative transfer, 139
    open, 138
    positive transfer, 139
    stabilisation, 139
Skin markers, 146, 147–148, 151
Sleeping posture, 228
Sleeplessness, 244
Sleep/wake cycle, 242
Slide, 88, **89**
Sliding filament theory, 11
Sling suspension, 102
Sociological approach, 2
Soft tissues
    apposition, 90
    contractures, 94
    elasticity, 94
    lesions, 92
    spinal protection, 211–213
    stress-strain curves, 98–99
Soleus muscle, 28, 184
Somatotypes, 108, 226
Span grip, 197
Specific gravity, 65
Spin, 88, **89**
Spinal cord, 70
    anterior horn, 78
    descending motor pathways, 76–77
    dorsolateral columns, 77
    organisation, 70–72
    protection, 211–212
    reflexes, 79
    sensory inputs, 70–71
Spinal motion segment, **205**, 213–214,
    215
    degrees of freedom, 218, **219**
Spine (vertebral column), 29–31
    age-related changes, 262
    end plates, 207
    function, 203–224
    functional anatomy, 30–31
    motion analysis, 222
    movements, 29–30, 215–221
    segmental stabilisation, 213–215
    shock absorbing function, 221–222

Spinous processes, **205**, 210
Stabilisers, 21
Stability, 52–53
  in fluids, 65–66
  limit, 53
  neutral, 53
  types, 53
Stable, 53
Stairs, walking up and down, 184–187
Stance phase, **176**, 177–178
  age-related changes, 263
  joint and muscle activity, 179–182
  rising from a chair, 188, 189–190
  sacroiliac joints, 221
  walking down stairs, 186–187
  walking up stairs, 184–185
Standing
  muscle activity, 214–215
  posture, 227, **228**
  rising from sitting to, 187–190
Step
  length, **176**, 179
  rate see Cadence
  width see Stride width
Stepping reactions, 231
Sternoclavicular joint, 31, 193, 200
Stick diagrams, 146, **147**
Stiffness, 61, 97, 98
Stimulus
  detection, 132
  identification, 131, 132–133
  interpretation, 132
  selection, 132–133
Straight leg raise, 25, 212
Strain, 61
  linear, 61–64
  rate, 96
Strap muscles, 19
Strength, 21, 106, 107–110
  age and gender differences, 107–108, 260
  body type and, 108
  development, 107
  endurance and, 111
  measurement, 108–110
    objective, 108–109
    subjective, 109–110
  peak, 107
Strength training, 113–117
  best types of exercise, 114–115
  changes during, 116–117
  for elderly, 107–108, 265, 266–267
  intensity, repetition and frequency, 116
  principles, **111**, 112
  programme types, 116
  specificity, 115–116
  types of muscle activity, 113–115
Stress (mechanical), 61
  forces, 24
  linear, 61–64
Stress (mental), 241, 242–243
  abnormal, 243–245
  definition, **242**

physiology, 243
  signs and symptoms, 244–245
Stress-strain curves, 63–64, 96
  biological materials, 97
  bone, 98
  soft tissue, 98–99
Stretching, 96–100
  ballistic, 100
  biological material, 96–99
  manual (auto), 100
  mechanical, 100
  static, 100
  therapeutic, 99–100, 126
Stretch reflex, 72, **73**, 74, 79
  functional, 73
  inverse, 73–74, 248
Striatum, 77
Stride length, **176**, 179
  age-related changes, 263
  kinematic analysis, 146–147
Stride width, **176**, 179
  age-related changes, 263
Subacromial bursa, 32
Subscapularis muscle, 32
Substantia nigra, 77
Subtalar joint, 28
Subthalamic nucleus, 77
Suggestion method (visualisation), 248, 249
Summation of force, 16, 40
Supine posture, 226
Supplementary motor area, 78
Supraspinatus muscle, 32
Supraspinous ligament, 210, **211**
Surface tension, 65
Sway back posture, 236–237
Swimming, 266
Swing phase, **176**, 178–179
  age-related changes, 263
  joint and muscle activity, 182
  walking down stairs, 187
  walking up stairs, 185–186
Symmetrical tonic neck reflex, **255**
Sympathetic nervous system, 243
Symphysis pubis, 211, 221
Synarthroses, 86
Synergist, 21
  helping, 21
  true, 21
Synovial fluid, 86, 90
Synovial joints, 24, 86
  classification, 86
  movements, 88

T

Tangent, 38
Teaching
  faults, 127
  therapeutic exercise, 124
Tectospinal pathways, 76–77
Telemetry, 150
Tendon reflex, 73–74

Tendons
  limits of flexibility, 90–91
  muscle attachments, 21, 24
  viscoelastic properties, 99
Tenodesis, 23
Tension (mechanical), **63**
  linear, 61, **62**
  muscle see Muscle(s), tension
  surface, 65
Tension (mental), 241–252
  definition, **242**
  see also Relaxation; Stress
Teres major muscle, 32
Teres minor muscle, 32
Tetanic contraction, 16
Thalamus, 77, 78, 79
Thenar eminence, 33
Thoracic cage, 30
  age-related changes, 259–260
  support, 210–211, 213
Thoracic muscles, spinal attachments, 213–215
Thoracic spine, **205**
  movements, 30, 216–217, 219
Thumb, 33, 34
Tibialis anterior muscles see Anterior tibial muscles
Tibialis posterior muscle, 28
Tip grip, 197
Tiredness see Fatigue
Toe off, **176**, 177–178
Toe strike, 184
Tonic neck reflexes, 232, **255**
Torque, 45, 106
  angle to peak, 152
  angle specific, 152
  measurement, 152, **153**
  peak, 152
Torque-velocity relationship, 152
Torsion, **62**
Training, 111–118
  circuit, 118
  definition, 111
  diminishing returns, 112–113
  for elderly, 265–267
  endurance see Endurance training
  general principles, 111–113
  learning and, 112
  motivation, 112
  overload, 111–112
  for power, 117
  reversibility, 112
  specificity, 112, 115
  strength see Strength training
  task specificity, 115–116
  warm-up, 113
  see also Exercise; Physical activity
Transfer
  cross, 122
  motor skills, 139
  in standing from a sitting position, 189–190
  wheelchair–toilet/bed, 195
Transforaminal ligaments, 213

Translation (linear motion), 47–49
Transverse plane, 86, **87**
Transverse processes, 210
Transversus abdominis muscle, 30, 215
Trapezius muscle, 31, 32–33, 215
Trendelenburg gait, 184
Triangle, trigonometry, 38
Triangular muscles, **19**
Triceps muscle, 33, 200
   long head, 32
Triceps surae muscle, 59, 60
Trick movements, 122–123
Trigonometry, 38
Tropomyosin, 10
Troponin (Tn), 10
Trunk
   control, development, 256, **258**
   movement during walking, 182
   muscles, 215
   in rising from a chair, 190
T (tubular) system, 9
Turbulence, 66, **67**
Turning moments, 25
Twitch, 16

U

Ultimate strength, 97
Unloading paths, 96–98
Upper limb, 193–202
   abduction, 32
   adduction, 32
   development, 193–194
   function, 195–202
      development, 194
      example analysis, 201–202
      structures permitting, 195–196
   movement during running, 184
   movement during walking, 182, 195
   sensory functions, 198–199
   spinal functions, 215, 221
   in standing from a sitting position,
      188, 190, 195
   support, 204–211
Utricle, 232

V

Validity, measurement scales, 162
Vastus medialis oblique muscle, 28
Vector quantities, 39
Velocity, 48–49
   angular, 49–50, 114
   definition, 48
   determinants, 20–21
   kinematic analysis, 146–147
   muscle contraction, 14–16, 107
   of shortening, maximal (Vmax), 15, 21
   specificity of training, 115–116
Venous circulation, maintaining, 94–95
Vertebrae, 204–205
Vertebral arch support, 210
Vertebral arteries, 213, **214**
Vertebral bodies, 29, 204
   function, 205–206
   trabeculae, 205, **206**
Vertebral canal, 211–212
Vertebral column *see* Spine
Vertebrobasilar insufficiency, 213
Vertical axis, 86, **87**
Vestibular apparatus, 80–81
Vestibular nuclei, 76
Vestibular system, 232
Vestibulospinal pathways (tracts), 76,
   232
Vibration, 126
Videotapes
   for kinematic analysis, 145–148
   as learning aids, 124
   for relaxation therapy, 246
Violin playing, 201–202
Viscoelastic materials, 96
Viscosity, 96
Vision, movement to enhance, 221
Visual cortex, 78
Visualisation (suggestion method),
   248, 249
Visual system, in postural
   maintenance, 232–233
V_{max}, 15, 21
VO_{2max}, 110

W

Wake, 68
Walking, 174–183
   age-related changes, 263
   aids, 201
   backwards, 184
   crutch, 195, 201
   for exercise, 266
   reflex, **255**, **258**
   up and down stairs, 184–187
   see also Gait
Warm-up, 113
Water
   intervertebral disc, 208
   mechanics, 64–68
Watts, 53, 106
Waves, **67**, 68
Weakness, 111, 260
Wheelchairs, 195, 201
Work, 53–54, 106
   linear, 53
   measurements, 152–153
   muscle, 13–14, 54
   rotational, 54
Wrist, 33–34, 199
   functional anatomy, 34
   movements, 33
Written instructions, 124

Y

Yield point, 64
Yield strength, 97
Young's modulus, 62, 64

Z

Z line, 9, **10**
Zygapophyseal (facet) joints, 210,
   216–217